Multiple Sclerosis Research in Europe

COMMISSION OF THE EUROPEAN COMMUNITIES

MULTIPLE SCLEROSIS RESEARCH IN EUROPE

Report of a Conference on Multiple Sclerosis Research in Europe, January 29th–31st 1985, Nijmegen, The Netherlands.

Sponsored by the Commission of the European Communities, as advised by the Committee on Medical Public Health Research

Editor
Otto R. Hommes

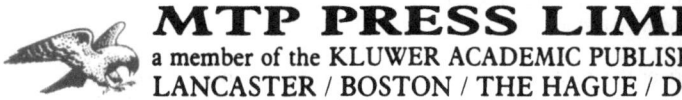
MTP PRESS LIMITED
a member of the KLUWER ACADEMIC PUBLISHERS GROUP
LANCASTER / BOSTON / THE HAGUE / DORDRECHT

for the Commission of the European Communities

Published in the UK and Europe by
MTP Press Limited
Falcon House
Lancaster, England

British Library Cataloguing in Publication Data

Multiple sclerosis research in Europe: report of
   a CEC Conference Nijmegen 29, 30, 31 January 1985.
   1. Multiple sclerosis—Research—Europe
   I. Hommes, Otto R.   II. Commission of the
   European Communities
   616.8'34'007204   RC377
   ISBN-13:978-94-010-8338-6   e-ISBN-13:978-94-009-4143-4
   DOI: 10.1007/978-94-009-4143-4

Published in the USA by
MTP Press
A division of Kluwer Boston Inc
190 Old Derby Street
Hingham, MA 02043, USA

Library of Congress Cataloging in Publication Data

Hommes, Otto R. (Otto Roelf)
   Multiple sclerosis research in Europe.
   At head of title: MSRE.
   Report to the Commission of the European Communities
of a Conference on Multiple Sclerosis Research in Europe.
   Includes bibliographies and index.
   1. Multiple sclerosis—Research—Europe—Congresses.
2. Multiple sclerosis—Congresses. 3. Conference on
Multiple Sclerosis Research in Europe (1985 : Nijmegen,
Netherlands) I. Commission of the European Communities.
II. Title. III. Title: MSRE. [DNLM: 1. Conference on
Multiple Sclerosis Research in Europe (1985 : Nijmegen,
Netherlands) 2. Multiple Sclerosis—occurrence—Europe.
WL 360 H768m 1985]
RC377.H66 1985   616.8'34'007204   85-24053
ISBN-13:978-94-010-8338-6
© ECSC, EEC, EAEC, Brussels and Luxembourg, 1986
Softcover reprint of the hardcover 1st edition 1986

EUR 10312 EN

Publication arranged by
Commission of the European Communities
Directorate-General Information Market and Innovation-
Scientific and Technical Communication
Brussels and Luxembourg.

Contents

Introduction   xi

Programme of the Conference   xv

List of Participants and Observers   xxv

SECTION I CLINICAL STUDIES

1 Clinical Studies in Multiple Sclerosis
S. Poser   3

2 Clinical Trials
P. Rudge   13

3 Onset, Course and Prognosis of Multiple Sclerosis
C. Confavreux   15

4 A Comparative Study Between Multiple Sclerosis Out-patients and
In-patients Staying at a Specialized Multiple Sclerosis Clinic
R. Medaer, M. Puystjens and H. Callaert   31

5 Incapacity and Disability in Multiple Sclerosis
J. M. Minderhoud, A. J. A. Prange and H. Dassel   41

6 Immunosuppression with Cyclophosphamide in Multiple Sclerosis
Patients
R. E. Gonsette and L. Demonty   45

7 Anti-lymphocyte Serum in Severe Multiple Sclerosis
   R. Marteau, F. Lhermitte and H. de Saxce   49

8 Long-term Prescription of Azathioprine in Multiple Sclerosis.
   A Review of Published Series
   O. Sabouraud and M. Mérienne   55

9 Azathioprine Assessment in Progressive Multiple Sclerosis.
   Clinical Aspects
   I. E. Zeeberg   61

10 Dietary Therapy in Multiple Sclerosis
    D. Bates   71

11 An Eight Years Follow-up Study of Transfer Factor Treatment on the
    Course of Multiple Sclerosis
    A. M. Nordenbo and I. Zeeberg   81

12 Compact Manual for Multiple Sclerosis Registration in Clinical
    Research
    O. Andersen, M. Andersson, T. Broman and I. Zeeberg   85

13 Comparison of Multiple Sclerosis Incidence Clinical and ABR Data
    Indicates a Higher Degree of Dissemination of Lesions in a
    Progressive than in a Remitting Course
    O. Andersen, U. Rosenhall and B. Runmarker   95

SECTION II IMMUNOLOGY

14 Multiple Sclerosis and Immunity: Facts, Fiction and Future
    Development
    J. Mertin   103

15 The Spectrum of Experimental Allergic Encephalomyelitis
    H. Lassmann and K. Vass   109

16 T Cell Subsets in Multiple Sclerosis
    M. A. Bach and E. Tournier-Lasserve   115

17 Functional Differences Between Cerebrospinal Fluid and Peripheral
    Blood T Cells in Multiple Sclerosis
    M. S. Wollheim and E. C. DeFreitas   123

18 Characterization of T Cell Subsets and Macrophages in Active
    Demyelinating Multiple Sclerosis Lesions
    H. Nyland, S. Mörk, R. Matre and A. Naess   131

19 Determination of Lymphocyte Subsets in Cerebrospinal Fluid (CSF)
    W. M. Nillesen and B. M. J. Uitdehaag   141

20 Ia-presenting Cells in Early Multiple Sclerosis Lesions and Adjacent
    Normal Looking White Matter; A Morphological Study
    H. J. ter Laak and O. R. Hommes   143

21 Developmental Aspects of Oligodendrocyte Structure and Function
    M. Schachner   153

22 Monoclonal Antibodies against Oligodendrocytes; A Morphological
    Study
    H. J. ter Laak, M. Schachner and O. R. Hommes   159

23 The Relationship of Immunological and Histological Abnormalities in
    Multiple Sclerosis
    I. V. Allen   163

24 Towards Cloning of Lymphoid Cells from Cerebrospinal Fluid
    F. Rotteveel, E. Braakman and C. J. Lucas   167

25 Activation of Natural Cytotoxic Activity *In Vitro* with Lymphocytes
    from Patients with Multiple Sclerosis
    E. Braakman, A. van Tunen and C. J. Lucas   175

26 Molecular and Cellular Basis of Autoimmune Encephalitogenesis
    H. Wekerle   185

27 Cytotoxic Antibodies in Multiple Sclerosis
    *L. Rumbach, J. M. Warter, M. M. Tongio, C. Marescaux, S. Mayer
    and M. Collard*   195

28 An Immunological Function for Astrocytes
    W. Fierz and A. Fontana   199

SECTION III BIOCHEMISTRY, NEUROBIOLOGY, MYELIN

29 The Biochemistry of Myelin
    J. M. Matthieu   209

30 The Cerebrospinal Fluid Immunoglobulins in Multiple Sclerosis
    P. Delmotte   217

31 Multiple Sclerosis: A Two Stage Process? Studies on the
    Abnormalities of Cerebral Spinal Fluid by Means of Isotopic
    Cisternography
    D. Inzitari, G. Volpi, A. Castagnoli and L. Amaducci   225

32 CSF Immunoglobulins and Clinical Course
    H. Link   231

33 Immunoglobulin Abnormalities for IgG, IgA and IgM in
    Cerebrospinal Fluid of Multiple Sclerosis Patients
    *K. J. B. Lamers, W. van Geel, J. C. N. Kok, O. R. Hommes and
    B. Feenstra*   241

34 Immunoglobulin IgG Abnormalities and the Oligoclonal Pattern of
    IgG in Multiple Sclerosis Brains
    K. J. B. Lamers, W. van Geel, R. A. Wevers and O. R. Hommes   251

35 IgG Synthesis in Multiple Sclerosis
    *D. Caputo, P. Ferrante, S. Procaccia, M. Zaffaroni and
    C. L. Cazzullo*   257

36 Antigenicity of Galactosylceramide
    B. Zalc, M. Monge, C. Lubetzki and N. A. Baumann   267

37 Immune Complexes and Complement in Multiple Sclerosis
    H. Jans   271

38 Myelin Basic Protein Like Reactivity in Normal Serum
    T. A. Out, P. C. Driedijk and J. Baas   277

39 Blood-brain Barrier in Experimental Allergic Encephalomyelitis and
    Multiple Sclerosis. A Minireview
    J. J. Hauw and J. M. Lefauconnier   283

40 The Possible Role of Viral Infections in Multiple Sclerosis
    V. ter Meulen   289

SECTION IV HLA, EPIDEMIOLOGY, GENETICS

41 Multiple Sclerosis Cooperative Etiological Study in Italy
   C. Fieschi   295

42 A Multicenter Study of the Incidence of Multiple Sclerosis in Italy.
   Design of the Study
   G. Comi   305

43 HLA Markers and Course of Disease in Multiple Sclerosis
   M. Merienne, O. Sabouraud, R. Fauchet, M. Madigand, G. Semana,
   M. Gueguen, G. Dejour and G. Morel   315

44 HLA Antigens in Multiple Sclerosis Patients in the Benelux
   H. Carton, I. van de Putte, J. M. Minderhoud, J. M. Balen,
   O. R. Hommes, P. Reekers, R. Medaer, M. de Bruyère, D. Latinne
   and A. Bouckaert   323

45 HLA Antigens and Multiple Sclerosis in Barbagia, Sardinia:
   Preliminary Results
   P. L. Mattiuz, C. Conighi, M. T. Grappa, R. Tola and G. Rosati   329

46 Clinical and Immunogenetic Data of 33 Double Case Families with
   Multiple Sclerosis: A Starting Point for Further Analyses on the
   DNA Level
   H. Zander   333

47 Twin Studies in Multiple Sclerosis
   A. Heltberg   337

SECTION V IMAGING AND NEUROPHYSIOLOGY

48 The Role of Imaging in the Diagnosis of Multiple Sclerosis
   W. I. McDonald   345

49 Nuclear Resonance Imaging of Multiple Sclerosis Brain Lesions
   L. Rumbach, M. C. Caires, C. Scheiber, J. M. Warter, J. Chambron
   and M. Collard   349

50 Neurophysiological Studies in Demyelination and Remyelination
   T. A. Sears   353

51 Horizontal Eye-movement Abnormalities in Multiple Sclerosis and
   Optic Neuritis
   E. A. C. M. Sanders and J. P. H. Reulen   357

52 The Vestibulo-ocular Reflex in Multiple Sclerosis
    P. L. M. Huygen, E. J. J. M. Theunissen and O. R. Hommes   363

53 New Possibilities in the Diagnosis of Multiple Sclerosis by Accurate
    Registration of Eye Movements with the DMI Method
    L. J. Bour and J. de Veth   373

54 A Parametric Study of Saccadic Eye Movements in Follow-up of
    Normals and Multiple Sclerosis Patients
    *E. T. L. van Munster, P. L. M. Huygen, L. J. Bour and
    O. R. Hommes*   383

55 Visual Evoked Responses in Definite and Suspected Multiple
    Sclerosis. Comparison of them to Cerebrospinal Fluid Oligoclonal
    Bands
    I. Milonas   393

    Index   399

Introduction

Multiple sclerosis is an unique disease with a tremendous impact on social life in countries with moderate climates. Its cause is unknown. In recent years however hopes have been raised that the disease might be fought, and possibly cured.

With the disappearance of poliomyelitis as the main paralyzing disease multiple sclerosis has taken its place as the single disease that is responsible for paralyzing the young with an incurable affliction of long duration, for social disruption and for an economic impact that is estimated to be higher than heart disease[1].

A multi-national, multi-disciplinary approach to this extremely disabling disease is urgently needed in this phase of hopeful scientific developments.

The Commission of the European Communities therefore sponsored a Conference on Multiple Sclerosis Research in Europe on 29, 30 and 31 January 1985 in Nijmegen, The Netherlands, with the aim of formulating practical proposals for such cooperation in the Communities. This volume contains the papers read at that conference.

An extensive report of the discussions and recommendations of the conference was presented to the Commission of the European Communities in March 1985[2].

It was felt that a general *rating scale* for use in clinical assessment of severity and course of the disease was urgently needed. Several of such scales already exist, but are not in general use[1].

In the last twenty years, prospects for treatment and even cure of multiple sclerosis have become more promising. However the *design and execution of treatment trials* were hampered by many flaws, so that the results have remained open to criticism. Recent years have brought new tools to clinicians to perform reliable clinical trials. These trials will need large numbers of patients and these numbers can be only collected in a short period of time by means of a coordinated effort on the part of a large number of clinical centers. European clinical centers could make a significant contribution.

Brain tissues, CSF and blood cells of multiple sclerosis patients are needed for nearly all studies. These materials have to be well preserved. Multinational *storage facilities for MS material* should be made available as soon as possible.

The conference felt that in this phase of clinical and basic studies in multiple sclerosis, the importance of some fundamental issues should be stressed. In particular *fundamental studies in neuro-immunology, remyelination, glial-axon-relationship and conduction block* should have priority. Many of the clinical questions are dependent for their solution on better insight into these fundamental problems.

Reliable markers for disease activity and disease course are still not known. It is one of the main problems in clinical studies and treatment trials. It should therefore be one of the aims of concerted action in MS research. Multiple sclerosis is not the only demyelinating disease present in Europe. The conference advocated that *other demyelinating* diseases of the central and peripheral nervous system should be studied in close relation to multiple sclerosis.

Neuropsychological studies in multiple sclerosis remain an underdeveloped area in MS research. Since NMR studies have demonstrated many lesions in so called 'silent' areas of the brain, attention should be directed to new methods to let these areas 'speak'. In recent years psycho-neuro-immunology has appeared as a new line of research with prospects of discoveries in the relation between human behaviour and man's immunological status.

The conference was divided into five sections.
- Clinical studies and therapeutic trials
- Immunology
- Biochemistry, neurobiology, myelin
- HLA, epidemiology, genetics
- Imaging and neurophysiology

Each of these sections formulated conclusions and proposals for coordinated research in Europe, that are briefly summarized here.

I CLINICAL STUDIES AND THERAPEUTIC TRIALS
Standardization of data collection is a prerequisite for all studies and trials. This should be used in an effort to improve protocol design in therapeutic trials.

Studies of placebo response, psychological aspects in response to treatment and other aspects of psycho-neuro-immunology should be examined.

II IMMUNOLOGY
Main emphasis should be directed to T cell clone and T cell line studies of the CSF. The morphology of CSF cells, their migration and traffic are of fundamental importance. Attention should be paid to neuromodulators and neuromediators in the immunological response. The specific cellular immunotherapy of experimental allergic encephalomyelitis (EAE) and neuritis (EAN) should also be stressed.

III BIOCHEMISTRY, NEUROBIOLOGY, MYELIN
In neuropathology the so called 'normal' white matter of MS brains should come under close scrutiny. Next should figure the early lesion in MS, the immuno-pathology of plaques and the pathology of peripheral nerves and the eye.

NMR findings in relation to pathology should be clarified in the coming years.

Biochemistry of myelin, myelinogenesis and remyelination is of basic importance for the understanding of the MS process. These studies should be linked to those of animal models of demyelination.

Viral studies in mechanisms of triggering auto-immune reactions in the brain and dysfunction of brain cells, neuro-virulence and viral persistence in the brain should be the focus of concerted action.

IV HLA, GENETICS, EPIDEMIOLOGY

With its migration of workers from southern to northern parts of the continent, Europe offers good opportunities to distinguish environmental aspects from genetic ones.

The HLA antigen frequencies should be studied in multicase families. Twin studies should offer even more opportunities to look into environmental and genetic causes of MS.

V NEUROPHYSIOLOGY AND IMAGING

Neurophysiology of conduction disturbances and their restoration are of prime importance. It may prove highly rewarding especially to study the improvement of conduction in the demyelinated state.

Early diagnosis should be made possible by new neurophysiological measuring techniques. Specific concentration of clinical neurophysiology on evoked potentials is advocated. The significance of progressive latency increase in multiple sclerosis related to morphological, biochemical and pharmacological aspects has to be elucidated. The study of central processing of the evoked potential may be especially rewarding.

NMR imaging has revolutionized insight in frequency and location of MS lesions in an early stage of the disease. Highly important investigations should be started in cooperation between various centers, especially on the relation between bio-chemistry and the NMR signal, on the tagging of cells that can be followed in NMR and the combination of NMR spectroscopy.

This conference kindled the hope that a cooperative effort and concerted action in Europe could greatly contribute to the understanding of the disease process in MS and to its treatment.

Otto R. Hommes,
Nijmegen, October 1985.

---

[1] Inman, R. P. (1984). Disability indices, the economic costs of illness, and social insurance: The case of multiple sclerosis. In: R. J. Slater and N. E. Raun (Editors), Symposium on a minimal record of disability for multiple sclerosis. A tribute to Torben Fog. *Acta Neur. Scand.*, suppl. 101, vol. 70, 46–55.
[2] Hommes, O. R. Report to the Commission of the European Communities of a Conference on Multiple Sclerosis Research in Europe held in Nijmegen, The Netherlands, 29, 30, 31 January 1985.

Conference on

MULTIPLE SCLEROSIS RESEARCH IN EUROPE

by entrustment of the

Commission of the European Communities

organized by Prof.Dr. O.R. Hommes

on 29, 30 and 31 January 1985

Belvoir Hotel, Nijmegen, The Netherlands

Organizing Committee in the Institute of Neurology:
Mrs. J.F.H. van Straten-Podgorski, secretary.
Mr. F.J.J. Dehue.
Drs. K.J.B. Lamers.

Institute of Neurology,   Secretariat:
Radboud University Hospital,   Reinier Postlaan 4,
Catholic University,   6525 GC Nijmegen.
Nijmegen, The Netherlands.   tel: 080-513970.

TUESDAY JANUARY 29, 1985

OPENING OF THE CONFERENCE

14.00 - 19.00 Registration

17.00 - 18.00 Chairmen's meeting

19.00 - 20.00 Official opening of the conference followed by reception

Speakers: Prof.Dr. O.R. Hommes, organizer.

              Prof.Dr. F.J.M. Daemen, Chairman Medical Faculty Nijmegen.

              Prof.Dr. B.P.M. Schulte, Director Institute of Neurology, Nijmegen.

              Dr. E. Levi, Director Joint Research Centre/CEC, Ispra, Italy.

20.00   Dinner.

WEDNESDAY JANUARY 30, 1985

PLENARY MORNING SESSION   Chairman: J.M. Minderhoud, Groningen

REVIEW

9.00 - 9.20	S. Poser, Göttingen	Clinical studies
9.20 - 9.40	P. Rudge, London	Clinical trials
9.40 - 10.00	J. Mertin, Mannheim	Immunology
10.00 - 10.20	P. Delmotte, Melsbroek	Immunoglobulins
10.20 - 10.40	H. Lassmann, Vienna	EAE

10.40 - 11.10 COFFEE BREAK

11.10 - 11.30	J.M. Matthieu, Lausanne	Myelin
11.30 - 11.50	R. Batchelor, London	HLA, genetics, epidemiology
11.50 - 12.10	A.M. Halliday, London	Pathophysiology and demyelination
12.10 - 12.30	W.I. McDonald, London	Imaging

12.30 - 14.00 LUNCH

WEDNESDAY JANUARY 30, 1985

PARALLEL AFTERNOON SESSIONS

SECTION I CLINICAL STUDIES   Chairman: Ch. Confavreux, Lyon

14.00 - 14.15   Ch. Confavreux, Lyon   Clinical characteristics of a
                                            hospital investigated MS
                                            population

14.15 - 14.30   R. Medaer, Overpelt   Incapacity and disability in MS

14.30 - 14.45   J. Minderhoud, Groningen   Incapacity and disability in MS

14.45 - 15.00   R. Gonsette, Melsbroek   Immunosuppressive treatment:
                                            cyclophosphamide

15.00 - 15.15   R. Marteau, Paris   Anti-lymphocyte globulin treatment

15.15 - 15.45   TEA BREAK

15.45 - 16.00   O. Sabouraud, Rennes   Azathioprine treatment

16.00 - 16.15   I. Zeeberg, Copenhagen   Azathioprine treatment

16.15 - 16.30   D. Dommasch, Würzburg   Cyclosporin A

16.30 - 17.00   D. Bates, New Castle   Dietary treatments
                                            Hyperbaric oxygen

17.00 - 18.30   Formulate proposals for coordinated research in Europe
                to be discussed in plenary sessions on Thursday
                    - expertise
                    - approach
                    - centers
                    - cooperation

WEDNESDAY JANUARY 30, 1985

PARALLEL AFTERNOON SESSIONS

SECTION II   IMMUNOLOGY   Chairman: C.J. Lucas, Amsterdam

14.00 - 14.15   M.A. Bach, Paris   T cell subsets

14.15 - 14.30   M. Sandberg-Wollheim,   Lymphocyte subpopulations in CSF
                Lund

14.30 - 14.45   H. Nyland, Bergen   T cell subsets in MS brain

14.45 - 15.00   O.R. Hommes, Nijmegen   T cell subsets in MS brain and CSF

15.00 - 15.15   C.J. Lucas, Amsterdam   Towards cloning of CSF cells

15.15 - 15.45   TEA BREAK

15.45 - 16.00   E. Braakman, Amsterdam   Cytotoxic activities

16.00 - 16.15   H. Wekerle, Würzburg   Modulation of T cells in EAE and MS

16.15 - 16.30   L. Rumbach, Strasbourg   Cytotoxic antibodies

16.30 - 17.00   W. Fierz, Zürich   Immunological functions of astrocytes

17.00 - 18.30   Formulate proposals for coordinated research in Europe
                to be discussed in plenary sessions on Thursday
                - expertise
                - approaches
                - centers
                - cooperation

WEDNESDAY JANUARY 30, 1985

PARALLEL AFTERNOON SESSIONS

SECTION III BIOCHEMISTRY, NEUROBIOLOGY, MYELIN

Chairman: I.V. Allen, Belfast

14.00 - 14.15	I.V. Allen, Belfast	Pathology of MS and EAE
14.15 - 14.30	J.J. Hauw, Paris	Blood brain barrier in MS and EAE
14.30 - 14.45	L. Amaducci, Florence	Spinal fluid dynamics
14.45 - 15.00	H. Link, Linköping	CSF immunoglobulins and clinical course
15.00 - 15.15	K. Lamers, Nijmegen	Immunoglobulin synthesis in brain and CSF
15.15 - 15.45	TEA BREAK	
15.45 - 16.00	D. Caputo, Milano	IgG synthesis in CSF
16.00 - 16.15	B. Zalc, Paris	MBP and galacto cerebroside as antigens
16.15 - 16.30	H. Jans, Copenhagen	Immune complexes and complement factors
16.30 - 16.45	Th. Out, Amsterdam	MBP like activity in normal serum
16.45 - 17.00	V. ter Meulen, Würzburg	Possible role of viral infections in MS
17.00 - 17.15	B. v.d. Zeijst, Utrecht	Murine corona virus and demyelination

17.15 - 18.30   Formulate proposals for coordinated research in Europe
to be discussed in plenary sessions on Thursday
- expertise
- approaches
- centers
- cooperation

WEDNESDAY JANUARY 30, 1985

PARALLEL AFTERNOON SESSIONS

SECTION IV   HLA, EPIDEMIOLOGY, GENETICS

Chairman: M. Merienne, Rennes

14.00 - 14.15	M. Merienne, Rennes	HLA and course of disease
14.15 - 14.30	C. Fieschi, Rome	Epidemiology in Italy
14.30 - 14.45	H. Carton, Melsbroek	HLA study in Benelux
14.45 - 15.00	A. Heltberg, Roskilde	Twin studies
15.00 - 15.15	H. Zander, München	Double case families
15.15 - 15.45	TEA BREAK	
15.45 - 16.00	G. Comi, Milano	Epidemiology in Italy
16.00 - 16.15	R. Batchelor, London	Cooperative HLA study program
16.15 - 16.30	P.L. Mattiuz, Ferrara	HLA study in Italy

16.30 - 18.30   Formulate proposals for coordinated research in Europe
to be discussed in plenary sessions on Thursday
- expertise
- approach
- centers
- cooperation

WEDNESDAY JANUARY 30, 1985

PARALLEL AFTERNOON SESSIONS

SECTION V   IMAGING AND NEUROPHYSIOLOGY

Chairman: T.A. Sears, London

14.00 - 14.15	E. Sanders, Leiden	Eye movement studies
14.15 - 14.30	P. Huygen, Nijmegen	The vestibulo-ocular reflex
14.30 - 14.45	E. van Munster, Nijmegen	Saccadic eye movement
14.45 - 15.00	L. Bour, Nijmegen	Double magnetic induction, a new approach to eye movement registration
15.00 - 15.15	T.A. Sears, London	Neurophysiological studies in de- and re-myelination
15.15 - 15.45	TEA BREAK	
15.45 - 16.00	I. Milonas, Thessaloniki	Evoked responses
16.00 - 16.15	A.M. Halliday. London	Evoked response studies in demyelination
16.15 - 16.30	W.I. McDonald, London	Imaging and NMR studies
16.30 - 16.45	M. Collard, Strasbourg	NMR in multiple sclerosis

16.45 - 18.30   Formulate proposals for coordinated research in Europe
to be discussed in plenary sessions on Thursday
- expertise
- approach
- centers
- cooperation

THURSDAY JANUARY 31, 1985

PLENARY MORNING SESSION

DISCUSSION OF PROPOSALS ON COORDINATION OF MS RESEARCH IN EUROPE

Chairmen: C. Fieschi, Rome and
J. Mertin, Mannheim

 9.00 - 10.00   Section I   : Clinical studies

10.00 - 11.00   Section II   : Immunology

11.00 - 11.30   COFFE BREAK

11.30 - 12.30   Section III : Biochemistry, neurobiology, myelin

12.30 - 14.00   LUNCH

PLENARY AFTERNOON SESSION   Chairmen: O.R. Hommes, Nijmegen and
H. Wekerle, Würzburg

14.00 - 15.00   Section IV   : HLA, epidemiology, genetics

15.00 - 16.00   Section V   : Imaging and neurophysiology

16.00 - 16.30   TEA BREAK

16.30 - 18.00   Final proposals for coordination of MS research in
Europe

18.00   Closing of the conference

LIST OF PARTICIPANTS

Names marked with ■ are observers

I.V. Allen
Institute of Pathology,
Grosvenor Road,
Belfast BT12 6BL, England.
tel. 240503 ext. 2019/2319.

L. Amaducci
Clinica Neurologica,
Viale Morgagni 85,
Firenze 50134, Italy.
tel. 0039-55-432224.

■ O. Anderson
Department of Neurology,
Sahlgren Hospital,
41345 Göteborg, Sweden.
tel. 46-31-601000/601570.

M.A. Bach
Institut Pasteur,
Unité de Pathologie de l'Immunité,
29 rue du Dr. Roux.
75724 Paris Cedex 15, France.
tel. 1-3061919 ext. 3260.

J.R. Batchelor
Department of Immunology,
Hammersmith Hospital,
Duncane Road,
London W12 OHS, England.
tel. 7432030 ext. 423.

D. Bates
The Royal Victoria Infirmary,
Queen Victoria Road,
New Castle upon Tyne NE1 4 LP, England.
tel. 325231.

■ N. Baumann
Laboratoire de Neurochimie,
INSERM U 134,
Hôpital de la Salpêtrière,
47 Boulevard de l'Hôpital,
75651 Paris Cedex 13, France.
tel. 1-5862012.

L.J. Bour
Radboud University Hospital,
Medical Physics and Biophysics,
Geert Grooteplein noord 21,
Nijmegen, The Netherlands

E. Braakman

Centraal Laboratorium van de Bloed-
transfusiedienst,
Afdeling Cel Immunologie,
Plesmanlaan 125,
1006 AD Amsterdam, The Netherlands.
tel. 020-5123317.

D. Caputo

Centro Studi Sclerosi Multipla,
Ospedale San Antonio,
Via Pastori 4,
21012 Gallarate (VA), Italy.
tel. 796616.

H. Carton

Centre National de la Sclérose en Plaques,
Vanheylenstraat 16,
B-1910 Melsbroek, Belgium.
tel. 7518030.

■M. Clanet

Centre Hospitalier Regional de Toulouse,
Service de Neurologie C,
C.H.U. Toulouse Purpan,
Place du Docteur Baylac,
31059 Toulouse Cedex, France.
tel. 491133.

M. Collard

Clinique Neurologique Hôpital Civil,
B.P. 42,
67091 Strasbourg Cedex, France.
tel. 88-367111.

■ E. Colon

Radboud University Hospital,
Department of Clinical Neurophysiology,
Reinier Postlaan 4,
6525 GC Nijmegen, The Netherlands.
tel. 31-80513973.

G. Comi

Department of Neurology,
Scientific Institute S. Raffaele,
University of Milan Medical School,
Milan, Italy.

Ch. Confavreux

Hôpital Neurologique,
59 Boulevard Pinel,
B.P. Lyon Montchat,
69003 Lyon Cedex, France.
tel. 7853-81-81 poste 34-36.

■ J-D. Degos

Hôpital Henri-Mondor,
Service de Neurologie,
94010 Créteil, France.
tel. 2075141 ext. 2301.

P. Delmotte

Centre National de la Sclérose en Plaques,
Vanheylenstraat 16,
B-1910 Melsbroek, Belgium.
tel. 02-7519742.

D. Dommasch

Neurologische Universitätsklinik und
Poliklinik im Kopfklinikum,
Josef Schneiderstrasse 11,
8700 Würzburg, G.F.R.
tel. 2012251.

W. Fierz

Section of Clinical Immunology,
University Hospital,
Häldeliweg 4,
CH-8044 Zürich, Switzerland.
tel. 01-2572863.

C. Fieschi

Dipartimento di Scienze Neurologiche,
00185 V. de dell'Universtià 30,
Rome, Italy.
tel. 06-490954.

R. Gonsette

Centre National de la Sclérose en Plaques,
Vanheylenstraat 16,
B-1910 Melsbroek, Belgium.
tel. 7518030.

A.M. Halliday

Institute of Neurology,
National Hospital for Nervous Diseases,
Queen Square,
London WC1, England.
tel. 01-8373611.

J.J. Hauw

Laboratoire de Neuropathologie Charles Fois,
Hôpital de la Salpêtrière,
47 Boulevard de l'Hôpital,
F 75651 Paris Cedex 13, France.
tel. 1-5703130.

A. Heltberg

Department of Neurology,
Amtssygehuset,
Køgevej 7-13,
4000 Roskilde, Denmark.
tel. 02-370337 ext. 502.

O.R. Hommes

Radboud University Hospital,
Department of Neurology,
Reinier Postlaan 4,
6525 GC Nijmegen, The Netherlands.
tel. 31-80513970.

P. Huygen   Radboud University Hospital,
                             Department of E.N.T.,
                             Philips van Leydenlaan 15,
                             6525 EX Nijmegen, The Netherlands.
                             tel. 31-8054944.

H. Jans   Medical Department C.,
                             County Hospital in Gentofte,
                             DK 2900 Hellerup, Denmark.
                             tel. 01-651200.
                             mailing address: Fogdens Plads 4,
                                              DK-2791 Dragør.
                                              Denmark.

■ J. Kesselring   Department of Neurology,
                             Inselspital,
                             3010 Bern, Switzerland.
                             tel. 031-643066

■ J.C. Koetsier   Valeriuskliniek,
                             Valeriusplein 9,
                             1075 BG Amsterdam, The Netherlands.
                             tel. 31-20788788.

■ M. Koolen   Fakulteit der Diergeneeskunde,
                             Rijksuniversiteit Utrecht,
                             Vakgroep Virologie,
                             Yalelaan 1,
                             Utrecht, The Netherlands.
                             tel. 31-30532486/532488.

■ J.J. Kuneman   Viviënstraat 27,
                             2582 RR Den Haag, The Netherlands.

■ H. ter Laak   Radboud University Hospital,
                             Department of Neurology, N4,
                             Reinier Postlaan 4,
                             6525 GC Nijmegen, The Netherlands.
                             31-80515294.

K. Lamers   Radboud University Hospital,
                             Laboratory of Clinical Chemistry,
                             Reinier Postlaan 4,
                             6525 GC Nijmegen, The Netherlands.
                             tel. 31-80514568.

H. Lassmann   Neurologisches Institut der Universität
                             Wien,
                             Schwarzspanierstrasse 17,
                             A-1090 Vienna, Austria.

■E. Levi

Biology Division D.G. XII,
Joint Research Centre CEC,
21020 Ispra (VA), Italy.
tel. 789349.

H. Link

Department of Neurology,
Karolinska Institutet,
Huddinge Hospital,
S-14186 Huddinge, Sweden.
tel. 08-7461000.

■G.E. Lovatt

Department of Clinical Investigation,
Wellcome Research Laboratories,
Langley Court,
Beckenham, Kent BR3 3BS, England.

■C. Lubetzki

Laboratoire de Neurochimie,
INSERM U 134,
Hôpital de la Salpêtrière,
47 Boulevard de l'Hôpital,
75651 Paris Cedex 13, France.
tel. 1-5862012.

C.J. Lucas

Centraal Laboratorium van de Bloed-
transfusiedienst,
Afdeling Cel Immunologie,
Plesmanlaan 125,
1006 AD Amsterdam, The Netherlands.
tel. 31-205123317.

■J. Luijten

Department of Neurology,
Nicolaas Beetsstraat 24,
3511 GV Utrecht, The Netherlands.
tel. 31-30379111 ext. 1364.

R. Marteau

Service de Neurologie,
Hôpital Saint-Antoine,
Pavillon Lemierre,
184 Rue du Faubourg St. Antoine,
75571 Paris Cedex 12, France.
tel. 3421807.

J-M. Matthieu

Laboratoire du Neurochemie,
Service de Pédiatrie,
Centre Hospitalier Universitaire Vaudois,
CH-1011 Lausanne, Switzerland.
tel. 21-411111/21-412570.

P.L. Mattiuz   Institute of Medical Genetics,
                           Via L. Borsari 46,
                           Ferrara 44100, Italy,
                           tel. 0532-35021.

W.I. McDonald   Institute of Neurology,
                           National Hospital for Nervous Diseases,
                           Queen Square,
                           London WC1, England.

R. Medaer   MS and Rehabilitation Clinic,
                           Boemerangstraat 2,
                           3583 Overpelt, Belgium.
                           tel. 011-640121.

M. Merienne   Service de Neurologie,
                           Hôpital Pontchaillou,
                           Rue Henri le Guillou,
                           35033 Rennes Cedex, France.

J. Mertin   Boehringer Mannheim GmbH,
                           Department of Immunopharmacology,
                           Sandhofer Strasse 116,
                           Postfach 31020,
                           6800 Mannheim 31, G.F.R.
                           tel. 0621-759-2416.

V. ter Meulen   Institut für Virologie und Immunobiologie,
                           Universität Würzburg,
                           Würzburg, G.F.R.
                           tel. 2013954.

I. Milonas   2nd Department of Neurology,
                           Agios Dimitrios Hospital,
                           University of Thessaloniki,
                           Thessaloniki, Greece.
                           tel. 204368.

J.M. Minderhoud   Academisch Ziekenhuis Groningen,
                           Afdeling Neurologie,
                           Oostersingel 59,
                           9713 EZ Groningen, The Netherlands.
                           tel. 31-50612430.

E. van Munster   Radboud University Hospital,
                           Department of Neurology,
                           Reinier Postlaan 4,
                           6525 GC Nijmegen, The Netherlands.

■W. Nillesen   Radboud University Hospital,
                           Department of Experimental Neurology,
                           Reinier Postlaan 4,
                           6525 GC Nijmegen, The Netherlands.
                           tel. 31-80515290.

 N. Nyland   Department of Neurology,
                           N-5016 Haukeland Sykehus,
                           Bergen, Norway.
                           tel. 05-298060 ext. 4000.

 Th. Out   Centraal Laboratorium van de Bloedtrans-
                           fusiedienst,
                           Postbus 9190,
                           1006 AD Amsterdam, The Netherlands.

■D.W. Paty   University of British Columbia,
                           Vancouver General Hospital,
                           Vancouver B.C., V5Z 3J5, Canada.
                           tel. 604-873-5441.

■C. Polman   Department of Neurology,
                           Academisch Ziekenhuis Vrije Universiteit,
                           De Boelelaan 1117,
                           1081 VV Amsterdam, The Netherlands.
                           tel. 31-205488006.

 S. Poser   Neurologische Universitätsklinik,
                           Robert Kochstrasse 40,
                           D 3400 Göttingen, G.F.R.
                           tel. 0551-396684.

■J. Raus and   Dr. L. Willems-Instituut vzw.,
■E. Bosmans   Universitaire Campus,
                           3610 Diepenbeek, Belgium.
                           tel. 011-226721.

 F. Rotteveel   Centraal Laboratorium van de Bloed-
                           transfusiedienst,
                           Afdeling Cel Immunologie,
                           Plesmanlaan 125,
                           1006 AD Amsterdam, The Netherlands.
                           tel. 31-205123317.

■E. Roullet   Service de Neurologie,
                           Hôpital St. Antoine,
                           184 Rue de Faubourg St. Antoine,
                           75012 Paris, France.
                           tel. 344.33.33.

P. Rudge   The National Hospitals for Nervous
                              Diseases,
                              Maida Vale Hospital, W.9,
                              Queen Square,
                              London W9 1TL, England.

L. Rumbach   Clinique Neurologique Hôpital Civil,
                              B.P. 42,
                              67091 Stasbourg Cedex, France.
                              tel. 88-367111.

O. Sabouraud   Service de Neurologie,
                              Hôpital Pontchaillou,
                              Rue Henri le Guillou,
                              35033 Rennes Cedex, France.
                              tel. 99-591604.

M. Sandberg-Wollheim   Department of Neurology,
                              University of Lund,
                              University Hospital,
                              S-211 85 Lund, Sweden.

E. Sanders   Academisch Ziekenhuis Leiden,
                              Department of Neurology,
                              Rijnsburgerweg 10,
                              2333 AA Leiden, The Netherlands.
                              tel. 31-71269111.

■ M. Schachner   Institut für Neurobiologie der
                              Universität Heidelberg,
                              Im Neuheimer Feld 504,
                              D-6900 Heidelberg, G.F.R.
                              tel. 06221-563827.

Th. Sears   Institute of Neurology,
                              National Hospital for Nervous Diseases,
                              Queen Square,
                              London WC1, England.
                              tel. 8373611.

■ A. Thompsen   St. Vincent's Consultants' Private Clinic,
                              Herbert Avenue, Merrion Road,
                              Dublin 4, Ireland.
                              tel. 695033.

■ E. Tournier Lasserve
Unité de Pathologie de l'Immunité,
Institut Pasteur,
28 rue du Dr. Roux,
75724 Paris Cedex 15, France.
tel. 1-306.19.19.

■ B. Uitdehaag
Radboud University Hospital,
Department of Experimental Neurology,
Reinier Postlaan 4,
6525 GC Nijmegen, The Netherlands.
tel. 31-80515289.

■ H. van Walbeek
Onze Lieve Vrouwe Gasthuis,
Department of Neurology,
le Oosterparkstraat 179,
1091 HA Amsterdam, The Netherlands.
tel. 31-205999111.

H. Wekerle
MGP-klinische Forschungsgruppe für
Multipele Sklerose,
Josef Schneiderstrasse 11,
Postfach 6120,
D-8700 Würzburg, G.F.R.
tel. 2012250.

B. Zalc
Laboratoire de Neurochimie,
INSERM U 134,
Hôpital de la Salpêtrière,
47 Boulevard de l'Hôpital,
75651 Paris Cedex 13, France.
tel. 1-5862012.

H. Zander
Labor für Immungenetik,
Kinderpoliklinik der Universität München,
Pettenkoferstrasse 8a,
D-8000 München 40, G.F.R.
tel. 089-5160-3713.

I. Zeeberg
Neuromed. Afd. 2081,
Rigshospitalet,
DK-2100 Copenhagen Ø, Denmark.
tel. 01-386633 ext. 2287.

B. van der Zeijst
Fakulteit der Diergeneeskunde,
Rijksuniversiteit Utrecht,
Vakgroep Virologie,
Yalelaan 1,
Utrecht-de Uithof, The Netherlands.
tel. 31-30532486/532488.

Section I
Clinical Studies

1

Clinical Studies in Multiple Sclerosis

S. POSER

Clinical studies in Multiple Sclerosis (MS) have a long tradition, the first clinical description being published over a century ago. But even earlier than this, a patient with MS, Augustus d'Este, recorded his symptoms in a detailed diary (Firth 1948). D'Este's handwriting gives more accurate account of his state of health than any medical description could: In 1822 it was extremely legible, but by 1848, shortly before his death, ataxia had deteriorated his penmanship considerably.

The classical description by Charcot is known to you all. He identified the key clinical features, among which scanning speech, nystagmus and intention tremor are known as the Charcot's triad. These early descriptions were biased toward the advanced cases and we still live under the impression of this unfavorable picture which contributes to the many prejudices connected with the diagnosis. R. Müller (1949) was one of the first to analyse a more representative sample of over 800 patients and to give a survey on the symptomatology, one which still appears in modern textbooks (table 1). The frequency of disturbances is comparable to the one we found in a sample of 3091 patients recorded recently (table 2). In addition to the present symptomatology the reversibility of signs and symptoms can be estimated from this table. Provided that patients who are examined during an acute bout are excluded, the comparison of the frequency during the total course and at present examination reflects the tendency of the particular sign to remit or the successful treatment of the disturbance. However, all these data were gathered from hospitalized patients and are therefore biased, again, towards the more severe mani-

3

festations.

Table 1 Frequency of symptoms in MS

Balance abnormalities	78%	Paraesthesiae	40%
Impaired sensation	71%	Giddiness	32%
Paraparesis	62%	Hemiparesis	18%
Micturition changes	62%	Facial palsy	15%
Optic neuritis	55%	Epilepsy	5%
Monoparesis	52%	Impotence	5%
Ataxia of limbs	45%	Hearing loss	4%
Diplopia	43%	Tic douloureux	2%

Müller (1949)
Published in Hallpike, J.F. (1983)

Table 2 Survey of the Symptomatology of 3091 MS Patients

              (mean duration of the disease 11.3 years)

disturbance	at present examination	during total course
spasticity	76.7%	84.7%
pareses	71.4%	84.7%
ataxia	71.2%	78.7%
sensory	68.9%	85.8%
sphincter/sexual	52.4%	61.1%
cerebral	33.4%	38.6%
trigeminal/facial	18.3%	30.5%
diplopia	13.9%	35.6%

We compared our own hospital statistics with results obtained by
examination of epidemiological patients and found that among the latter,
the frequency of disturbances was less in all functional systems (table
3). This more favorable picture also appeared when we considered the disability present after a certain duration of the disease (figure 1). The
traditional Kurtzke disability scale with its full steps between 0 and 10
was used to characterize the hospital and the epidemiological sample.
There are many different rating scales available at present and an effort
is being made to come to an agreement in respect to a minimal record of
disability for international comparisons (Slater and Raun 1984). Besides
the disability status scale, the functional system scales of Kurtzke, an
incapacity and a socioeconomic scale are included. These efforts are important prerequisites for rehabilitation research and planning committees
and if there is to be European agreement on clinical research an adequate
documentation system has to be developed. It is not possible to use a
universal system for all aspects of MS. For therapeutic trials, for instance, it has to be more detailed than the minimal data set.

Table 3   Present symptomatology of different MS-samples

	Epidemiological Group N = 221	Hospital Group N = 1837
Mean Duration of Disease	12.1 years	10.5 years
DISTURBANCES		
Spasticity/Babinski	61 %	80 %
Paresis	57 %	78 %
Sensitivity	69 %	73 %
Eye motility	11 %	14 %
Trig./Facial	14 %	15 %
Brainstem/cerebellum	63 %	77 %
Cerebral	33 %	36 %
Vegetative	49 %	56 %

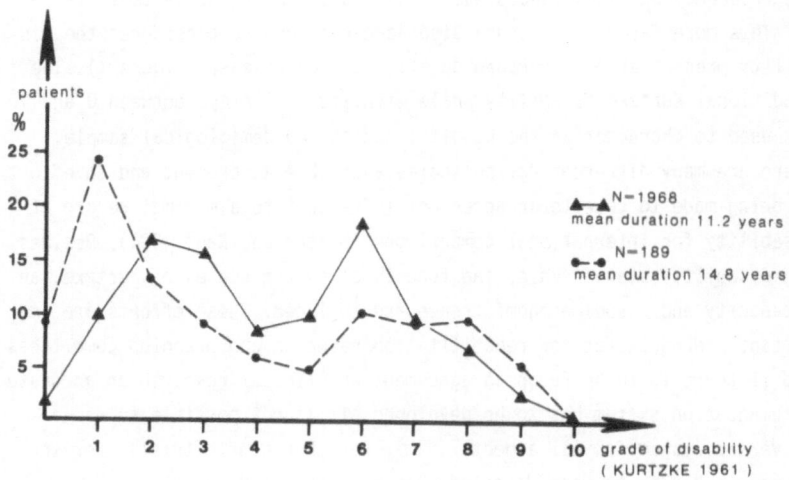

figure 1   Distribution of disability in MS.
Comparison of a hospital▲——▲ and an epidemiological •——•
sample.

Sipe et al. (1984) recently published a neurological rating scale
based on a detailed neurological examination, and Mickey et al. (1984)
proposed an illness severity score in which the disability scale, the
functional systems and course characteristics are combined to form a total score. Whether these attempts are better than the ones used by Fog
(1965) remains open at the moment. He was one of the first who tried to
gain information pertaining to the natural course of the disease by recording the neurological signs and symptoms over time in individual patients. With this method he was able to recognize different types of the
course and predicted the future course by the use of computer programs
(figure 2). Most of the results on course and prognosis were later confirmed and they are essentials for planning clinical studies; e.g. it is

important to realize that the frequency of bouts is of lesser significance for the eventual prognosis than the progression which develops in
between or underlying the bouts.

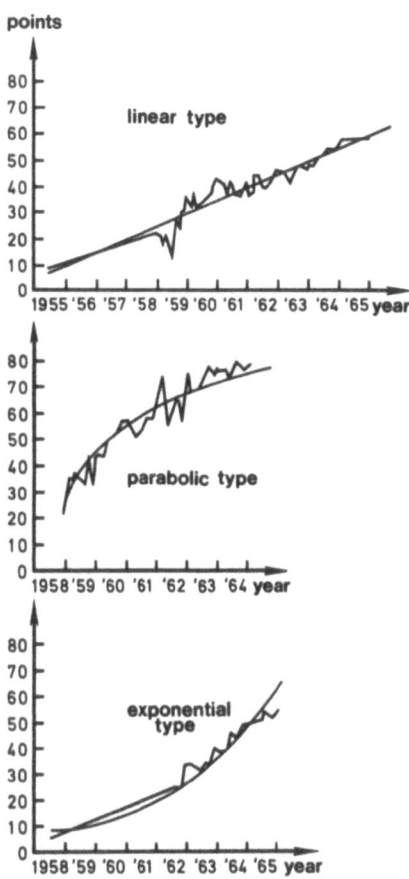

figure 2   The different types of course in MS according to Fog, T., 1966
            (Acta Neurol. Scand. 42: 608-611).

Among the many factors which have been analysed in respect to prognosis only 4 or 5 are generally accepted as predictors:

1. The pyramidal and cerebellar signs present after 5 years are a good prognostic parameter for the future course (Kurtzke et al. 1977).

2. The lower the age at onset, the better the prognosis. There is disagreement, however, whether the age at onset per se or the course of the disease is the decisive factor.

3. The remitting course has a better prognosis than the chronic progressive form (figure 3). Patients who are older at the onset more often have a chronic progressive course. From figure 4 it is evident that the remitting form has a good prognosis irrespective of the age at onset. The course seems to be a more significant factor than the age at onset.

4. The symptomatology at onset has a correlation to the prognosis: In a recent study by Visscher et al. (1984) earlier findings were confirmed that initial sensory signs and symptoms identify patients with a benign prognosis irrespective whether they are combined with other signs. Optic neuritis as initial sign was found to indicate a good prognosis by some authors, but not by others.

5. The area of residence seems to influence the prognosis: Clark et al. (1982) found that patients in the Los Angeles County (latitude 34°) had a worse prognosis compared to patients living in the King and Pierce Counties in the state of Washington (latitude 47°). This finding is in agreement with data from Asia. Although MS is rare in these regions it runs a more severe course in the individuals affected. In Clark's study the malignant cases more often reported adverse responses to heat exposure and favorable responses to cold exposure. Although temperature changes are usually considered to influence the disease only temporarily, the authors discuss the possibility that adverse effects associated with exposure to heat were in some cases irreversible. The well-known deteriorations connected with infections -particularly of the upper respiratory tract- can be caused by even minor temperature increases. Antipyretics can help to prevent these exacerbations.

Among the various factors which were claimed to influence the prognosis are emotional difficulties, trauma, vaccinations and gestational processes. All these may precipitate a temporary deterioration but do not influence the long-term prognosis. With respect to pregnancy we were recently able to confirm the findings of previous studies that onset and

cumulative frequency of patients

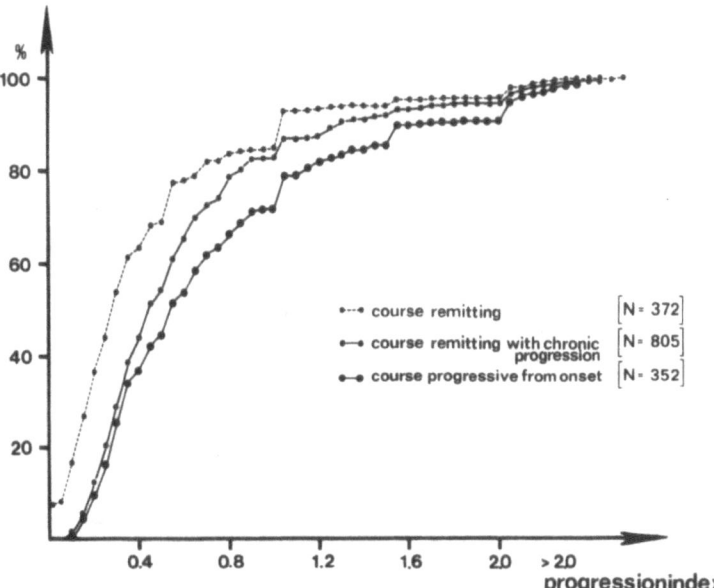

figure 3   Comparison of the prognosis for different courses of MS.

$$\text{Progressionindex} = \frac{\text{grade of disability}}{\text{duration of disease}}$$

deterioration occur more often during puerperium than during pregnancy (table 4), but that the final prognosis is not influenced by these bouts and deteriorations.

The accumulation of bouts after childbirth is a complex and poorly understood phenomenon and I think it is deserving of more research. A co-operative clinical study would enable the prospective follow-up of pregnant MS-patients including a monitoring of immunological parameters. It is known that several substances which are produced or increased during pregnancy, such as alpha-fetoprotein, are immunologically active and could protect the mother against deterioration of established or suspected autoimmune disease -an event which is well documentated in patients with rheumatoid arthritis and often observed in myasthenia gravis.

cumulative frequency of patients

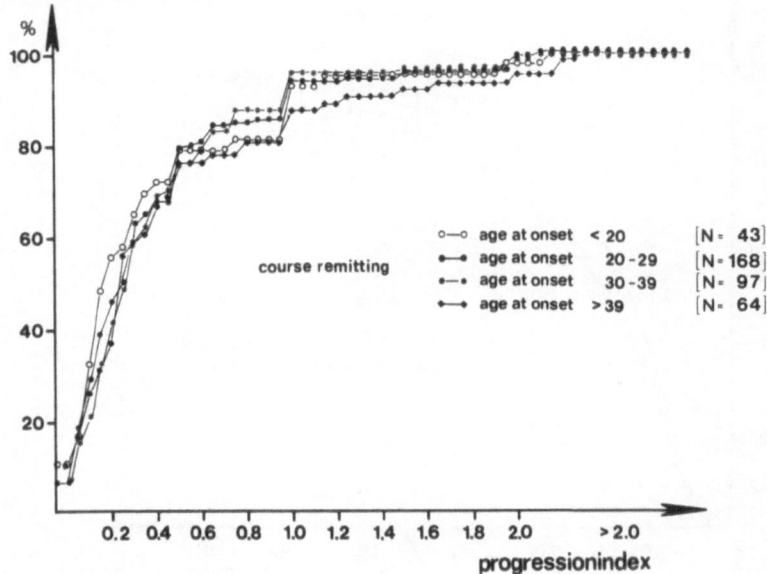

figure 4   Comparison of the prognosis for different ages at onset of
remitting MS.

$$\text{Progressionindex} = \frac{\text{grade of disability}}{\text{duration of disease}}$$

Table 4   Significance of Pregnancy and Childbirth
in Relation to Multiple Sclerosis

Patients pregnant before onset of disease	345
Onset during pregnancy	19 (5.5%)
Onset during 6 months after childbirth	59 (17.1%)
Patients pregnant during the disease	110
Deterioration during pregnancy	13 (11.8%)
Deterioration during 6 months after childbirth	28 (25.5%)

My final remark on clinical studies relates to diagnostic classification. An agreement on what we consider to be multiple sclerosis or what
we refer to as definite, probable or possible MS is a prerequisite for
any cooperative research. Fortunately the book on "Diagnosis of Multiple
Sclerosis" edited by Ch. M. Poser et al., who is my namesake but no relative, was published a few weeks ago. The guidelines for research protocols given in chapter 19 and the comparison of the different diagnostic
criteria in chapter 20 form a good basis for any committee working on the
diagnostic criteria in a European study. On the whole it seems to be accepted that csf-findings should be included within the criteria, a proposal which was made by Bauer over 10 years ago (table 5).

I believe that this agreement makes our goal of cooperative research
easier to attain.

Table 5 Diagnostic Criteria of Multiple Sclerosis   (Bauer 1972)

I. Definite
   A. 2 or more episodes of worsening in remitting cases, or a slow or
      a stepwise progression of signs and symptoms over at least one
      year
   B. Dissemination in space
   C. Typical csf-findings: mononuclear pleocytosis up to 50 cells/mm³,
      total protein normal or elevated slightly up to 100 mg/100 ml,
      left colloidal reaction, elevation of globulin fraction (IgG)

II. Probable
    Not all of the criteria of I are fulfilled, but at least two groups
    are present (A+B, B+C, A+C)
    In initial bout: I B+C present, typical csf-changes outlasting the
    clinical symptomatology
    In progression from onset: I B+C present, steady progression over at
    least 6 months, typical csf-changes persisting.

III. Possible
     A physician competent in clinical neurology should decide that the
     patients condition could not be better explained on the basis of
     some other disease. Course and symptomatology are not sufficiently
     characteristic of MS (I B+C), however.
     Monosymptomatic retrobulbar neuritis is located here

Clark, V.A., Detels, R., Visscher, B.R., Valdiviezo, N.L., Malmgren,
    R.M. and Dudley, J.P., 1982. Factors associated with a malignant or
    benign course of multiple sclerosis. JAMA, 248: 856-860.
Firth, D. 1948. The case of Augustus D'Este. Cambrigde University Press,
    Cambrigde.
Fog, T., 1965. A Scoring System for Neurologic Impairment in Multiple
    Sclerosis. Acta Neurol. Scand. 41, Suppl. 13: 551-555.
Kurtzke, J.F., Beebe, G.W., Nagler, B., Kurland, L.T. and Auth, Th.L.,
    1977. Studies on the natural history of multiple sclerosis 8. J.
    chron. Dis. 30: 819-830.
Mickey, M.R., Ellison, G.W. and Myers, L.W., 1984. An illness severity
    score for multiple sclerosis. Neurology 34: 1343-1347.
Müller, R., 1949. Studies on disseminated sclerosis. Acta Med. Scand.
    Suppl. 222: 1-214.
Poser, Ch.M., Paty, D.W., Scheinberg, L., McDonald, W.I. and Ebers, G.C.,
    (eds.) 1984. The Diagnosis of Multiple Sclerosis. New York, Thieme-
    Stratton.
Sipe, J.C., Knobler, R.L., Braheny, Sh.L., Rice, G.P.A., Panitch, H.S.
    and Oldstone, M.B.A., 1984. A neurologic rating scale (NRS) for use
    in multiple sclerosis. Neurology 34: 1368-1372.
Slater, R.J. and Raun, N.E. (eds.), 1984. Symposium on a Minimal Record
    of Disability for multiple sclerosis. Acta Neurol. Scand. 70, Suppl.
    '101: 1-217.
Visscher, B.R., Liu, K-S., Clark, V.A., Detels, R., Malmgren, R.M. and
    Dudley, J.P., 1984. Onset symptoms as predictors of mortality and
    disability in multiple sclerosis. Acta Neurol. Scand. 70: 321-328.

2

Clinical Trials

PETER RUDGE

Multiple sclerosis is a heterogeneous disorder. One group of patients
has repeated relapses, followed in some by progression, others are
progressive from the onset. Both the relapse rate and progression of
the disease alters in a non-linear way with time. For these reasons it
is not possible to assess the effect of any putative therapy without an
adequate control group of patients. Ideally a study of therapy should
involve a large population randomly assigned to the test and placebo
groups. In addition, if possible, the trial should be double blind to
avoid the substantial placebo response known to occur during trials of
multiple sclerosis therapy.

Four important points need emphasis:

1. The methods of selection, assessment and end points of any trial
should be clearly stated at the outset.

2. The acceptable false positive rate (type I error) should be stated
prior to the outset. If the therapy is potentially dangerous this error
should be smaller, say 1%, than if the therapy is harmless.

3. The acceptable false negative rate (type II error) for a given type
I error should be estimated prior to the outset making reasonable
assumptions as to the likely benefit to accrue from a treatment. This
will enable the experimenter to estimate the size of the two groups to
be recruited.

4. Do not repeatedly analyse the accumulating data and terminate the trial on this basis. This grossly underestimates the false positive value in the final analysis.

No trial of therapy in multiple sclerosis to date has fulfilled these criteria.

3

Onset, Course and Prognosis of Multiple Sclerosis

C. CONFAVREUX

INTRODUCTION.

By reviewing the 349 Multiple Sclerosis (M S) cases examined in a
Neurological Department over a twenty-year period (1957-1976), the purpose
was to give a general view on the onset and the course of M S and to identify characteristics which may serve as pronostic markers and assist in
therapeutic decisions (1).

MATERIEL AND METHODS.

All of the cases examined in the Department for a suspicion of M S
were reviewed in 1976. The only 349 cases satisfying our diagnostic classification (1) were selected. This classification is based upon the Mac
Alpine's with "dissemination in space" and "dissemination in time" criteria,
but it takes into account paraclinical data, notably Evoked Potentials and
C T Scan for the demonstration of the space dissemination. It also uses
Cerebro Spinal Fluid (C S F) alterations for the definition of a biological
criteria.

Definitions of relapses and progression, pure relapses and relapses
with sequelae, remittent phase and progressive phase, have already been
given (1). Similarly, three types of clinical course were defined (1) : the
remittent, the remittent-progressive and the progressive types. Symptomatology was classified as follows : long tracts dysfunction (L T) which
refered either to upper or lower limbs dysfunction, sensory symptoms or
sphincteric disturbances; optic neuritis (O N); brainstem dysfunction (B S),

15

i.e. diplopia, "tic douloureux", dizziness...; when at least two of these three categories were present in the same individual, the clinical picture was considered as plurisymptomatic and further subdivided in two categories according to the presence of O N or not. Three levels of non-reversible disability were defined : none; moderate, still ambulatory; severe, not ambulatory. An "outcome index" was used : "hyperacute", "acute", "subacute", and "intermediate" forms had severe non-reversible disability with a disease duration of less than 5 years, 5 to 10 years, 10 to 15 years, and more than 15 years, respectively. "Benign" forms had no disability after 10 years of disease duration or a moderate disability after 15 years. "Not classified" forms had no severe disability and a too short follow-up.

Data were collected on standardized documents. Since 1976, this was made prospectively. Analysis was made by computerized data processing. Chi-Square test and Variance analysis were used for statistical evaluation.

BASIC DATA.

Among the 349 M S cases, 50 per cent were "definite", 30 per cent "probable" and 20 per cent "possible" forms. Females were 60 per cent of the total. In 1976, the mean period of follow-up was 9.0 years.

ONSET.

Mean age at onset was 31.3 ± 10.1 years. In 10 per cent of the cases, the onset was before the age of 20 years, in 70 per cent from ages 20 to 40 years and in 20 per cent after the age of 40 years. The mode of onset was remittent in 82 per cent of the cases and progressive in 18 per cent. Symptomatology at onset is presentend in TABLE 1.

TABLE 1 :   DISTRIBUTION (%) of 349 M S patients
ACCORDING TO SYMPTOMATOLOGY AT ONSET

L T only	52
O N only	16
B S only	10
Plurisymptomatic without O N ...	14
Plurisymptomatic with O N	6
Varia	2

(For abbreviations, see text).

Age, mode and symptomatology at onset had tight correlations. Mean age at onset was 30.0 years for cases with a remittent onset compared to 37.3 years in progressive forms. The difference was significant. This was still observed when ages at onset were compared by distributions (Figure 1). Inside each category of age at onset, the proportion of cases with a progres-

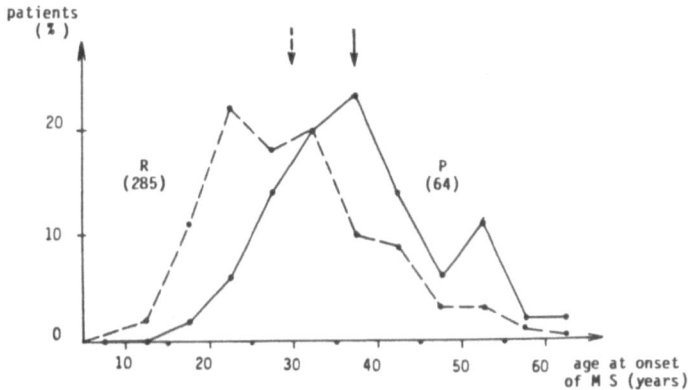

Figure 1.   Distributions (%) of the 285 patients with a
             remittent onset (R) and the 64 patients with
             a progressive onset (P), according to age
             at the onset of M S.

sive onset among the total of M S cases increased with advancing age (Figure 2). It must be noted, however, that this proportion reached only 50 per cent for cases with onset at the age of 60 years. Frequency of long tracts lesions increased while optic nerve and brainstem lesions decreased significantly with advancing age (TABLE 2) and progressive onset compared to remittent onset (TABLE 3).

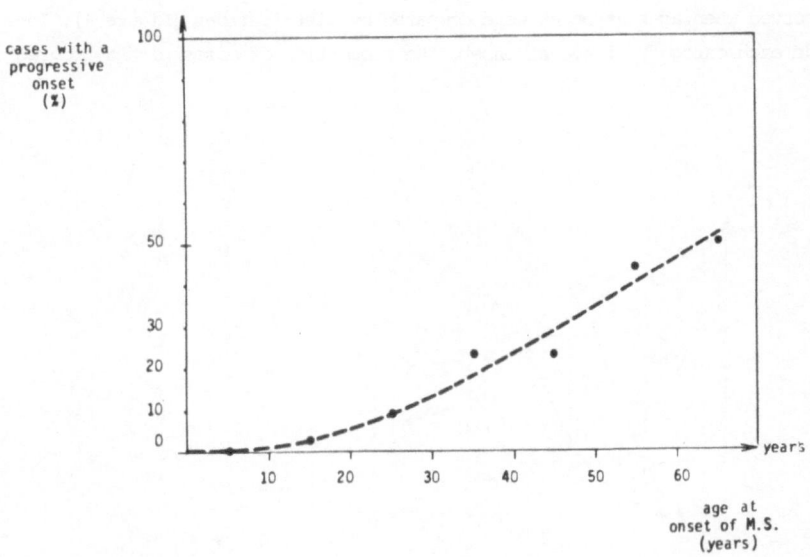

Figure 2.   Percentages of cases with a progressive onset
             among M S cases within each category of age
             at onset.

TABLE 2 :   SYMPTOMATOLOGY AND AGE AT ONSET.

The distribution (%) of the 349 M S patients according to symptomatology
at onset is presented inside each category of age at onset.

	< 20 years	20-40 years	≥ 40 years
L T only	33	53	61
O N only	12	19	8
B S only	29	8	9
Plurisymptomatic without O N	12	13	15
Plurisymptomatic with O N	10	5	8

$(X^2 = 25.6; p < 0.005)$.

(For abbreviations, see text).

TABLE 3 :   SYMPTOMATOLOGY AND MODE AT ONSET.

The distribution (%) of the 349 M S patients according to symptomatology at onset is presented inside each category of mode at onset.

	Remittent		Progressive
L T only	47	....	78
O N only	18	....	5
B S only	12	....	2
Plurisymptomatic without O N ...	14	....	14
Plurisymptomatic with O N	8	....	O

(X^2 = 23.9 ; p < 0.001).

(For abbreviations, see text).

COURSE.

Remittent forms and remittent-progressive forms were marked by ages at onset (1) and symptomatology at onset (data not shown) not significantly different. Nevertheless, the mean period of follow-up was significantly higher for remittent-progressive cases (1). It was concluded that remittent-progressive forms were remittent forms which have had "time to grow older".

The age of the patient seemed to be decisive concerning the stages of the disease (Figure 3). Whatever the detailed clinical course, mean age at onset of the pure relapses was not significantly different. The same observation was true for age at onset of relapses with sequelae and for age at onset of progression. Moreover, mean ages at onset for these three stages were significantly different from each other (variance analysis p < 0.001).

The chronology of relapses was studied for the remittent phase only since relapses were often difficult to identify during the progressive phase. The probability for a new relapse to occur was highest immediately following a relapse and then fell exponentially (Figure 4). The interval between consecutive relapses tended to shorten (Figure 5). In fact, this reflected shorter intervals between relapses for cases with higher number of relapses (data not shown).

For the remittent-progressive cases, the mean period before onset of progression was 6.8 years. Actuarial analysis (Figure 6) showed that patients affected by progression were 18 per cent at the onset of M S, 30 per cent at five years and 50 per cent at eleven years of duration of the disease.

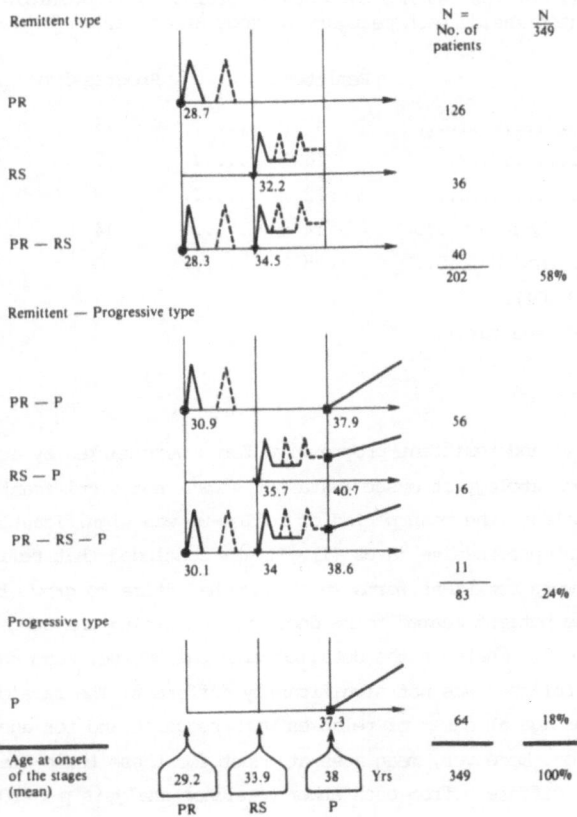

<u>Figure 3.</u>   Ages at onset of the different stages during
the course of M S. P R = pure relapses.
R S = relapses with sequelae. P = progressive
phase.

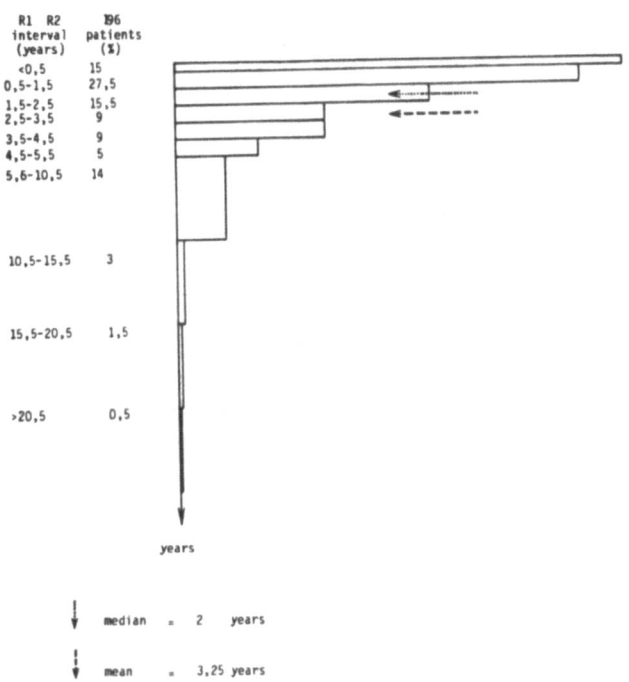

Figure 4.   Distribution (%) of the 196 M S patients with
at least two relapses during the remittent phase
according to the interval (years) between the
first and the second relapses (R_1 R_2 interval).

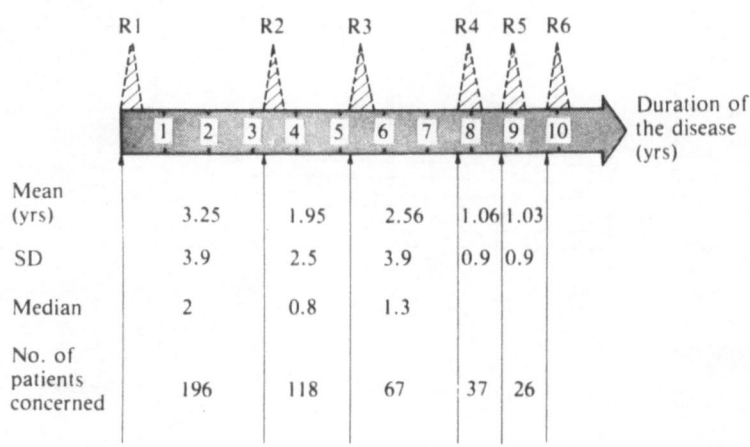

Figure 5.   Interval between consecutive relapses during
the remittent phase. S D = standard deviation.
R = numbered relapse

FUNCTIONAL OUTCOME.

The mean interval from onset of the disease to moderate disability was
3.45 years. It was 9.5 years for severe disability. From actuarial analysis,
it could be noted that half of the M S patients were moderately disabled
or severaly disabled or dead after six, eighteen and thirty years of
duration of the disease, respectively (Figure 7).

FACTORS AFFECTING PROGNOSIS.

Three criteria were used : the period from disease onset to moderate
and severe disabilities, the outcome index and the actuarial method for
onset of disability. The sex of the patient had no influence. The older the
age at M S onset, the faster the M S course. Mean intervals to moderate and
severe disabilities were 7.9 and 14.3 years for M S onset before the age of

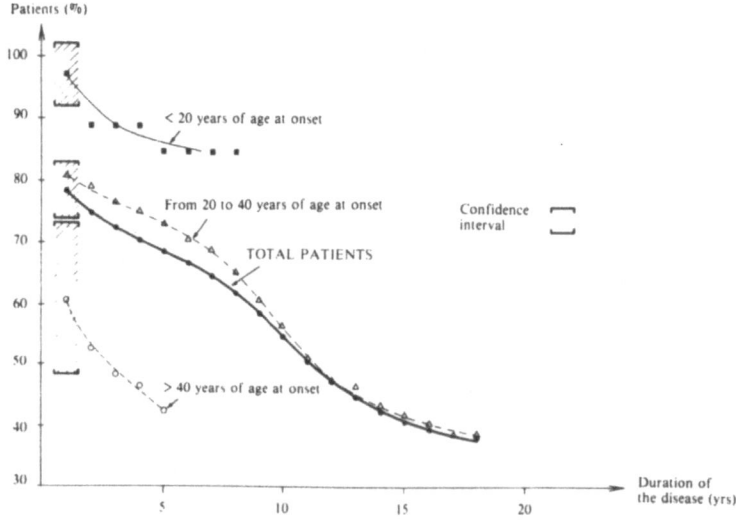

Figure 6.   Actuarial curve of progression for the 349 M S
             patients. It represents the percentage of patients
             not yet in the progressive phase according to
             disease duration. Curves for three categories of
             age at onset are also presented. Confidence
             intervals (hatched) : for upper curve, ± 5.0;
             for middle curves, ± 4.5; for lower curve, ± 12.0

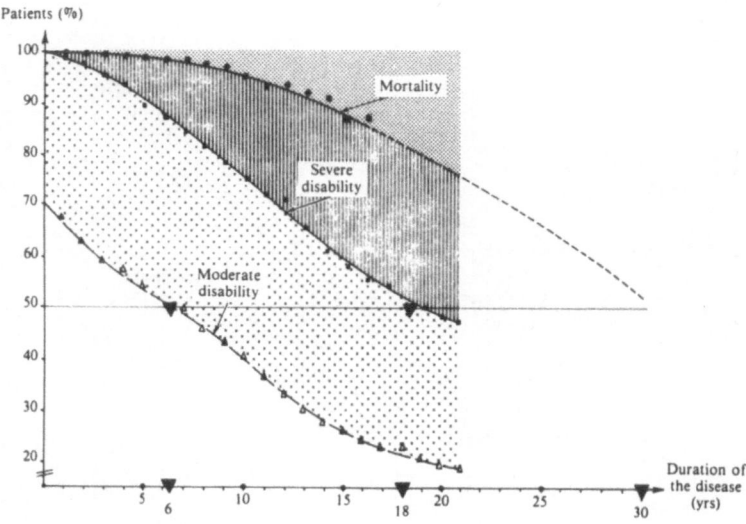

<u>Figure 7</u>.   Actuarial curve of functional outcome for the
349 M S patients. It represents the percentage
of patients not moderately disabled or severely
disabled or dead according to disease duration.

20 years; they were 0.8 and 4.8 years, respectively, for M S onset from
ages 50 to 60 years (Figure 8). The influence of age was also clear from
the actuarial curves for moderate (Figure 9) and severe disabilities
(Figure 10) and from the outcome index (TABLE 4). Progressive mode of onset
was correlated with poor outcome. Intervals to moderate and severe disabilities were 0.34 and 5.8 for progressive forms compared to 4.8 and 10.9
for cases with a remittent onset. There were three times more hyperacute
cases and three times less benign cases in progressive forms compared to
cases with remittent onset (TABLE 5). Symptomatology at onset had no
pronostic value. The interval between the first two relapses in the remittent phase had a significant relationship to M S outcome : the shorter the
interval, the poorer the prognosis (TABLES 6 and 7). The same result was
observed, in the remittent-progressive cases, for the interval from the
onset of the disease to the onset of the progression (TABLE 8). Lumbar
puncture data had little prognostic value (1).

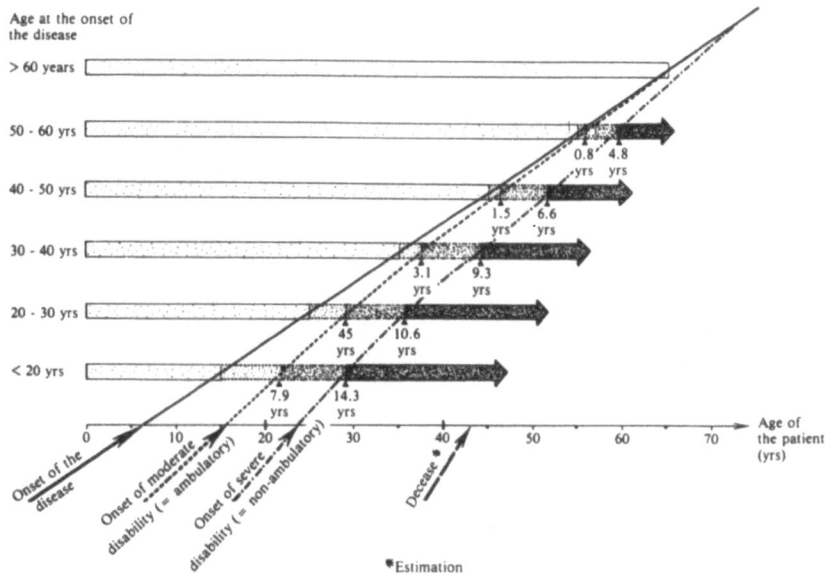

Figure 8.   Age at onset of M S and the functional outcome.
For each category of age at M S onset, the ages
at M S onset, moderate disability onset, severe
disability onset and decease are graphically
shown with reference to abscissae which represents
the age of the patient.

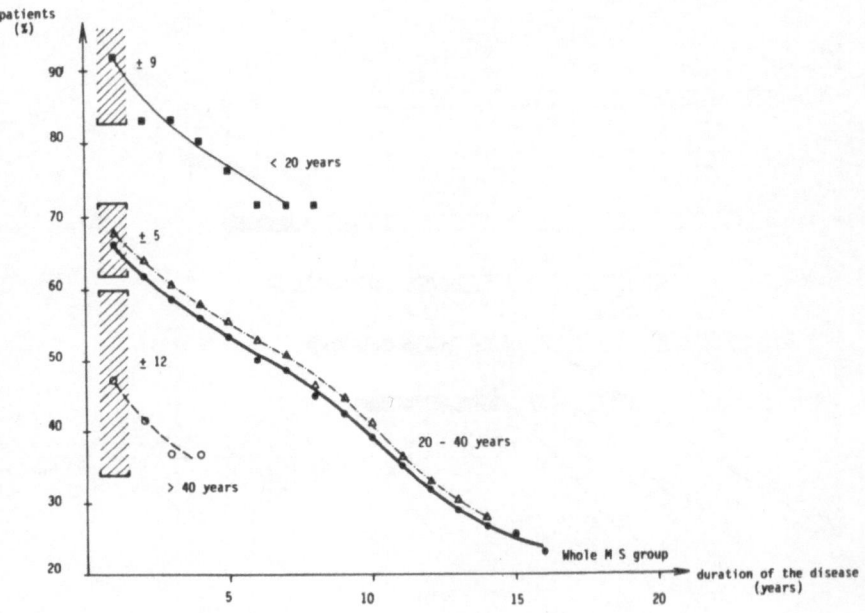

<u>Figure 9</u>.   Actuarial curve of moderate disability for the
349 M S patients. Curves for three categories
of age at onset are also presented. Confidence
intervals (hatched).

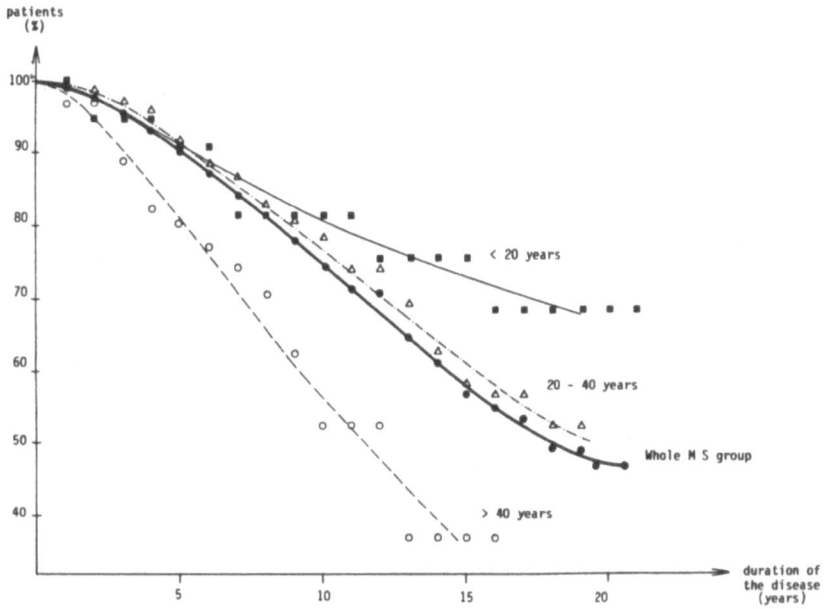

Figure 10.   Actuarial curve of severe disability for the
349 M S patients. Curves for three categories
of age at onset are also presented.

TABLE 4 :   AGE AT M S ONSET AND OUTCOME INDEX.

Outcome index	Age at M S onset (mean ± S D)
Hyperacute	35.7 ± 10.3
Acute	34.1 ± 9.2
Subacute	29.2 ± 7.2
Intermediate	26.6 ± 11.4
Benign	27.6 ± 7
Not classified	31.7 ± 10.4

(Variance analysis; $p < 0.001$).

TABLE 5 :   MODE OF ONSET AND OUTCOME INDEX.

Outcome index	Remittent onset (%)	Progressive onset (%)
Hyperacute	6	20
Acute	6	14
Subacute	6	5
Intermediate	5	0
Benign	16	6
Not classified	61	55

$(X^2 = 177 ; p < 0.001)$.

TABLE 6 :   INTERVAL BETWEEN THE FIRST TWO RELAPSES IN THE REMITTENT PHASE (R1 R2 interval) AND INTERVALS FROM M S ONSET TO MODERATE AND SEVERE DISABILITIES (mean ± S D)[x]

R1 R2 interval (years)	Interval to moderate disability (years)	Interval to severe disability (years)
< 1	2.1 ± 2.5	8.1 ± 6.9
1 - 5	6.8 ± 5.5	10.0 ± 3.8
5 - 10	11.8 ± 5.4	17.0 ± 5.1
≥ 10	19.2 ± 7.7	31.7 ± 8.4
	(variance analysis ; $p < 0.001$)	(variance analysis : $p < 0.001$)

[x] calculated from 1984's available data.

TABLE 7 :   INTERVAL BETWEEN THE FIRST TWO RELAPSES
IN THE REMITTENT PHASE (R1 R2 interval)
(mean ± S D) AND OUTCOME INDEX.

Outcome index	R1 R2 interval (years)
Hyperacute	0.9 ± 1.9
Acute	2.4 ± 1.3
Subacute	3.7 ± 3.5
Intermediate	6.6 ± 5.8
Benign	6.2 ± 5.6
Not classified	2.1 ± 1.9

(Variance analysis; $p < 0.001$).

TABLE 8 :   INTERVAL FROM THE ONSET OF THE DISEASE
TO THE ONSET OF PROGRESSION (mean ± S D)
AND OUTCOME INDEX FOR THE REMITTENT -
PROGRESSIVE FORMS OF M S .

Outcome index	Interval to progression (years)
Hyperacute	1.7 ± 1.1
Acute	6.0 ± 3.9
Subacute	8.4 ± 3.4
Intermediate	13.3 ± 6
Benign	10.6 ± 3.7
Not classified	4.3 ± 3.4

(Variance analysis ; $p < 0.001$).

CONCLUSION.

Whatever strong are correlations between some clinical characteristics and prognosis, it must be noted that it is not yet possible to correctly predict outcome facing individual M S patients. Therefore, data collection from any M S case examined in the Department is going on, and, to date, there are more than 800 such cases. Further evaluation of lumbar puncture data, notably C S F cytology and genetic markers is currently investigated. Stochastic models of the course of M S are in elaboration.

AKNOWLEDGEMENTS.

We are greatful to Professors Michel Devic and Gilbert Aimard for continuous help; Jean-Jacques Ventre for data collection; Albert Biron and Philippe Messy for computerized data processing; Simone Droguet for technical assistance; Association pour la Recherche sur la Sclérose En Plaques (A.R.S.E.P.) for financial support.

(1) Confavreux C., Aimard G., Devic M., 1980. Course and Prognosis of
      Multiple Sclerosis assessed by the computerized data processing
      of 349 patients. Brain, 103, 282-300.

4

A Comparative Study between Multiple Sclerosis Out-patients and In-patients staying at a specialized Multiple Sclerosis Clinic

R. MEDAER, M. PUYSTJENS and H. CALLAERT

INTRODUCTION

Data concerning the disability and the home situation of M.S. patients are virtually non-existing. Therefore, regional and national planning of resources is difficult. There are no statistical data concerning the reasons of admission in a specialized M.S. clinic.

In 1983, an investigation was initiated in order to make up a profile of multiple sclerosis in- and out-patients. The goal was to trace differences between the two populations. The role of a M.S. clinic should become more clear; also, advices could be formulated to promote a longer stay in a home environment.

MATERIAL AND METHODS

The study was carried out from July 1983 to July 1984. In the M.S. and Rehabilitation Center Overpelt, 105 M.S. patients were evaluated. At home, social workers of the M.S. Society evaluated 319 M.S. patients, at random, across Flanders. In order to quantify the patient parameters, the Minimal Record of Disability (Slater, 1984) was used. In the M.S. clinic, the MRD was scored by a neurologist (E.D.S.S.), a nurse (I.S.S.) and a social worker (E.S.S.) For the in-patients, the MRD was entirely scored by a social worker. (Table 1-2-5-6).

31

By means of statistical analysis, a search for differences between out- and in-patients has been carried out by use of t-tests and Wilcoxon-Mann-Whitney tests. The level of significance was set at 5 percent. The dependence between E.D.S.S. level and residence is studied by means of a contingency table. An analogous study was performed on the progression rate and the population subgroups.

RESULTS

Demographic data

In all, 427 patients were examined (table 1). The mean age was 51.0 years.

Table 1 - Demographic data

Populat. Items	Outpatients ♂ n=125 X̄	 s.d.	Outpatients ♀ n=194 X̄	 s.d.	Inpatients ♂ n=50 X̄	 s.d.	Inpatients ♀ n=55 X̄	 s.d.	Total Population n=427 X̄	 s.d.
Age	51.1	11.8	50.6	11.8	50.0	10.7	51.5	11.7	51.0	11.61
Duration of illness	20.4	10.6	20.0	11.2	19.9	9.2	19.5	11.8	20.1	10.9
Age beginn. of illness	31.1	10.2	30.6	9.6	30.1	9.1	32.0	10.1	30.9	9.8
EDSS (Kurtzke)	6.7	1.8	6.7	1.7	7.4	1.6	7.3	1.6	6.9	1.7
Progression rate	0.45	0.34	0.49	0.45	0.46	0.3	0.56	0.44	0.48	0.4
Sex Ratio F/M	1.55				1.10				1.42	

There were no significant differences between both populations, and between sexes. This was also true for the mean duration of illness (20.1 years) and the distribution of the mean age of onset (30.9 years). The sex ratio for the in-patients was 1.55, and for the out-patients 1.1. The difference between the two values is statistically significant.

The Expanded Disability Status Scale (E.D.S.S.) and Progression Index

Between the two populations the difference concerning the mean score for the E.D.S.S. was highly significant (table 2.) For in-patients, the mean score is 7.4, indicating that the patient is "unable to take more than a few steps; restricted to wheel-chair; may need aid in transfer; may require motorized wheel-chair". For the out-patient, the mean score is 6.7, meaning that the patient is "in need for constant bilateral assistance to walk about 20 meters without resting". This applies for both male and female patients.

Table 2 - E.D.S.S. and Progression Index

| | Home patients | | | | MS clinic | | | | Total population | |
| | ♂ | | ♀ | | ♂ | | ♀ | | | |
	$\overline{x}$	s.d.	$\overline{x}$	s.d.	$\overline{x}$	s.d.	$\overline{x}$	s.d.	$\overline{x}$	s.d.
EDSS (Kurtzke)	6.7	1.8	6.7	1.7	7.4	1.6	7.3	1.6	6.9	1.7
Progression Index	0.45	0.34	0.49	0.45	0.46	0.3	0.56	0.44	0.48	0.4

Significant difference for Kurtzke score (p = 0.0003)
No significant difference for progression index (p $\leqslant$ 0.05)

When the E.D.S.S. is further split up, a highly significant relationship is found between the degree of disability and being at home or staying in the clinic. (chi^2 = 19.05 with d.f. = 3). The group scoring higher than 8 is overrepresented in the in-patients (table 3.) The course of the disease was investigated using the progression index (Poser et al., 1982) : E.D.S.S. score divided by disease duration in years.

Table 3 - Relation between E.D.S.S. and home - clinic

E.D.S.S.

	0-4	4.5-6	6.5-7.5	8-10	Total
Home	31 (9.7%)	77 (24.1%)	104 (32.5%)	108 (33.7%)	320 (100%)
Clinic	6 (5.7%)	15 (14.1%)	24 (22.6%)	61 (57.5%)	106 (100%)
Total	37	92	128	169	426

Chi^2 = 19.05 with d.f. = 3
Highly significant relationship.

For the total population, the progression index was 0.48. There is no statistically significant difference between in- and out-patients (chi^2 = 7.13 with d.f. = 6) (table 4.)

Table 4 - Population subgroups according to Progression Index

Progression Index	Population subgroups				
	♂ home	♂ clinic	♀ home	♀ clinic	Total
≤ 0.3	45	16	76	16	153
0.3 < p.i. < 0.6	58	23	76	21	178
≥ 0.6	22	10	39	18	89
total	125	49	191	55	420

chi^2 = 7.13 with d.f. = 6
No significant relationship between progression index and subgroups.

The cumulative frequency of the progression index is showed in figure 1 and 2. The steeper the rise, the better the evolution. For the statistically revelant interval of 0.3-0.7 for the progression index, the mean difference is 3% for males and 10% for females in the favour of the out-patients. Thus, the more benign cases with a slower progression are found in a higher proportion in the out-patients.

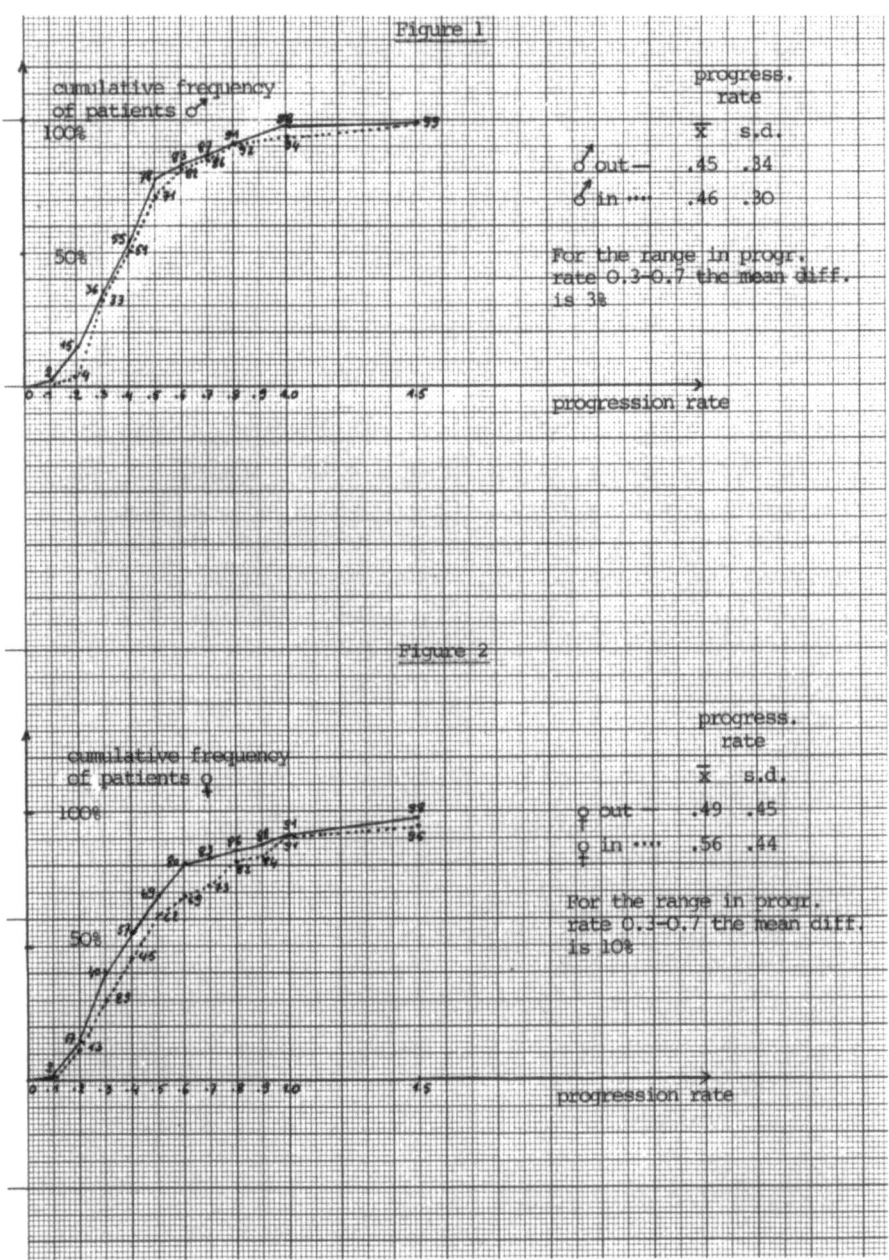

The Incapacity Status Scale (I.S.S.)

The data are summarized in table 5. There are highly significant differences ($p \ll 0.01$) for stair climbing, ambulation, grooming and medical problems. The difference is significant ($p < 0.05$) for transfers, bowel function, dressing and feeding. There were no significant differences for bladder function, vision and mentation. A clear similarity was found for bathing, speech and hearing, fatigability and sound function.

Table 5 - Incapacity Status Scale

Populat. Items	Outpatients ♂ n=125		Outpatients ♀ n=194		Inpatients ♂ n=50		Inpatients ♀ n=55		Total popul. n=427		Significance out/in
	X̄	s.d.	X̄	s.d.	X̄	s.d.	X̄	s.d.	X̄	s.d.	
Stair climbing	2.9	1.2	2.9	1.1	3.3	1.2	3.3	1.1	3.0	1.14	h.s.
Ambulation	2.8	1.3	2.7	1.2	3.3	1.2	3.1	1.3	2.8	1.3	h.s.
Transfers	2.1	1.2	2.1	1.2	2.4	1.4	2.5	1.5	2.2	1.3	s.
Bowel funct.	1.1	1.2	1.3	1.2	1.6	1.4	1.5	1.4	1.3	1.2	s.
Bladder funct.	1.2	1.1	1.5	1.2	1.6	1.5	1.9	1.4	1.5	1.3	n.s.
Bathing	2.7	1.3	2.5	1.3	2.6	1.4	2.7	1.3	2.6	1.3	n.s.
Dressing	2.3	1.6	1.9	1.5	2.6	1.4	2.5	1.6	2.2	1.6	s.
Grooming	1.6	1.6	1.4	1.5	1.9	1.5	2.0	1.6	1.6	1.6	h.s.
Feeding	1.2	1.2	1.1	1.2	1.5	1.3	1.5	1.4	1.2	1.9	s.
Vision	1.3	0.8	1.2	0.9	1.3	0.9	1.5	0.8	1.3	0.9	n.s.
Speech+hearing	0.6	0.9	0.5	0.8	0.4	0.6	0.5	1.0	0.5	0.8	n.s.
Medical probl.	1.7	1.1	1.8	1.2	2.7	1.5	3.0	1.3	2.0	1.3	h.s.
Psych. funct.	1.0	0.9	1.0	0.9	1.2	1.2	1.4	1.3	1.1	1.0	n.s.
Fatigability	2.5	1.3	2.7	1.0	2.3	1.2	2.9	1.2	2.6	1.2	n.s.
Sexual funct.	2.9	1.5	2.6	1.6	2.8	1.5	2.8	1.6	2.7	1.5	n.s.

h.s. = highly significant
s.   = significant
n.s. = not significant

The Environmental Status Scale (E.S.S.)

Three major differences were found at the expense of the inpatients (table 6) : personal residence/home, actual work status and

community services (for each item p≪0.01). On the average, in-patients
are out of work and are indeed no longer capable of working, their home
needs major modifications, e.g. central heating, extensive ramps,
renovation of several rooms, elevator ... More than 3 hours of community
services per day are required. The out-patients show another picture :
a job up to one quarter time is possible, only moderate modifications
of the home are needed, such as replacing doors, renovation of a room,
installing a simple ramp, and the community services required are limited
on the average to one hour per day.

Smaller, but still statistically significant differences (p < 0.05)
are found for financial/economic status, personal assistance required
and transportation. The situation for the in-patients is worse :
he is financially more dependent, he needs more help from others in the
activities of daily living (on the average three hours instead of one
hour for the out-patients) and transportation should be especially
adapted. The out-patient on the other hand is able to use standard
private transport. Public transport is not suitable for both populations.

Table 6 - Environmental Status Scale

Population	Outpatients		Inpatients		Total populat.	Signific. out/in
	♂ n=125	♀ n=194	♂ n=50	♀ n=55	n=427	
Items	$\overline{x}$ s.d.	$\overline{x}$ s.d.	$\overline{x}$ s.d.	$\overline{x}$ s.d.	$\overline{x}$ s.d.	
Work	4.2 1.5	3.9 1.5	4.7 1.3	4.5 1.2	4.2 1.5	h.s.
Financ./Econom.	2.3 1.3	2.1 1.3	3.0 1.6	2.2 1.5	2.3 1.4	s.
Home	1.6 1.5	1.5 1.6	3.0 1.7	2.8 1.9	1.8 1.7	h.s.
Pers. ass. req.	2.4 1.5	2.9 1.3	3.0 1.5	3.1 1.6	2.8 1.4	s.
Transportation	2.8 1.2	2.8 0.9	3.1 1.1	3.2 1.2	2.9 1.1	s.
Comm. health s.	2.0 1.4	1.9 1.5	2.7 1.3	3.3 1.1	2.2 1.5	h.s.
Societal role	2.7 1.0	2.6 1.0	2.8 1.4	2.8 1.4	2.7 1.1	n.s.

CONCLUSIONS

The population we investigated showed a higher mean age and
longer mean duration of illness compared with epidemiological studies
focused on case-finding, and is therefore probably not representative
for the total M.S. population in Flanders; patients with recent

diagnosis and benign cases do not often stay at a M.S. clinic, and are
obviously seldomly member of the M.S. Society. Nevertheless in our study
out- and in-patients can be compared quite well : they have the same
mean age, duration of illness, age at onset. The mean age of onset falls
in the same range of those found in other reports (Acheson, 1977;
La Rocca et al, 1984; Madonna et al., 1984; Sheperd, 1979).
The sex ratio confirms the preponderance of females in M.S. (La Rocca
et al., 1984; Madonna et al., 1984; Poser et al., 1982; Sheperd, 1979).
Although not statistically significant, there is a clinical trend
towards more men being present in the in-patients.
The progression index has the same dimensions as mentioned by other
sources (Lauer et al., 1984a-b. Again there is a clinical trend towards
more rapid progression for the in-patients.
Analysis of the different items of the I.S.S. and E.S.S. demonstrate
quite important differences.

     The problem profile of the in-patient is as follows : he is
restricted to a wheel-chair - stair climbing is impossible. The risk
for complications such as bedsores, contractures, and urinary tract
infections is quite severe. Working is no longer possible. Staying at
home would require major structural home renovation. Community services
are required up to 5 hours per day. Also worth mentioning is that
activities such as transfers, defecation, dressing and eating are
somewhat more difficult for in-patients. The financial status is worse
and transport requires a specially adapted vehicle.
The out-patient has a quite different profile : he is able to walk 5
meters, longer distances require crutches or a wheel-chair. A doctor' s
call every three months suffices. Working is possible, although limited
to one quarter time at the most. The home requires only moderate
alterations. One hour of community services per week is sufficient.
Assistance in activities of daily living are needed for about one hour
per day. Transportation is possible by a standard car.
Apart from the differences, there are some points of similarity that
are quite striking. Disturbances of sexual function and bladder
function are as frequent in the out-patients as in the in-patients.
This confirms other investigations where no correlation was found
between disturbances of sexual function on the one hand and disability,
age or duration of illness on the other hand (Minderhoud et al., 1984).

In conclusion we would like to propose advices in order to permit a longer stay of M.S. patients at home or in a sheltered environment. Points that should be stressed are :

° adaptation of the home : this will have to be extensive and requires expert opinion.

° assistance in activities of daily living by ADL workers at home.

° more attention towards prevention of complications such as decubite, contractions and urinary tract infections.

° more treatment at home by nurses, social workers, physiotherapists, ... acting as a team.

° adapted means of transportation, e.g. by means of special vans.

Realisation of these advices requires extensive efforts from both society and home environment.

If acquaintance with a M.S. clinic could be made possible in the earlier stages of illness, information about the actual therapeutical possibilities would possibly limit the group with very severe medical and social problems.

ACKNOWLEDGEMENT

The autors would like to express their gratitude to the social workers of the Flemish M.S. Society for their extensive field work, and to Ms. L. Bringmans, Mrs. J. Vandeweyer and Mrs. A. Vanherck for the preparation of the manusscript.

REFERENCES

Acheson, E.D., 1977. Epidemiology of multiple sclerosis. Br.Med.Bull., 33(1):9.14.

La Rocca, N.G., Scheinberg, L.C., Slater, R.J., 1984. Field testing of a minimal record of disability in multiple sclerosis : The United States and Canada. Acta Neurologica Scandinavica, 101(70):126-137.

Lauer, K., Firnhaber, W., Reining, R. and Leuchtweis, B., 1984a. Epidemiological investigations into multiple sclerosis in Southern Hesse (I). Acta Neurologica Scandinavica, 70:257-265.

Lauer, K., Firnhaber, W., Reining, R. and Leuchtweis, B., 1984b. Epidemiological investigations into multiple sclerosis in Southern Hesse (II). Acta Neurologica Scandinavica, 70:266-273.

Madonna, M.G., Hannah, B., La Rocca, N.G., 1984. Experience in the use of the minimal record of disability in multiple sclerosis chapters and community settings. Acta Neurologica Scandinavica, 101(70):139-142.

Minderhoud, J.M., Leenhuis, J.G., 1984. Sexual disturbances arising from multiple sclerosis. Acta Neurologica Scandinavica, 70:299-306.

Poser, S., Bauer, H.J. and Poser, W., 1982. Prognosis of multiple

sclerosis. Acta Neurologica Scandinavica, 65:347-354.
Poser, S., Raun, N.E. and Poser, W., 1982. Age at onset, inital sympto-
    matology and the course of multiple sclerosis. Acta Neurologica
    Scandinavica, 66:355-362.
Shepherd, D.I., 1979. Clinical features of multiple sclerosis in nord-
    east Scotland. Acta Neurologica Scandinavica, 60:128-230.
Slater, R.J., 1984. Criteria and uses of the minimal record of dis-
    ability in multiple sclerosis. Acta Neurologica Scandinavica, 101
    (70):16-20.

5

Incapacity and Disability in Multiple Sclerosis

J. M. MINDERHOUD, A. J. A. PRANGE and H. DASSEL

INTRODUCTION

The data used in this paper on the incapacity and disability caused by multiple sclerosis, were obtained from an epidemiological study in the province of Groningen, in the northern part of The Netherlands. All known patients with a definite and probable diagnosis MS in this area, with about 560.000 inhabitants, were examined and scored. This included their history, the neurological examination (Poser, 1978), the Disability Status and the Functional Disabilities (Kurtzke, 1961, 1975) and the Incapacity and Environmental Status (IFMMS).
With a prevalence of 56.25 per 100.000 inhabitants and a mean incidence of 2.16, 315 patients could be included in this study.

RESULTS

In contrast to many other studies we did not find a bell-shaped distribution of the frequencies of the DSS, as was stated by Kurtzke also, but a double bell-shaped distribution around DSS 2 and DSS 7 respectively (fig. 1 and fig. 2).

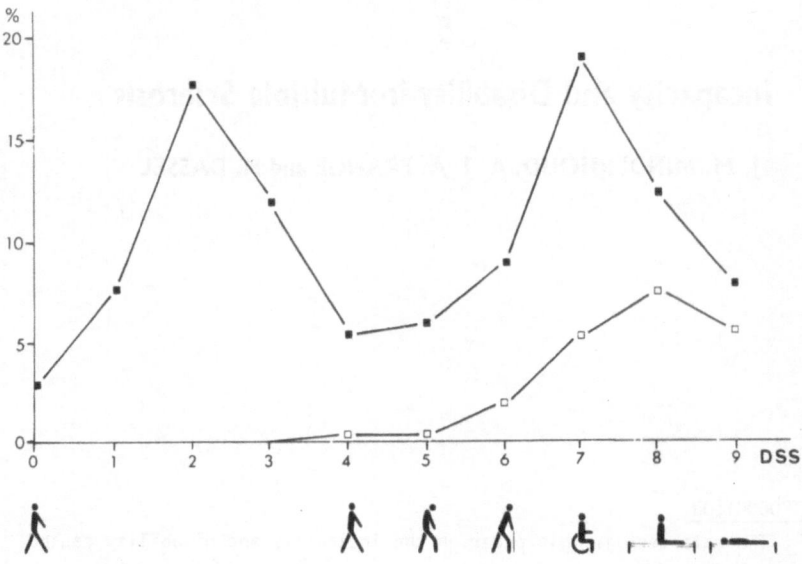

Fig. 1   Distribution of DSS of all MS patients (n=315) included in the
epidemiologic study (■). ◻: the percentages of patients staying
in nursing homes, rehabilitation centres or hospitals.

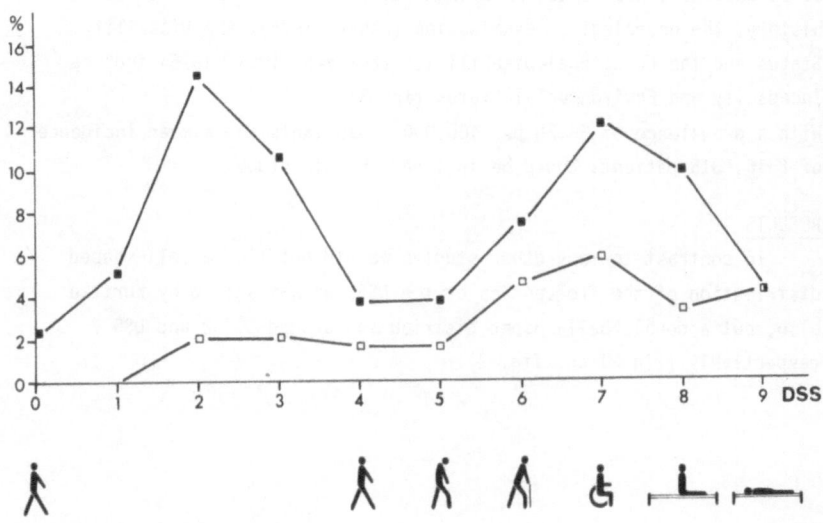

Fig. 2   Distribution of DSS of MS patients with an intermittent/progres-
sive course (■), and those with a progressive course of the
disease only (◻).

Patients were divided into a group starting their signs and symptoms with a course with ups and downs, and a group with a progressive course of the disease only. The first signs and symptoms of MS in these groups were found respectively at the mean age of 30.1 years and at the mean age of 36.7 years. The fact that the patients as well as their examiners could exactly determine the year in which the progression of the handicap started to be continuously in patients with an intermittent course before, and that the mean age of the patients at which this happened did not differ clearly from the mean age at which signs and symptoms of the patients with a progressive course only had started, stressed the hypothesis that multiple sclerosis is a disease with a progressive course and handicap, although about two-third of the patients encountered an intermittent onset.

TABLE 1   Data of the groups of patients included in this study

	Intermittent course	Progressive course
Number of patients	224 (71.1%)	91 (28.9%)
Mean age of first signs and symptoms	30.1 years	36.7 years
Mean age of start of continuous progression	36.5 years	36.7 years
Males:females	1:1.73	1:1.11

Even prior to the onset of clinical signs, fatiguability could be present for many years.
Factoranalysis of the scores of the Incapacity Scale resulted in for factors determining the handicap of MS patients (Minderhoud et al., 1984). These factors were related to motor functions (mostly lesions of the spinal cord), to lesions in the brainstem, cerebellum, optic nerve and the cerebral hemispheres - taken together as supra-spinal lesions -, to lesions causing bladder, bowel and sexual functions - probably caused by separate lesions in the lumbo-sacral part of the spinal cord - and to fatiguability. The majority of the scores of the Environmental Scale correlated with the motor group of handicaps, although in patients with a low DSS supra-spinal signs and symptoms and especial fatiguability played an important role in their actual work status and their social

activity. Also defects in the cluster of bladder, bowel and sexual functions caused major problems related to social activity of the patients with a low DSS (Minderhoud et al., 1984).

In patients with a higher DSS (more than 4) spinal-motor as well as supraspinal lesions play an important role in the total handicap in patients with a progressive course only, as well as in patients who had an intermittent course of the disease before changing to a progressive course.

CONCLUSIONS

    In this study the results of the scoring of handicaps and disability were used to study the pattern of handicaps in MS patients. Although individual patients show various patterns of signs and symptoms, on the whole an uniform pattern of the course of the handicaps in MS can be found. This pattern shows that the basis of the course of the disease is a progressive one, although this is preceded in many patients by an intermittent onset and even by fatiguability which is often present before any sign of the disease. Because of this pattern the progression rate can better be calculated starting from the beginning of the progressive course of the disease than from the beginning of the intermittent phase.

REFERENCES

Poser, S., 1978. Multiple sclerosis. Springer Verlag, Berlin-Heidelberg-New York.
Kurtzke, J.F., 1961. On the evaluation of disability in multiple sclerosis. Neurology, 11: 686-694.
Kurtzke, J.F., 1975. A reassessment of the distribution of multiple sclerosis. Acta Neurol. Scand., 51: 110-136, 137-157.
Minderhoud, J.M., Dassel, H. and Prange, A.J.A., 1984. Proposal for summing the incapacity status or environmental status scores. Acta Neurol. Scand., suppl. 101, vol. 70, 87-91.
Minderhoud, J.M., Leemhuis, J.G., Kremer, J., Laban, E. and Smits, P.M., 1984. Sexual disturbances arising from multiple sclerosis. Acta Neurol. Scand., 70: 299-306.

6

Immunosuppression with Cyclophosphamide in Multiple Sclerosis Patients

R. E. GONSETTE and L. DEMONTY

INTRODUCTION

In a first clinical study (Gonsette et al. 1977), a short-term (2-3 weeks) intensive immunosuppression was induced by intravenous injection of high doses of cyclophosphamide (CY) in multiple sclerosis (MS) patients with a remitting-progressive form. After a follow-up for 2-6 years, it appeared that a marked reduction of the annual relapse rate (ARR) as well as a stabilization of neurological and functional disability were observed respectively in 70 and 62 % of the patients. The same beneficial effect of intensive CY immunosuppression on the progressive form of the disease has been observed by Hommes et al. (1980) and Hauser et al. (1983).

It was evident however that the beneficial influence of CY on the ARR as well as on the long-term deterioration was transient and did not exceed 2-3 years in most patients. In order to extend the remission period, a second protocol was designed, associating immune effects of intensive and chronic administration of CY.

MATERIAL AND METHODS

According to the second protocol, a maintained oral immunotherapy
with CY was instaured soon after the acute treatment. A daily dose of
50 mg CY was adopted since this dosage has proved immunologically effective in autoimmune diseases. Since intensive CY immunosuppression appeared more effective in active forms of the disease, the recruitement was
limited to patients experiencing frequent relapses (mean ARR : 1.39), with
a short evolution (mean : 4 years) and a disability no greater than 6 on
Kurtzke scale (mean : 2.27). Blood tests determinations as well as neurological and functional evaluations (Kurtzke DSS) were performed every 2
months. From January 1984, lymphocytes subsets longitudinal studies and
magnetic nuclear resonance examinations were included in the protocol.

The most frequently observed adverse reactions were gastritis, leuko-
penia, hepatotoxicity and secondary infections. Symptoms of cystitis were
taken seriously and in those cases CY was tapered or even stopped. A drop
out was observed in 43 patients (38 %) mainly due to gastric intolerance
and cystitis. A follow-up for 2 years and over was possible in 59 cases
(males : 36, females : 23) and the mean follow-up period at the present
time is 4.76 years.

CY dosage was 50 mg a day in 25 patients, and 50 mg every other day
in 34, totalizing 281 patient years observation (cumulative annual dose
9 to 18 g).

Side-effects of CY make blinded studies quite difficult. The group of
59 patients treated with combined acute and chronic CY immunosuppression
was therefore compared to 59 patients treated according to our first protocol with a single short-term immunosuppression. In both groups,
patients were matched as close as possible according to sex, age at onset,
duration of disease, handicap at entry, etc...

RESULTS

After a mean follow-up period of 4.76 years, the handicap remained
unchanged in 47/59 chronically treated patients (80 %) compared to 23/59
in the control group (39 %). The difference between both groups is significant at the level $p < 0.01$.

The stabilization of the disease was confirmed by the mild increase
of the Kurtzke DSS in patients with a chronic immunosuppression (2.44 at
the end of the mean observation period versus 2.27 at entry).

In the same way, a marked influence of the ARR was observed (0.25 during immunotherapy versus 1.39 before treatment).

Immune effects of CY in treated patients were studied in longitudinal determinations of lymphocytes subsets populations. The H/S ratio was definitely lower in the 21 CY treated patients (1.24) than in 33 non CY treated patients (2.78). This restaured normal H/S ratio in CY treated patients resulted from a decrease of H cells populations (treated : 36.57 %, untreated : 45.92 %) as well as from an increase of the S cells subset (treated : 30.34 %, untreated : 19.14 %). Differences concerning H/S ratio and subsets populations are significant at the level $p < 0.05$. In opposition no significant changes were noted concerning panlymphocytes, NK and B cells.

Magnetic nuclear resonance control examinations are currently under way but it is too early to draw any firm conclusion.

CONCLUSIONS

It has been shown in various clinical studies that the evolution of MS disease can be temporarily arrested by an intensive, short-term CY immunosuppression. Our recent results with a combined, acute and chronic, CY immunotherapy show that this treatment is able to prolong the beneficial effect of a short-term immunosuppression in 80 % of the patients.

Potential immune effects of CY make this drug particularly suitable in correcting immunological disturbances observed in MS. In our experience, CY appears capable to restaure a normal H/S ratio by decreasing H cell and increasing S cell populations. The same has been found by Hauser et al. (1983) and Brinkman et al. (1984).

Moreover it has been demonstrated by Feringa et al. (1978) that after complete spinal cord transection, a statistically significant increased regeneration of descending motor axons was found in animals treated with CY. This effect could be favourable in MS lesions too.

However, the risk of cancer has always been a major deterrent to widespread use of CY. Three thousand clinical files of non-immunosuppressed MS patients have been reviewed in our department. Among 330 reported deaths, the cause was established in 257 cases and malignancies were found in 27 (10.5 %). Out of 265 CY treated patients (296 patient-years), death was reported in 37 and malignancies in 4 (10.8 %). According to our experience, cancer incidence appears to be the same in CY treated patients as in non-immunosuppressed MS population.

Subjective adverse reactions make chronic administration of CY quite difficult. There is a hope however that lower doses or intermittent administration produce the same benefit and less unwanted effects.

Interestingly enough it has been recently demonstrated by Lublin (1984) that repetitive low doses of CY are definitely more effective than higher doses in decreasing the incidence of relapsing EAE.

Even though CY is not the final treatment of MS, it appears that the favorable results observed with this substance by several authors make immune basis of MS a virtual certainty and are a strong incentive for further researches in this direction.

REFERENCES

Brinkman, C.J.J., Nillesen, W.M., and Hommes, O.R., 1984. The effect of cyclophosphamide on T lymphocytes and T lymphocyte subsets in patients with chronic progressive multiple sclerosis. Acta Neurol. Scand., 69 : 90-96.

Feringa, E.R., Davis, S.W., Vahlsing, H.L., and Shuer, L.M., 1978. Fink-Heimer/Nauta demonstration of regenerating axons in the rat spinal cord. Arch. Neurol., 35 : 522-526.

Gonsette, R.E., Demonty, L., and Delmotte, P., 1977. Intensive immunosuppression with cyclophosphamide in multiple sclerosis. Follow-up of 110 patients for 2-6 years. J. Neurol., 214 : 173-181.

Hauser, S.L., Dawson, D.M., Lehrich, J.R., Beal, M.F., Kevy, S.V., Propper, R.D., Mills, J.A., and Weiner, H.L., 1983. Intensive immunosuppression in progressive multiple sclerosis. A randomized, three-arm study of high-dose intravenous cyclophosphamide, plasma exchange, and ACTH. New Engl. J. Med., 308 : 173-180.

Hommes, O.R., Lamers, K.J.B., and Reekers, P., 1980. Effect of intensive immunosuppression on the course of chronic progressive multiple sclerosis. J. Neurol., 223 : 177-190.

Lublin, F.D., 1984. Immunomodulation of relapsing experimental allergic encephalomyelitis. Neurol., 34 : 1615-1617.

7

Anti-Lymphocyte Serum in Severe Multiple Sclerosis

R. MARTEAU, F. LHERMITTE and H. DE SAXCE

We present here the results of one-year treatment by anti-lymphocyte serum (ALS) of severe progressive MS patients allocated randomly. This study was made in the years 1978-1984. All these patients were followed 4 years.

MATERIAL AND METHODS

Patient selection: patients suffering of recent ($\leqslant$ 5 years), strongly progressive multiple sclerosis were selected. The diagnostic criteria were those internationally used. The gravity and progressiveness of the disease were decided based upon the frequency of relapses and the prompt deterioration of the functional handicap. All these patients had at first been treated with steroids, with no effect on the progressiveness of the disease. Group 1 included 45 patients treated with antilymphocyte serum; 39 patients suffered of incompletely remitting relapses, with permanent deterioration after each relapse; 6 patients suffered of directly progressive multiple sclerosis. There were 20 men and 25 women, 30 years old on average. Group 2 included 22 patients, 17 with relapsing forms and 5 directly progressive. There were 12 men and 10 women, 31 years old on average. Patients were first selected at random to be in one or the other group.

Treatment: Group 1: patients were treated by the combined application of antilymphocyte serum, azathioprine (2 mg/kg/day) and prednisone (20 mg/day). Group 2: patients were treated with azathioprine and prednisone only, same dosage. Antilymphocyte serum was prepared by Institut Mérieux. A 5 ml vial contained 62.5 mg of active proteins; several lots were used, which are now standardized. The serum was applied through slow intravenous infusion, taking 4 to 6 hours. Infusions were made every day for the first 2 weeks, 3 times a week for the following 2 weeks. The 1-year continuous treatment consisted of 1 infusion per week or 4 infusions in one week per month. The average dose was 2 to 3 vials per infusion, depending on the clinical and biological tolerance. Group 2 was treated with the same quantities of azathioprine and prednisone for 1 year. The 2 groups remained on azathioprine during the 4 years of follow-up.

RESULTS

Treatment had to be discontinued in 7 patients: in 5 of them for 10-th day serum disease (11% of the patients), in 2 for clinical and psychic intolerance. Treatment was never discontinued for technical reasons. Various transitory fever and skin reactions were also noted on the day of infusion cured by intravenous injection of prednisolone. Biological tolerance: the total lymphocyte count decreased temporarily. The platelet count decreased during the treatment due to antiplatelet effect of the antilymphocyte serum. This transient decrease was readily adjusted through dosage reduction or momentary interruption of the treatment. Proteinuria was always negative. Equine antiglobuline antibodies (see table III): 35 files were examined. The antibody titer was measured before, during, at the end of the initial treatment and monthly thereafter. For 21 patients, titers remained negative, regardless of the sampling period. For 12 patients, antibody titers increased sharply between day-10 and day-20. For 2 patients, titers increased slightly. 5 of the patients showing positive increase in their antibody titer had a day-12 serum disease. Treatment was maintained for the other patients. The level of E-rosette was regular before treatment for all files. After treatment this level decreased in 10 cases. The level of the C3 and C4 complement was normal in 31 out of 32 cases before treatment. Therapeutical results were always evaluated based upon the frequency of bouts (table I) and the disability scale (table II).

CONCLUSIONS

Our former pilot study (Lhermitte et al., 1979) about 50 patients treated during 6 weeks by ALS, corticosteroids and azathioprine showed low incidence of side-effect, effective immunosuppression, as measured by cutaneous tests during treatment and lasted 2 months after; 4 years after treatment 22% of patients were still improved (only recent patients (≤ 5 years).

This randomized study confirms that the adjunction of intravenous ALS improves significantly the effects of corticosteroids and azathioprine at 1 and 4 years after, as evaluated by disability scale: all the improved patients have no equine antiglobuline antibodies. If no equine antibodies appears, duration of treatment can be up to 1 year. As suggested by different authors (Brendel et al., 1974, Frick et al., 1974, Lance et al., 1975, Seland et al., 1974) ALS treatment can alter the rate of progression of severe MS unresponding to classical immunosuppression and can be used under strict medical monitoring for patients suffering of recent MS (≤ 5 years).

Table I. Bouts-rate.

There is no significative difference in the 2 groups

	1 year	2 years	4 years
Group I	11	14	7
A.L.S. + C + A			
Group II	8	11	9
C + A			

Table II

Comparative analysis of disability scale, patients followed 4 years :
improvement is significatively higher at 1 and 3 years.

Years		Improved	Stable	Aggravated	
1	I	18	11	9	x_2 = 4.25
	II	3	9	10	p<0.05
2	I	13	8	17	
	II	2	5	15	
3	I	7 — 22 — 15		16	x_2 = 6.12
	II	2 — 5 — 3		17	p<0.01
4	I	7 — 16 — 9		22	
	II	2 — 6 — 4		15	

Table III

Equine antiglobuline antibodies. All the patients improved have no
equine antiglobuline antibodies.

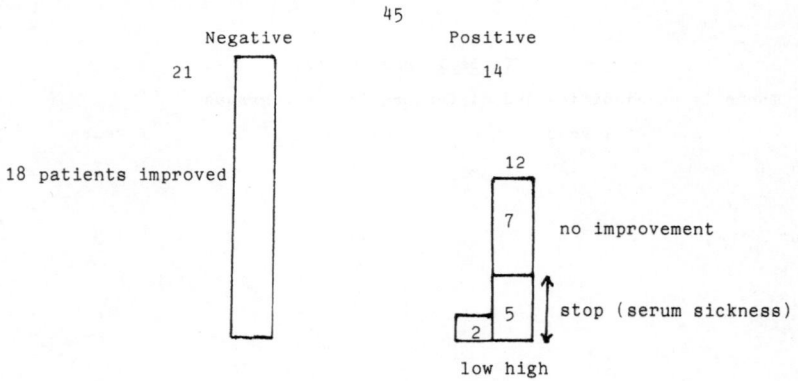

45

Negative   Positive

21   14

18 patients improved

12

7   no improvement

5   stop (serum sickness)

2

low high

REFERENCES

Brendel, W., Ring, J. and Seifert, J., 1974. Immunosuppressive treatment of MS with ALG and or thoracic-duct-drainage. Neurology, 25: 490.

Frick, E., Angstwurm, H. and Strauss, G., 1974. Immunosuppressive therapy of multiple sclerosis. Münch. Med. Wochenschr., 116: 2105-2112.

Lance, E., Abbosh, J., Kremer, M., Jones, V., Knight, S. and Medawar, P., 1975. Intensive immunosuppression in multiple sclerosis. Neurology, 25: 491.

Lhermitte, F., Marteau, R. and de Saxce, H., 1975. Traitement de la sclérose en plaques par le sérum antilymphocytaire. Immunopathologie dy système nerveux. In: M.E. Schuller (editor) INSERM, Paris, 134: 281-300.

Lhermitte, F. Marteau, R. and de Saxce, H., 1979. Treatment of multiple sclerosis with antilymphocyte serum: Results of a pilot study on 50 patients followed-up over a 4 year period. Rev. Neurol., 135: 389-400.

Marteau, R., Lhermitte, F. and de Saxce, H., 1977. Treatment of multiple sclerosis using antilymphocyte serum. Abstracts XIth World Congress of Neurology, International Congress series no. 427: pp. 332, Excerpta Medica, Amsterdam.

Reveillard, J.P., 1972. Immunosuppression par les sérums antilymphocytaires dans l'espèce humaine. Nouv. Rev. Fr. Hématol., 12: 9.

Ring, J., Lob, G., Angstwurm, H., Bross, B., Backmund, H., Seifert, J., Coulior, K., Frick, E., Mertin, J., Brendel, W., 1974. Intensive immunosupprssion in the treatment of multiple sclerosis. Lancet II: 1094-1096.

Seland, T.P., Pherson, M.C., Grace, M., Lamoureux, G. and Blain J.G., 1974. Evaluation of antilymphocyte globuline in acute relapses of multiple sclerosis. Neurology, 24: 34-40.

8

Long-term Prescription of Azathioprine in Multiple Sclerosis. A Review of Published Series

O. SABOURAUD and M. MÉRIENNE

INTRODUCTION

The interest of Neurologists for the utilisation of continuous immunosuppression during many years in the treatment of Multiple Sclerosis
arouse even before Azathioprine was available. Around 1968 Azathioprine
became the major prescription in this field. It was supported by the
clinical observation of severe cases, with frequent attacks and uninterrupted progress of the physical disability, who under treatment were
apparently stabilized for years with no further worsening of their neurological status. Such results were collected in a few centers and seemed
to deserve further studies. Randomized double blind studies have been
achieved during the period 1978-1982 ; but they failed to show clear
differences between the treated patients and the control untreated group.
The question then had to be considered : were the first clinical observations a false evaluation through multiple biases, as it occurs too easily
with open, non formalized trials ? or was there some limitation in the
randomized double-blind procedures ? This questioning is justified on
two important points. 1) The double-blind studies are of relatively short
duration, one or two years, much shorter than the pilot studies. 2) The
cases entered in the double-blind series look relatively mild if compared
to those selected for the open trials. For instance the control cases did
not deteriorate during the period of the study or did so very moderately
(one step in the scale), some of them even improving their score. The cases
in most of the open studies were selected on the basis of a permanent

deterioration ot the clinical state, with an increasingly severe disabi-
lity.Following these remarks, the assessment about a possible therapeutic
effect of Azathioprine should not be considered as brought to an end by
the published double-blind trials. Another source of information is to be
found in some reports on treatments started in the years 1968-1972 and
continued for many years.

The long-term experience with Azathioprine

Studies have been published, whose main interest is the long period of
treatment (4 to 10 years or even more) and the duration of observation
from 4 to 15 years or more. Four studies belong to this group :
Rosen (1979), Aimard et al. (1980), Sabouraud et al. (1983), Lhermitte et
al. (1984). All of them bring arguments in favour of some efficacy of
the treatment, at least on some forms of Multiple Sclerosis. Nevertheless
this agreement has to be discussed as the studies are not truely comparable. The report by Rosen accounts for two studies. The first is a
pilot study on 85 patients treated with azathioprine for 6 to 14 years
(average 9 years) All were selected because their neurological state
deteriorated in the pre-treatment period on at least three semi-annual
examinations. The assessment was on the basis of Mc Alpine mobility scale.
Less than 10 % of patients under treatment had progressed from an ambulatory to an immobile status, which was considered different from the
evolution predictable according to the natural history of M.S.   The
second study deals with a population of 42 patients (different from the
preceding group), aged 35-50 years, randomised into treatment and control
groups, all of them selected on the basis of the progressive course of
the M.S. for 3 years. At the end of 3 to 6 years, 65 % of the untreated
cases were in wheel-chairs or worse, as compared to 9 % of the treated
group. In these data, we can underline the large group and the long
duration of the pilot study, and the realization of a long randomised
trial.

        Aimard et al (1983) have conducted a prospective study on 175
patients, treated between 1977 and 1980, Of the 175, 128 had a remittent
course (i.e. attacks clearly identified) with an average of 4, 7 years
of pre-therapeutic observation, and of 4 years under Azathioprine. They
were compared to another group of 78 patients, with the same duration
and characteristics of the disease, but not selected at random. The

results were judged on the occurrence or absence of a worsening of the
symptoms during the period of trial (worsening either through the evolution of attacks, or following a continuous course) 53 % of the control
group has deteriorated, as compared to 18% of the treated group. Among
these 18%, 10% of the whole population (128) has shifted from an intermittent to a continuous course. Aimard et al. conclude that treatment
started at the remittent period of the disease increases delays
between attacks, decreases the percentage of cases presenting with a
worsening of disability, decreases the percentage of cases shifting to
a continuous progression. Treatment at the continuous progressive phase
seems to slow down the rate of progression of the disease.

Our own series (Sabouraud et al. 1983) concerns the follow-up of an
open study initiated in 1968. 102 cases were started on Azathioprine
before Dec. 1972. They were selected on the basis of a worsening of
their neurological status established through an observation of 12
months minimum. 35 stopped during the first years. 67 cases have maintained the treatment during 5 to 10 years. The evolution was evaluated
with the Kurtzke disability scale, with no control group.27 cases deteriorated, following a continuously progressive course. 40 cases remained
stable during years of treatment : all had followed a remittent course
(although with incomplete remissions) until the treatment started. A
deterioration through a series of attacks was not observed under treatment

Lhermitte et al. have published the evaluation of 145 cases treated
with Azathioprine for an average of 5 years 8 months : 71 over 5 years,
32 over 10 years. The observation leads to separate the cases with attacks
(97) and the cases with a progressive course and no attacks (48). In the
first group (remittent forms), 63 (65%) are stabilized, 34 (35%) are in
a worsened state. In the second group (continuously progressive) 17(35%)
are stabilized, 31 (65%) are worse. The evaluation is made through a
scale of neurological state and disability described by the authors.
The conclusion is in favor of an efficacy of Azathioprine on the course
and aggravation of M.S. in the remittent forms. No effect is recognized
in the continuously progressive form.

Discussion

These 4 attempts to assess the effect of prolonged Azathioprine administration show differences on many points. 1) There appears to be a dis-
crepancy between the study by Rosen and the three French series. The

first one stresses the non-remittent evolution of the cases during the
pre-treatment period of the whole group treated (with favourable effect).
The other three separate remittent forms with good results, from conti-
nously progressive evolution with no results or difficult to demonstrate.
In fact this difference may be mainly a matter of terminology. As studies
2 and 3 insist on the aggravative course of the cases treated, "remittent"
forms designate cases of M.S. where exacerbations can still be identified leading to permanent symptoms in a stepwise fashion. In the presentation by Rosen, no mention is made of exacerbations, so that "non remittent"
probably indicates the end of true and complete remissions often chara-
teristic in the first phase of M.S. evolution. Actually the number of
cases collected by Rosen may give an indication that remittent forms
which continue to experience episodic exacerbations while in a secondary
worsening phase are included in the study. (continuously progressive
cases being much less frequent). 2) The selection of severe cases is part
of the methodology in studies 1, 3, and 4.Aimard et al in the 1983 publication stand apart as they do not mention this criterion ; their group
is also somewhat different from the orther 3 because treated earlier in
the course of the disease. 3) The duration of treatment is limited in
Rosen's randomized study and in Aimard's group. It covers a wide range
in the group published by Lhermitte.It is prolonged (average around 9
years) in Rosen's pilot study and in our own.
Thus the group of patients and the evolution are defined in different
ways, Nevertheless all four studies happen to consider as the essential
parameter the duration of a stabilization, i.e. a stop in the progression of symptoms. The arrest in deterioration is appreciated through
a comparison of the scores along different disability scales. It seems
remarkable that the duration of stabilization has appeared as the most
easily appreciable parameter. This conclusion justifies the prolongation
of the survey : as the number of years with no evolution grows, the
efficacy of the treatment becomes more probable. A consequence of prolonged trials is that the use of placebo for years or the attitude of no
treatment for controls may be open to critics. Related to this very long-
lasting observation the change in evolutive modality, described as ente -
ring a continuous progressive deterioration, with no more exacerbation,
stands as a major event. This point has been particularly emphasized by
Confavreux in the description of 349 untreated patients. It becomes

perhaps more important with Azathioprine treatment, as this type of deterioration does'nt seem much accessible, if at all, to the therapeutic
effect. This remark may have an incidence on the physio-pathologic
hypotheses.

If the effect of a permanent treatment with Azathioprine needs 10 years or
more to be recognized, the final issue will ask even a longer period of
observation to be established, the question being whether the treatment
post-pones or suppresses the risk of entering a severe and progressive
deterioration.

Finally the probability that Azathioprine may bring the lesions of
M.S. to an inactive state does not mean that this kind of treatment can
be generalized. Among the complications, some are only difficulties in
continuing the treatment : the digestive troubles and pain are in this
category. Some happened to be rare and controllable, such as infections
or transitory drops in blood cell counts. The consequences of long
treatment with Azathioprine in the development of malignant tumors and
hemopathies cannot be ignored : it is sufficiently rare to be inapparent
in studies 1 and 2 summarized above. It is documented in the study by
Lhermitte et al. and in our own casuistic. Patients must be informed of
the risk. And treatment should be strictly reserved to severe cases
when a severe disability is threatening.

References

Aimard,G. Confavreux,C. Ventre,J.J. Devic,M. - 1983. Etude de 213 cas
de Sclérose en Plaques traités par l'azathioprine de 1967 à 1982. Rev.
Neurol. 139, 8-9, 509-514

Lhermitte,F. Marteau,R. Roullet,E. de Saxcé,H. Loridan,M.1984. Traitement prolongé de la Sclérose en Plaques par l'azathioprine à doses
moyennes. Bilan de quinze années d'expérience. Rev. Neurol. 140, 10,
553-558.

Rosen,J.A. 1979 - Prolonged azathioprine treatment of non-remitting
multiple sclerosis - J. Neurol. Neurosurg. Psych. 42, 4, 338-344.

Sabouraud,O. Oger, J. Menault,F. Madigand,M. Mérienne,M. 1984
Traitement immunosuppresseur au long cours dans la Sclérose en Plaques
Evaluation de 67 traitements par azathioprine commencés avant 1972.
Rev. Neurol. 140, 2, 125-130.

9

Azathioprine Assessment in Progressive Multiple Sclerosis. Clinical Aspects

I. E. ZEEBERG

INTRODUCTION

The picture of multiple sclerosis (MS) can be specified in terms of clinical type and clinical course, but few diseases offer greater difficulties in prognosis.

Established parameters of disease activity and progression in the individual patients are limited and because of the unpredictable course of MS as a whole, the assessment of treatment is notoriously difficult.

Investigators of MS generally recognize that treatment should affect both relapses and progression. If treatment is used for the acute relapse, we expect the frequency, severity and duration of the relapses to be diminished. However, in the long term, slow progression of neurologic signs and symptoms may become more significant than relapses.

Although there has been a number of trials of immunosuppression with azathioprine in MS, its value is not conclusively established and indications not yet defined.

To give a full review of this controversial field is an impossible task on an occasion such as this. I have decided, therefore, to concentrate my presentation on one aspect only, namely the number of patients exhibiting chronic progression and the rate at which this progression occur. In my opinion this is the most precise measurement of efficacy and if conducted on allocated groups in a double-blind trial the most reliable guide for possible effectivenes of treatment. It is my hope, that this restricted aspect may provide a framework for the discussion not only for the indication of azathioprine, but even more to clinical and methodological questions and the interpretation of immunosuppression.

Notable negative studies are recorded (fig. 1 and 2).Cendrowski 1971 in his prospective controlled trial reported 10 patients with a slowly progressive course which had identical mean disability status score before and immediately after immunosuppression, but 5 of them suffered afterward from continous progression within the first year.

Silberberg et al.1973 mentioned the condition of five out of six patients with chronic progressive course prior to administration of azathioprine, who continued to deteriorate.

Mertens et al. 1977 acknowledged that 7 out of 10 chronic progressive patients continued to worsen in spite of the therapy.

Aimard et al. 1980 reported on 27 patients treated with immunosuppression during progressive phase. In all patients disability worsened and three patients died. The authors emphasized that treatment was given in advanced cases and lack of efficacy still needs to be demonstrated in initial progressive forms.

Dommasch et al. 1980 have reported no influence on secondary chronic progression (11 patients) and no change in primary chronic progression (7 patients).

Frick et al. 1980 treated 24 patients with chronic progressive course. Deterioration occurred in 14, 10 remained unchanged and expected progression ceased, which might be regarded as a favorable effect.

In a summary of 213 cases of MS treated with azathioprine by Aimard et al. 1983. 47 patients with the progressive forms was evaluated. The ratio of total disability scores to number of years of observation was reported reduced in treated when compared with control patients.

Patzold et al. 1980 in there open controlled prospective study of 107 MS patients, randomly allocated into two groups, in which one group of 56 patients was treated with azathioprine for two years or more. Deterioration of control group was here found twice as rapid as the treated group over a period of at least one year. Duration of MS in each patient, however, had an important influence on response to drug. Those with a history of MS longer than two years prior to start of therapy had no significant change in the course of their disease.

On the other hand, the goal of halting progression in an open study has been reported by Rosen 1979 where only 2 out of 22 chronic progressive

AZATHIOPRINE
(chronic progressive multiple sclerosis)

Fig. 1.

INVESTIGATOR	dose	average treatment	numbers of progressive MS patients	unchanged or allivia- ted course	deteriorated course
1971 Cendrowski N = 21	125–200 mg/day	9–14 weeks	10 azathioprine 2 placebo	10	(5 after the trial)
1973 Silberberg et al N = 15	2–4.7 mg/kg/day	15 months	6		5
1977 Mertens et al N = 101	100–200 mg/day	2½ years	41 remitting/progressive 10 primarily progressive	(15) (3)	26 7
1980 Aimard et al N = 77	150 mg/day	5 years	27		27
1980 Dommasch et al N = 52	100–100 mg/day	3 years	11 relapsing/chronic progressive 7 primarily progressive		11 7
1980 Frich et al N = 88	100–150 mg/day	34 months	24	10	14

AZATHIOPRINE
(chronic progressive multiple sclerosis)

Fig. 2.

INVESTIGATOR	dose	average treatment	numbers of progressive MS patients	unchanged or allivia- ted course	deteriorated
1983 Aimard et al N = 175	150 mg/day	4 years	31 remittant/progressive 16 progressive	on average: alliviation of progression-index during treatment	
1980 Patzold et al N = 56	2 mg/kg/day	732 days	27 intermittant/progressive 8 progressive	on average: therapy allivia- ted the course of the disease	
1979 Rosen N = 22	100–200 mg/day	6 years	22 (last randomized study)	20	2

MS patients went from a "markedly restricted mobility" to "immobile - confined to wheelchair" status while receiving azathioprine. Ten out of twenty untreated patients made such a change, 1 died and 2 became bedridden.

Concerning our own double-blind, group comparison study, the results
surprisingly appeared to be more than a "holding action", both for the
placebo and the azathioprine treated patients. No serious side-effect occured but the risk of adverse effects in the azathioprine treated patients
has otherwise been considerable in nearly all of the studies quoted.

MATERIAL AND METHODS

The material potentially covered all clinically definite MS patients
(according to the diagnostic criteria of Schumacher) in regular control at
a neurological department. The 36 patients ($\female$: 18, $\male$: 18, mean age 37.4)
all had symptoms of non primary progressive course of MS as demonstrated
and statistically evaluated in monthly repeated neurological examinations
through at least a one year pre-treatment period. The patients were allocated into comparable groups for azathioprine or placebo treatment according to pre-trial progression coefficient, histocompatibility (DR2), sex,
duration of illness, age and neurological deficit. The patients were admitted into treatment in parallel over eight weeks during autumn 1979 (17
patients), 1980 (7 patients) and 1981 (12 patients). During the trial, the
prior drug treatment was continued and changes were made only according to
the indications usually practiced in the department.

The cytostatically treated patients received a daily dosage of 2-2½
mg/kg body weight azathioprine in order to maintain a white blood cell
count $< 5 \times 10^3$ (wBD)/microl. Therapeutic management was handled from another department and independent of the clinical examination as well as unknown to the neurologist. Each patient was examined at intervals of approximately 4 weeks using a neurological scoring system, where each sign and
symptom was graded clinically and converted by a computer program into a
total neurological deficit, expressed as a percentage of a hypothetical
maximal deficit, which quantified the state of the disease. For each patient the neurological deficit was plotted against time, and the rate of
change of neurological deficit - regression coefficient - was calculated.
The regression coefficient for patients treated with azathioprine of placebo were compared by the Mann-Whitney rank sum test and the mean rate of

progression in the two groups was calculated from square root transformed values.

RESULTS

The clinical course of the 36 patients (17 azathioprine, 19 placebo) calculated after 12 months of treatment, was compared and found without significant difference concerning the progression coefficient for the placebo and azathioprine treated group (fig. 3). For the individual course in the one year pre-treatment period, compared with one year of treatment, mean rate of progression changed from 2.89 to 1.26 (percent of total neurological deficit per year). So regardless of treatment given a remarkable statistically reduction in the rate of progression was found for the patients in the trail. For the selected part of the patients who recieved more than two years of treatment, similar calculations were equal in general outcome. Further in these patientgroups, by use of Kurtzke disability status score after the termination of the trial 1982/83, no difference could be demonstrated and even though a posttrial overall significant change in disability deterioration in the placebo was shown (fig. 4) at least two years azathioprine treatment did not offer significant effect over placebo in the first 15-18 months period after the treatment (fig. 5).

CONCLUSION

Although the experience with azathioprine appears to have some beneficial effect on the progressive course in MS, no significant difference to placebo has been demonstrated in a double-blind trial with allocated MS patients, in pretrial steady progress and treated for a period of one to three years. Azathioprine is suitable to carefully controlled clinical evaluation in order to determine as closely as possible what the efficacy might be, but other approaches to symptomatic and curative treatment must continue.

Fig. 3.

<u>BASIC STUDY:</u>

Group-comparison, double blind trial 1979–1982
(azathioprine versus placebo)
with open medication control.

MEAN PROGRESSIONKOEFFICIENT

	pretrial	after one years treatment
2.39	-0.65
3.75	0.27

Azathioprine treated group   (N = 17)
Placebo treated gruop   (N = 19)
                             ─────────
                              N = 37

No significant difference 5%
level between the two groups

Fig. 4.

THE VARIABLE IN KURTZKE DISABILITY SCORE FOR 1979 AND 1980 ALLOCATED GROUPS

DURING TOTAL PERIOD

Friedman two-way
Analysis of variance

	AT THE BEGINNING OF TREATMENT	AT THE END OF TREATMENT	AT THE PRESENT FOLLOW UP STATE	
SUM OF RANKS	AZATHIOPRINE	15.5	20.5	24.0	P > 0.3
	PLACEBO	15.5	20.5	30.0	P < 0.05

Fig. 5.

CHANGE IN KURTZKE DISABILITY SCORE FOR THE 1979 AND 1980 ALLOCATED GROUPS

DURING FOLLOW UP PERIOD   (>15 - ≤18 MONTHS)

	DETERIORATION	UNCHANGED OR IMPROVED	
AZATHIOPRINE	4	6	10
PLACEBO	7	4	11
	11	10	N = 21

Fisher fourhold table test: no significant difference (5% level) between the two groups in terms of deterioration assessed by disability system

REFERENCES

Aimard, G., Confavreux, C., Devic, M., 1980. Long term immunosuppressive treatment with azathioprine in multiple sclerosis. A 10 years trial with 77 patients. In: H. Bauer (Editor), Progress in Multiple Sclerosis. Berlin. Springer-Verlag, pp. 371-375.

Aimard, G., Confavreux, C., Ventre, J.J., Guillot, M., Devic, M., 1983: A study of 213 cases of multiple sclerosis treated with azathioprine from 1967 to 1982. Rev. Neurol., 139, 8-9: 509-513.

Cendrowski, W.S., 1971: Therapeutic trial of Imuran (azathioprine) in multiple sclerosis. Acta neurol. Scand., 47: 254-60.

Dommasch, D., Lurati, M., Albert, E., Mertens, H.G., 1980: Long-term azathioprine therapy in multiple sclerosis. In: H.Bauer (Editor), Progress in Multiple Sclerosis. Berlin. Springer-Verlag, pp. 381-387.

Frick, E., Angstwurm, H., Blomer, R., Strauss, G., 1980: Long-term treatment of multiple sclerosis with azathioprine. In: H. Bauer (Editor), Progress in Multiple Sclerosis. Berlin. Springer-Verlag, pp. 376-380.

Mertens, H.G., Dommasch, D., 1977: Long term study of immunosuppressive therapy in multiple sclerosis, comparison of periods of the disease before and during treatment. In: P. Delmotte, O.R. Hommes, R. Gonsette (Editors), Immunosuppressive Treatment in Multiple Sclerosis. Ghent, Belgium, European Press, pp. 198-211.

Patzold, U., Pocklington, P., 1980: Azathioprine in multiple sclerosis - A 3 years study of its effectiveness. J. Neurol., 223, pp. 97-117.

Rosen, J.A., 1979: Prolonged azathioprine treatment of non-remitting multiple sclerosis. J. Neurol. Neurosurg. Psychiatry, 42: pp. 338-344.

Silberberg, D., Lisak, R., Zweiman, B., 1973: Multiple sclerosis unaffected by azathioprine in pilot study. Arch. Neurol., 28: 210-212.

10

Dietary Therapy in Multiple Sclerosis

D. BATES

Introduction

Epidemiological data provided the first evidence of an association between multiple sclerosis (MS) and the consumption of dietary fats (Swank, 1950). More recent reports have confirmed a higher prevalence of MS in populations consuming diets rich in saturated fatty acids and low in polyunsaturates (Alter et al, 1974). Biochemical studies of brain, serum and red blood cells have shown a deficiency of polyunsaturated fatty acids, particularly linoleic acid, in patients with MS (Thompson, 1966).

This biochemical and epidemiological evidence prompted controlled trials of dietary supplementation with linoleic acid during the 1970's (Millar et al, 1973, Bates et al, 1978 and Paty et al, 1978). Although two of these trials appeared to show some significant benefit for the treated group, the third failed to show any effect. The suggestion was made that the variation in results might be due to different characteristics of the patients in the trials at the time of admission. Those patients in the two trials showing benefit were, on average, less disabled and had disease of shorter duration than those in the trial which gave negative results. The present report is the result of a reassessment of the combined results.

Patients and Methods

(a) Patients

In all three trials only patients who were able to walk with or without aids were included (Kurtzke D.S.S. 6 or less). A total of 172 patients were identified of whom 87 were treated and 85 were in the placebo group (Table I). Sixty eight patients were male and 104 female with a mean age of onset of disease of 29.4 years and a mean duration of disease of 11.0 years. The mean age at entry to the trial was 40.4 years and the average of the Kurtzke D.S.S. at entry to the trial was 3.2.

Patients were assessed neurologically at intervals of six to 26 weeks and relapses documented and scored (Millar et al, 1967). Patients were followed for 24 to 30 months.

TABLE 1

Patient Characteristics

	Treated	Control
Number of patients	87	85
Men	31	37
Women	56	48
Mean age at onset of MS	30.2	28.5
Mean age at entry to trial	40.8	40.0
Mean duration of disease	10.6	11.5
Mean Kurtzke DSS at entry	3.3	3.2

(b) Treatment

Patients in each of the three trials were randomly allocated to a treatment group receiving linoleic acid in a dose of 17.2 to 23 g daily or to a control group receiving oleic acid in a dose of 7.6 to 16 g daily. Assessment of serum lipids was made in certain patients at admission to the trial, 12 and 24 months. No other dietary advice was given to patients and other treatments were prescribed as necessary.

(c) Analysis

The cohort was divided into two groups with respect to disability at admission and duration of disease. In terms of disability the group with minimal disability had Kurtzke D.S.S. scores of two or less and the other scores between three and six. In terms of duration groups were identified with disease of less than five years, between six and 10 years and over 11 years. For each level of disability and duration of disease the statistical significant of differences between the control and treated groups were tested for each of three variables; change in Kurtzke D.S.S. during the trial, number of relapses occurring and severity of relapses. Mann Whitney U Tests were performed because of the ordinal level of measurement.

Results

The data with respect to change in Kurtzke score, number of attacks and severity is shown in Table II. There is little difference in overall disability or attack rate between the treated and untreated groups though the severity of attacks is less in patients taking therapy.

TABLE II

Final Assessments

	Treated	Control
Mean Kurtzke DSS at end	3.8	3.9
Percentage of patients with relapses	63	59
Mean relapse score	15.3	26.5
Mean number of relapses/year	0.7	0.6
Mean duration of trial in months	28.1	28.2

(a) Change in Disability Scores

The mean changes in Kurtzke D.S.S. scores from admission to the end of the trial for the two groups at each of the two levels of disability on entry are shown in Table III. Patients with minimal disability treated with linoleic acid have significantly less deterioration over the two and a half years than those in the control group. Patients with moderate to severe disability (Kurtzke three to six) show no significant difference.

Table IV shows the mean D.S.S. at entry and at the end of the trial for each of the two different disability groups and again whereas the patients with moderate disability show a significant deterioration whether treated or not, those with mild disability show no significant change in the treatment group and a significant deterioration in the control group.

In Table V is shown the change in disability scores for patients in each of the three duration of disease categories where there is no significant difference between the treated and control groups.

TABLE   III

Change in Disability Scores

	Mean Change		
Disability at entry	Treated	Control	
0 - 2	0.12	0.81	p < 0.05
3 - 6	0.71	0.76	ns

TABLE   IV

DSS As a Function of Disability at Entry

Mean DSS

Disability at entry	Entry	End	
0 - 2			
Treat.	1.4	1.5	ns
Control	1.4	2.2	p = 0.03
3 - 6			
Treat.	4.8	5.5	p < 0.0001
Control	4.6	5.4	p < 0.0001

TABLE   V

Change in Disability Scores

Mean Change

Duration at Entry (years)	Treatment	Control	
0 - 5	0.1	0.6	ns
6 - 10	0.5	1.0	ns
> 11	0.6	0.7	ns

(b) Relapse Scores

In Table VI the mean of the relapse scores for each patient duration the course of the trial in both the treated and untreated groups are expressed in relation to the two levels of disability at entry. There is a significant difference between treated and untreated groups in both the mildly and more severely affected patients. In Table VII assessing the mean relapse score for different durations of disease again confirms a significant difference that the relapse score is always lower in the group treated with linoleic acid.

TABLE   VI

Relapse Scores Related to Disability

Disability at entry	Mean Relapse Score		
	Treatment	Control	
0 – 2	12.2	22.8	p < 0.001
3 – 6	18.8	32.5	p < 0.01

TABLE   VII

Relapse Scores Related to Duration

Duration at entry (years)	Mean Relapse Score		
	Treatment	Control	
0 – 5	12.6	25.4	p < 0.05
6 – 10	18.4	29.6	p < 0.01
> 11	14.9	24.9	p < 0.03

(c) Number of Relapses

Comparison of the number of relapses in groups with differing severity and different duration fo disease reveals that there is no statistically significant difference at any level of initial disability or duration of illness (Table VIII).

Discussion

The re-analysis of the data from the original trials of linoleic acid in MS confirms the suggestion that patients with minimal disability at entry to the trials who were given active treatment showed significantly less deterioration over the course of the trial than did controls. In addition, it appears that treatment with linoleic acid significantly reduces the severity and duration of relapses regardless of

TABLE VIII

Number of Relapses

Mean number of relapses per year

	Treatment	Control	
Disability			
0 - 2	0.8	0.9	ns
3 - 6	0.6	0.3	ns
Duration			
0 - 5	1.0	0.9	ns
6 - 11	0.8	0.6	ns
> 11	0.5	0.5	ns

the disability and duration of the illness but that there is no significant effect on the frequency of relapses (Dworkin et al, 1984).

The reason for the apparent beneficial effect of linoleic acid on the progression of multiple sclerosis and on the severity and duration of relapses remains a mystery. One hyopthesis would suggest that linoleic acid is involved in the regulation of cell mediated immunity (Mertin et al 1977) and, since multiple sclerosis may have an auto-immune basis (McFarlin et al, 1982), the linoleic acid may have an immunosuppressive effect. Linoleic acid reduces the severity of experimental allergic encephalomyelitis (Mead et al, 1978) which effect may be mediated by prostaglandin derivatives. It has been suggested that the effectiveness of linoleic acid in reducing EAE is related to disease severity (Hughes D et al, 1980).

Other studies of multiple sclerosis have reported a differential response to immunosupressive treatment as a function of disability or duration of illness. One uncontrolled clinical trial of intensive immunosuppression with cyclophosphamide (Gonsette et al, 1977) showed that response to treatment was greatest in patients with shortest duration of illness. Hommes et al (1980) also found that patients whose

disability at the start of treatment was low or who had the shortest
duration of illness showed the best response to treatment with
cyclophosphamide. These results are also in agreement with those of the
uncontrolled clinical trial of low animal fat and high polyunsaturated
fat diet reported by Swank (1970) who reported that patients with minimal
disability or who began treatment early in the course of their illness
showed little deterioration over a 20 year period of the disease.

The advantage of linoleic acid as a dietary supplement in multiple
sclerosis is that it is non-toxic, inexpensive and unlikely to cause the
patient hardship. Although potential benefit may be small, it would seem
worth encouraging the patient to take a diet high in linoleic acid and it
is evident that further studies to explain the nature of its action are
indicated and that other studies investigating different polyunsaturated
fatty acids may also be relevant.

References

Swank, R.L., 1950 Multiple sclerosis: a correlation of its incidence
   with dietary fat. Am. J. Med. Sci. 220: 421-430

Alter, M., Yamoor, M. and Harshe, M., 1974 Multiple sclerosis and
   nutrition. Arch. Neurol. 31: 267-272

Thompson, R.H.S., 1966 A biochemical approach to the problem of
   multiple sclerosis. Proc. R. Soc. Med. 59: 269-276

Millar, J.H.D., Zilkha, K.J., Langman, M.J.S., 1973 Double blind
   trial of linoleic supplementation of the diet in multiple sclerosis.
   Br. Med. J. 1: 765-768

Bates, D., Fawcett, P.R.W., Shaw, D.A., Weightman, D. 1978 Polyunsaturated
   fatty acids in the treatment of acute remitting multiple sclerosis.
   Br. Med. J. 2: 1390-1391

Paty, D.W., Cousin, H.K., Reed, S. Adlakha, K. 1978 Linoleic acid in
   multiple sclerosis: failure to show any therapeutic benefit.
   Acta. Neurol. Scand. 58: 53-58

Dworkin, R.H., Bates, D. , Millar, J.H.D., Paty, D.W. 1984 Linoleic
   acid in multiple sclerosis. Neurology, 34 1441-1445

Mertin, J., Meade, C.J., 1977 Relevance of fatty acids in multiple
   sclerosis. Br. Med. Bull. 33: 67-71

McFarlin, D.E., McFarland, H.F., 1982 Multiple sclerosis. N. Engl. J. Med
370: 1246-1251

Meade, C.J., Mertin, J., Sheena, J., Hunt, R. 1978 Reduction by linoleic
acid of the severity of experimental allergic encephalomyelitis in the
guinea pig. J. Neurol. Sci. 35: 291-308

Gonsette, R.E., Demo.tt, L., Delmotte, P., 1977 Intensive immunosuppresion
with cyclophosphamide in multiple sclerosis. J. Neurol. 214: 173-181

Hommes, O.R., Lammers, K.J.B., Reckers, P. 1980 Effect of intensive
immunosuppression on the course of chronic progressive multiple sclerosis.
J. Neurol. 223: 177-190

Swank, R.L., 1970 Multiple sclerosis: 20 years on low fat diet. Arch.
Neurol. 23: 460-474

11

An 8 Years Follow-up Study of Transfer Factor Treatment on the Course of Multiple Sclerosis

A. M. NORDENBO and I. ZEEBERG

INTRODUCTION

Transfer factor (TF) has been given to patients with multiple sclerosis (MS) in several trials hoping to modulate the course of the disease. The rationale of these trials was based on the theory which relates MS to a selective immuno-deficient state with a probable viral etiology, and the fact, that TF enhances the in vitro immunological response in MS patients (Zabriskie et al., 1975).

In the study of Behan et al. (1976) TF was given in a double-blind trial comprising 30 patients who received treatment over 6 months. No effect of TF versus placebo was found. No scoring system was used, but each neurological deficit found on the initial examination was contrasted and compared with that found on the final assessment. The patients chosen was not defined as to type or course of the disease. Fog et al. (1978), encouraged by a previous study (Fog et al., 1977) carried out a double-blind trial of TF versus placebo. The study was planned to last 2 years, but was stopped after 13 months, since no significant effect was found by use of computerized scoring system and group comparison. Details of these patients, who comprise our follow-up material, are listed below. Neither Collins et al. (1978) were able to demonstrate any significant difference between TF and placebo treated, carefully matched patients with MS. The treatment period was here 12 months.

So far, controlled double-blind studies of TF versus placebo proved negative, but in 1980 Basten et al. published the results of a 2 years treatment study in 58 patients. They reported a significant retardation of the progression of the disease after 18 months of TF treatment. Less than 10% improved in each group.

No follow-up study have been presented in the literature. We have therefore carried out an 8 years follow-up study to see whether previous given treatment with TF had any long-term effect on the course of the progressive forms of MS.

MATERIAL AND METHODS

The 32 patients (18 females, 14 males, age 19-34 years) who in 1976 participated in a double-blind controlled trial (Fog et al., 1978) all had MS of the progressive type, but were at the time of entry in the study not restricted to a wheelchair. The patients in the TF and placebo treated groups were matched according to disability, age, sex and HLA-type. The TF was prepared from random donors.

Follow up 1984. All patients were contacted through their general practitioner. One patient living far away was interviewed by phone and information was obtained from her nurse and doctor. Hospital records were also obtained on those deceased at the time of follow-up. The patients were examined by one of us and scored according to the Kurtzke's disability status scale and functional systems (Kurtzke 1983). The list of the treatment given was delivered to us after the scoring of all patients.

RESULTS

In table 1 are listed the disability status scores of the patients at the time of follow up. No significant difference between the two groups can be demonstrated (Mann Whitney rank sum test).

Table 1

Disability status score at time of follow-up.

Kurtzke's DSS	Placebo	TF
$5.0 \leq DSS \leq 6.5$	7	6
$7.0 \leq DSS \leq 7.5$	1	3
$8.0 \leq DSS \leq 9.5$	6	5
DSS = 10 (dead)	2	2
	N=16	N=16

CONCLUSION

From the present study nothing indicates that TF prepared from random donors given for 13 months to patients with progressive MS has any effect on the further course of the disease. Whether TF prepared from relatives offers anything in favour of TF prepared from random donors is being tested in the ongoing trial of van Haver et al. (1984). At present the studies published concerning the possible therapeutic effect of TF in any form of MS is not encouraging as well as the validity of the theoretical foundation for the treatment still is questionable.

ACKNOWLEDGEMENT

We are grateful to Chief Neurologist T. Fog for valuable informations making this study possible.

REFERENCES

Basten, A., McLeod, J.G., Pollard, J.D., Valsh, J.C., Stewart, Q.J., Ganick, R., Frith, J.A., Van Der Brink, C.M., 1980. Transfer factor in treatment of multiple sclerosis. Lancet, ii: pp. 931-934.

Behan, P.O., Meluille, I.D., Durward, W.F., McGeorge, A.P., Behan, W.M.H., 1976. Transfer factor therapy in multiple sclerosis. Lancet, i, pp. 988-990.

Collins, R.C., Espinoza, L.R., Plank, C.R., Ebers, G.C., Rosenberg, R.A., Zabriskie, J.B., 1978. A double-blind trial of transfer factor vs placebo in multiple sclerosis patients. Clin. Exp. Immunol., 33, pp. 1-11.

Fog, T., Jersild, C., Platz, P., Svejgaard, A., Pedersen, L., Kam-Hansen, S., Raun, N.E., Mellerup, E., Jacobsen, B., Linnemann, F., West, P., 1977. Acta Neurol. Scand., suppl. 63, 55: pp. 253.

Fog, T., Pedersen, L., Raun, N.E., Kam-Hansen, S., Mellerup, E., Platz, P., Ryder, P.L., Jacobsen, B.K., Grob, P., 1978. Long-term transfer-factor treatment for multiple sclerosis. Lancet, i, pp. 851-853.

Van Haver, H., Lissoir, F., Theys, P., Droissart, C., Van Hees, J., Ketelaer, P., Carton, H., Gautama, K., Vandeputte, I., Vermylen, C., 1984. Transfer factor treatment in MS: A 3 year prospective double-blind study (1982-85) In: R.E. Gonsette and P. Delmotte (Editors), Immunological and clinical aspects of multiple sclerosis. MTP Press Limited. Lancaster/Boston/The Hague/Dordrecht, pp. 161-165.

Kurtzke, J., 1983. Rating neurologic impairment in multiple sclerosis: An expanded disability status scale (EDSS). Neurology, 33: pp. 1444-1452.

Zabriskie, J.B., Utermohlen, V., Espinosa, L.R., Plank, C.R., Collins, R.C., 1975. Immunologic studies with transfer factor in multiple sclerosis patients. Neurology, 25: pp. 490.

12

Compact Manual for Multiple Sclerosis Registration in Clinical Research

O. ANDERSEN, M. ANDERSSON, T. BROMAN and I. ZEEBERG

INTRODUCTION

It has, since Charcot's time, been almost unanimously recognized that the course of MS may take the form of bouts, or it may be chronically progressive, either from the onset or after a number of bouts. The essential histological and immunological difference, if any, between bouts and progress is still a matter of debate. Apart from this genuine problem, different interpretations of terms create new problems. The parameters discussed below have been amply tested in the Göteborg incidence material (Andersen 1980).

MS DIAGNOSTIC CATEGORIES

Part 1. Discussion on use of "paraclinical methods".

Computerized tomography or evoked response data are, according to the diagnostic criteria of Poser et al. (1983), allowed to substitute for one MS-compatible clinical lesion in clinically definite MS as well as in clinically probable MS. Computerized tomography is useful for morphological assessment although the frequency of positive findings probably is lower when the clinical diagnostic probability is low (Vinuela et al., 1982, Ebers et al., 1984). Although certain individual evoked responce lesions (e.g. optic nerve) could be almost as MS-typical as the corresponding clinical lesions, they are not generally disease-specific (Sedgwick 1983). Nuclear magnetic resonance yield new data on distribution and biology of plaques although the specificity was not high in the report of Ormerod et al., 1984.

CSF data are not used in the Schumacher criteria (1965), but are required in the criteria compiled by Bauer (1980). The criteria proposed by Poser et al. (1983) provide two alternatives: Clinical MS diagnosis independent of CSF data, and "laboratory-supported" MS diagnosis supported by CSF specific oligoclonal bands or quantitatively increased IgG production evidenced in the CSF. Basically, intrathecal immunological reactions are not etiologically specific (Link et al., 1971). Studies of the differential diagnosis of intrathecal immunoglobulin production (Olsson et al., 1976, Frydén et al., 1978, Hershey et al., 1979) reveal low frequencies of differential diagnostic conditions other than inflammatory, but to the best of our knowledge no long-term studies have been performed. However, as some time relationships in MS differential diagnoses tend to increase the specificity of a CSF specimen investigated more than two years after onset of symptoms, we discuss the following conditions:

1. One monofocal attack with intrathecal gamma globulin production. After mumps meningitis, the intrathecal immunological reaction may persist for 12 months, but only in a minority of patients and with diminishing intensity (Vandvik et al., 1978). With focal CMV lesions of the CNS, e.g. myelopathy problems of differential diagnosis and nosology seem unsolved. Some cerebrovascular lesions are associated with an intrathecal immunological reaction which subsided within one year in 11/17 cases (Roström 1981). In MS the intrathecal immunoglobulin production usually persists for years, probably for a lifetime.

2. One multifocal attack with intrathecal gamma globulin production. There is no persistent intrathecal immunological activity subsequent to postinfectious encephalomyelopathy, but experience seems to be scarce.

3. Repeated multifocal attacks with intrathecal gamma globulin production. Although neurosarcoidosis and collagenoses may elicit an intrathecal immunological reaction which may be located primarily to the intrathecal compartment, it is usually associated with a pronounced blood-brain barrier lesion, and in sarcoidosis with a characteristic cytology. After treatment of neurolues, a diminishing intrathecal immunoglobulin production may persist for more than two years (Löwhagen et al., 1983).

4. Progressive lesion with intrathecal gamma globulin production. This is known to occur with e.g. some ependymomas. If conclusions from CSF analysis are postponed for 2 years, the tumour may reveal itself through its focal and progressive symptomatology.

Part 2. Diagnostic categories. Experience from the Göteborg MS incidence material.

In each example it is understood that the age of the patient, the neurological syndrome and the course of the symptoms are compatible with MS. Well-documented retrospective data may be used for supportive analysis of initial phases of the disease, but personal longitudinal follow-up data are obligatory for the use of detailed clinical information exemplified below. In incidence studies, personal follow-up during decennia is expected. The present diagnostic classification is not designed to be used with less than two years of personal follow-up in any case.

MS QUESTIONABLE

This file is a base for future follow-up in prevalence and indicence studies and a means of keeping retrospective data.

Subgroup 1 : Example 1 : An acute lesion of one of the nerves of the extraocular muscles or its nucleus, but without evidence of a brain stem lesion.

Exampel 2 : An acute vestibular syndrome without evidence of a brain stem lesion.

Subgroup 2 : Example 1 : Two acute lesions separated by at least one month, each of which affects one of the nerves to the extraocular muscles or its nucleus, however without evidence of a brain stem lesion, and with the first lesion in a state of remission when the second lesion occurs. (Reservation for syndromes compatible with painful ophthalmoplegia and the sinus cavernosus syndrome).

Example 2 : Trigeminal neuralgia below 40 years of age.

Example 3 : A slowly progressing central paraparesis and a moderate parahypesthesia without a sensory level, often with a "posterior cord" predominance.

POSSIBLE MS

The minimal requirements for this category are certain focal lesions with a typical MS symptomatology, or MS QUESTIONABLE SUBGROUP 2 cases ha-

ving a typical intrathecal immunological reaction as determined by CSF
analysis MORE THAN TWO YEARS AFTER ONSET OF MS.

Example 1 : A typical acute optic or retrobulbar neuritis as evidenced by
immediate or residual signs. The diagnosis is acceptable with
subtle residuals such as slightly reduced unilateral color vision with the Boström-Kugelberg pseudosisochromatic plates if
there was a typical anamnesis, in particular including pain on
eye movement, and appropriate investigation is performed to
exclude retinopathy as a cause of the color vision defect.

Example 2 : A typical acute focal myelopathy as evidenced by appropriate
signs. The syndrome diagnosis of myelopathy may be considered
reliable if based on a convincing personally obtained history
with details concerning sensory quality and level.

Example 3 : A typical central vestibular syndrome verified by brain stem
signs, particularly the signs of internuclear ophthalmoplegia.

Example 4 : Typical tonic seizures.
NOTE: Generally, a mere recurrence of one of the symptoms listed here does not per se justify a higher diagnostic probability level.

Example 5 : A slowly progressive central paraparesis and moderate parahypesthesia combined with convincing signs of lower motor neuron
lesion of bladder or lower extremities, in particular sluggish
reflexes previously noted to be exaggerated (reservation for a
number of longitudinal myelopathies including that of dural
A-V fistula).

Example 6 : QUESTIONABLE MS SUBGROUP 2 cases having a typical intrathecal
immunological reaction as determined by CSF analysis MORE THAN
TWO YEARS AFTER ONSET OF SYMPTOMS. This category may be treated as MS questionable in special statistics. See discussion
on CSF analysis in part one.

PROBABLE MS

The minimal requirements for this category are one POSSIBLE MS lesion
with an added MS QUESTIONABLE lesion, or one POSSIBLE MS lesion with an
added lesion essentially of the same (POSSIBLE) category, judged to be reliable from personally checked anamnestic details but without the documen-

tation outlined in the examples. Accepted as PROBABLE MS are also clinically POSSIBLE MS cases having a typical intrathecal immunological reaction as determined by CSF analysis MORE THAN TWO YEARS AFTER ONSET OF SYMP-
TOMS. The PROBABLE category does not contain cases with multiple vague
symptoms or signs none of which is an absolutely significant CNS manifestation.

Example 1 : A progressive para-and tetraparesis with a contingent "posterior cord" syndrome which ultimately, after years of steady
progress, is complicated by an internuclear ophthalmoplegia.

Example 2 : An acute remitting attack of focal myelopathy with sensory
predominance followed by a non-focal progressive lesion of
central motor neurons with a para- or tetraparesis, sometimes
also a moderate diffuse sensory pendant.

Example 3 : More than two attacks of combined brain stem focal and long
tract lesions with at least five years of follow-up without
progression, provided the brain stem symptoms are slight and
variable, and the long tract symptoms pronounced and varying.
NOTE: The identification of a steadily progressive course in
MS is feasible within a few months in acute cases, and within
two years of follow-up in the majority of patients. However,
in some chronic cases the diagnosis of steady progress has to
be postponed for up to 10 years after onset.

Example 4 : A typical "migrating" lesion within one CNS region, i.e. a series of MS predilection symptoms (e.g. bilateral partial internuclear ophthalmoplegia) occurring in a typical subacute
sequence during weeks, with the first lesion in a continuous
state of evident remission at the time of appearance of the
second phase, and a similar relationship between occasional
subsequent phases. In myelopathy, a second phase with a bilateral sensory hand ataxia may evolve while a truncal sensory
level subsides.
NOTE: The differential diagnosis between MS and postinfectious
encephalomyelitis is a clinical problem fraught with unsolved
definition problems. Histologically, the lesions of acute disseminated encephalomyelitis are all of the same age, whereas
there is a considerable variation in the age of the lesions
present in MS (Prineas 1970).

Example 5 : The statement in example 4 is also valid for analogous migratory phenomena between right- and left-sided useless hand
without a sensory level, or between typical acute optic or retrobulbar neuritis on the right and left side, when the contralateral "migration" occurs after a delay of at least one month,
following or during the remission.

CLINICALLY DEFINITE MS

The minimum requirement for this category is the combination of two
separate POSSIBLE MS lesions in a bout or migrating pattern, with one lesion in either a stationary phase after remission or in a process of continuous remission at the time of appearance of the next lesion, alternatively in a combined bout and subsequent progression pattern, or in a successive multifocal progression pattern. An alternative minimal requirement
is a clinically probable MS case having a typical intrathecal immunological reaction as determined by CSF analysis MORE THAN TWO YEARS AFTER ONSET
OF SYMPTOMS.

VERIFIED MS

Only qualified neuropathological investigations are accepted for the post-
mortem diagnosis of MS. In cases with tiny or shadow plaques, histology is
essential to verify or exclude the diagnosis.

MS BASIC COURSE PARAMETERS

A BOUT is defined as the development within days to weeks of MS-compatible symptoms provided that the condition has been essentially unchanged or improving during the previous month.

It is necessary to distinguish between bouts and another transient
type of deterioration, designed the "pseudobout", and furthermore to define two subtypes of bouts, the polyphasic and the prolonged bouts, in order
to avoid gross error in bout frequency computations.

A PSEUDOBOUT is a clinical deterioration believed to represent functional changes in pre-existing (partially) demyelinated lesions rather
than new inflammatory or demyelinating MS activity. Its duration is often
confined to a few days or less. It characteristically fluctuates with the

eliciting factor, which may be fever, passive heating or physical activity, tiredness or emotional stress, often in varying combinations.

A POLYPHASIC BOUT is a manifestation that fulfils the bout criteria except that the interval after the preceding bout is less than one month. The bout-like phases attack different regions of the central nervous system. A MIGRATING bout is analogous to a polyphasic bout except that the bout-like phases seem to attack different parts of the same region.

A PROLONGED BOUT: Bout activity, with new symptoms occurring at intervals of days or weeks continues during several months relentlessly, or with only very short periods or remission. The next phase may be almost stationary, or, more often, severely progressive.

STEADY PROGRESS is defined as the development of MS-compatible symptoms so insidious as to be undetectable at weekly examinations and not necessarily detectable at monthly examinations. To describe the steady progress a time scale unit of at least one year is required. This insidious progression may occur from onset or after a remitting course. Particularly in the latter event, the progression may be periodic, and it may be impossible to distinguish between periodic progression and added bouts.

TYPES OF CLINICAL MS COURSE

A. EXACERBATING - REMITTING 1. Without sequele.
2. With sequele.
3. Sequele difficult to differentiate from progress, "Stepwise pseudoprogress".

B. PROGRESSIVE 1. Steadily progressive from onset.
2. Steadily progressive after previous exacerbating - remitting course. Most often no bouts, but new bouts may occur.
3. Periodically progressive.

COMMENTS

Should the clinical symptomatology be nothing but the top of the iceberg, still the amount of myelin lesions would be stochastically related to the sum of neurological deficit. More controversial is the statement that clinical bouts do reflect a particular type of spread while the progress may represent a different pathological progress perhaps with more extensive autoimmunity. Anyhow, for patients with acute well-defined bouts and intervening years of well-being, BOUT FREQUENCY (Andersen 1980) is certainly a relevant measure of disease activity. In many clear-cut cases the EVENT OF STEADY PROGRESS indicates a decisive turning-point of the disease. However, for patients with complicated progress and bouts manifestations from the same tracts, no reliable bout frequency can be computed, and DEFICIT SCORE is the most relevant parameter.

REGISTRATION

Semantics will optimally be uniform enough to allow modem total data transfer between centers.

Systems for registration of score, detailed symptomatology or integrated neuroanatomy are available for different purposes of research.

REFERENCES

Andersen, O., 1980. Restricted dissemination of clinically defined attacks in an MS incidence material. Acta Neurol. Scand., 62, Suppl. 77.

Bauer, H.S., 1980. IMAB-Enquête Concerning the Diagnostic Criteria for MS. In: Bauer, Poser, Ritter: Progress in Multiple Sclerosis Research. Springer Berlin, pp. 555-563.

Ebers, G.C., Finuela F.V., Feasby, T., Bass, B., 1984. Multifocal CT enhancement in MS. Neurology, 34: pp. 341-346.

Frydén, A., Link, H., Norrby, E., 1978. Cerebrospinal Fluid and Serum Immunoglobulins and Antibody Titers in Mumps Meningitis and Aseptic Meningitis of Other Etiology. Infection and Immunity, 21: pp. 852-861.

Hershey, L.A., Trotter, J.L., 1980. The Use and Abuse of the Cerebrospinal Fluid IgG Profile in the Adult: A Practical Evaluation. Ann. Neurol., 8: pp. 426-434.

Link, H., Müller, R., 1971. Immunoglobulins in Multiple Sclerosis and infections of the nervous system. Arch. Neurol., 25: pp. 326-343.

Löwhagen, G., Andersson, M., Blomstrand, C., Roupe, G., 1983. Central Nervous System Involvement in Early Syphilis. Acta Derm. Venereol., 63: pp. 409-417.

Olsson, J., Pettersson, B., 1976. Comparison between agar gel electrophoresis and CSF serum quotients of IgG and albumin in neurological diseases. Acta Neurol. Scand., 53: pp. 308-322.

Ormerod, I.E.C., du Boulay, E.P.G.H., Callanan, M.M., Johnson, G., Logsdail S.J., Moseley, I.S., Rudge, P., Roberts, R.C., McDonald, W.I., Halliday A.M., Kendall, B.E., Macmanus, D.G., Ron, M.A., Zilka, K.J., 1984. NMR in multiple sclerosis and cerebral vascular disease. Lancet, II: pp. 1334-1335.

Poser, C.M., Paty, D.W., Scheinberg, L., McDonald, W.I., Davis, F.A., Ebers, G.C., Johnson, K.P., Sibley, W.A., Silberberg, D.H., Tourtellotte, W.W., 1983. New diagnostic criteria for multiple sclerosis: Guidelines for research protocols. Ann. Neurol., 13: pp. 227-231.

Prineas, J.W., 1970. Etiology of multiple sclerosis. In: Handbook of Clinical Neurology. North-Holland, Amsterdam, vol. 9, pp. 107-160.

Roström, B.: 1981. Specificity of Antibodies in Oligoclonal Bands in Patients with Multiple Sclerosis and Cerebrovascular Disease. Thesis. Linköping University.

Schumacher, G.A., Beebe, B., Kibler, R., Kurland, L.T., Kurtzke, J.F., McDowell, F., Nagler, B., Sibley, W.A., Tourtellotte, W.W., Willmann, T.L., 1965. Problems of experimental trials of therapy in multiple sclerosis: Report by the panel on the evaluation of experimental trials of therapy in multiple sclerosis. Ann. N.Y. Acad. Sci., 122: pp. 552-568.

Sedgwick, E.M., 1983. Pathophysiology and Evoked Potentials in Multiple Sclerosis. In: Hallpike, Adams, Tourtellotte: Multiple sclerosis. Pathology, diagnosis and management. Chapman and Hall, London, pp. 177-201.

Vandvik, B., Norrby, E., Steen-Johnsen, J., Stensvold, K., 1978. Mumps Meningitis: Prolonged Pleocytosis and Occurrence of Mumps Virus-specific Oligoclonal IgG in the Cerebrospinal Fluid. Eur. Neurol., 17: pp. 13-22.

Vinuela, F.V., Fox, A.J., Debrun, G.M., Feasby, T.E., Ebers, G.C., 1982. New perspectives in computed tomography of multiple sclerosis. AJR, 139: pp. 123-127.

13

Comparison of Multiple Sclerosis Incidence Clinical and ABR Data Indicates a Higher Degree of Dissemination of Lesions in a Progressive than in a Remitting Course

O. ANDERSEN, U. ROSENHALL and B. RUNMARKER

INTRODUCTION

Robinson and Rudge (1977, 1980) found that patients with definite MS often (24/32) have ABR (Auditory Brain Stem Response) pathology. The proportion was lower (9/20) in the MS probable group, and much lower in the patients without a brain stem lesion. However, 70-80% of MS patients with brain stem lesions had pathological ABR independent of their diagnostic probability. ABR seems to be somewhat more sensitive to demyelinating than to vascular lesions (Rudge 1983). Matthews et al. (1977) found a very low incidence of abnormal evoked potentials with a single episode of acute neurological (AN) disease resembling MS. Chiappa et al. (1980) reported on normal ABR in optic neuritis and in transverse myelitis. Rudge (1983) stated that MS patients without relapses have a remarkably stable ABR. However, high frequencies of evoked response abnormalities in suspected and possible MS (52%) were reported by Kjaer (1983). Such discrepancies are difficult to evaluate without detailed longtudinal clinical data. A relationship has been found between increased duration or severity of MS and increased incidence of ABR pathology (Kjaer 1980). We designed

the present study to study a further possible relationship,
between MS course parameters - bout and progress - and ABR
pathology.

MATERIAL

        All data in the present study were derived from a single
source, a 15 year incidence material of 312 MS cases, of whom
283 belong to the probable, definite or verified categories.
We have 21 - 35 years of personal follow-up of survivors, with
examination intervals of some years in latent or steadily progressive phases, generally with good compliance. The value of
the material is its potential for long-term prognosis. From
this incidence material 3 subgroups were selected: 1) Patients
in a progressive phase with progressing brain stem lesions,
e.g. internuclear ophtalmoplegia. 2) Patients in the progressive phase without any brain stem lesion. Progress is from onset or with only a focal myelopathy preceding the onset of
progress. 3) Patients with a remitting course now in latent or
stationary phase, with at least one previous brain stem bout.
For comparison, a fourth group of 7 non-incidence definite MS
cases were investigated with ABR within one month of onset of
an acute brain stem bout. Not all patients who were by 1980
eligible according to the above categories were finally
examinated by ABR. In group 1), 20 of 43, in group 2), 7 of 17,
and group 3), 12 of 43 were investigated. Losses were due to
some deaths, continued disease activity changing the category,
revised diagnosis, patients moving away or refusing ABR, and
in one case hearing loss unrelated to MS. No obvious systematic selection has occurred, and we believe the subgroups still
represent the very unbiased incidence material.

METHODS

        ABR audiometry was performed in a sound proof room. One
thousand and twenty-four clicks with alternating phase were
presented monaurally by TDH-39 earphones with a repetition rate
of 25 stimuli/s. The intensity level was 80 db HL (115 db peak
equivalent SPL). Surface self-adhesive silver/silver chloride
electrodes were placed on the forehead, on the ear lobes and

on the nose (ground electrode). The signals were band pass
filtered of 150 Hz, with a high cut-off frequency of 2500 Hz.
The signals were conveyed to a Nicolet 527 signal averager.
One averaged response consisted of 1024 individual sweeps.
Identical tests procedures were repeated many times to ensure
reproducability. The averaged responses of two identical
stimulus round were superimposed on a graph, using an X-Y
plotter. The latency of wave V was measured and the I-V interval was calculated. The results were compared with age and sex
matched control groups with normal hearing and no signs of any
vestibular or neurological disturbances. The mean values of
the wave V latencies and the I-V intervals +2SD of the control
group were considered as normal. The interaural time difference of wave V (II_5) between the right and left ears from the
same individual was also calculated. An II_5 of 0.4 ms or more
was evaluated as pathological.

RESULTS

The most striking finding was the normal ABR in 11 of the
12 group 3 cases with previous clinical brain stem lesions.
The results from comparison of the groups are shown in table
1. Diagnostic categories had no significant influence on the

Table 1

ABR	Number of patients		
	ABR normal	ABR pathological	P, Fishers exact test
Group 1	3	17	
Group 3	11	1	0.000059
Group 2	2	5	
Group 3	11	1	0.0191
Group 1+2	5	22	
Group 3	11	1	0.000052
MS probable	4	2	
MS definite	12	21	0.3438
Score below 92	14	5	
Score above 91	2	18	0.00012
Definite MS			
Group 1+2	5	20	
Group 3	7	1	0.0025

occurrence of ABR pathology in this study. The variation of
duration is limited by the incidence character of the material.
Evidently, the transition from bout to progressive phase does
significantly increase the risk for ABR pathology. However,
the severity of the disease is a confounding factor. The
theoretical maximum score of the non-parametric system used is
700, and the present material was bisected by the median 91.
Re-evaluation of the material, levelling out the confounding
factor, shows that neither high score nor progressive course
independently has a significant relationship to ABR pathology,
although the relationship is near-significant for progressive
course, table 2. Phase audiometry pathology has a relationship

Table 2

ABR

For score below 92	Number of patients		
	ABR normal	ABR pathological	P, Fishers exact test
Group 1+2	3	4	0.0759
Group 3	11	1	
For group 1+2			
Score below 92	3	4	0.2028
Score above 91	2	17	

to progressive course similar to but somewhat weaker than that
of ABR, table 3. Of the 7 cases investigated during bout
activity, with a median score of 26, 6 patients had a pathological ABR.

Table 3

Phase audiometry

	Number of patients		
	PhA normal	PhA pathological	P, Fishers exact test
Group 1+2	8	12	0.0091
Group 3	11	1	

CONCLUSIONS

It is believed that an acute development of ABR pathology may reflect lesions of the auditory pathways, or influence from neighbouring brain stem lesions (Kjaer 1980). In this study, the ABR was used as a probe to detect dissemination of MS lesions in bout and progressive phases. The results indicate that a progressive course is more related to ABR pathology than a previous bout, even a brain stem bout. The normal ABR, probably indicating a low density of MS lesions, in benign intermittent cases seem to correspond to the low bout frequency in such cases. The notion is supported that lesions in this major type of MS are focal and limited in number, while the lesions in a progressive course are multifocal. The study needs confirmation by morphological methods.

REFERENCES

Chiappa, K.H., Harrison, J.L., Brooks, E.B., Young, R.R. 1980. Brainstem Auditory Evoked Responses in 200 Patients with Multiple Sclerosis. Ann. Neurol. 7:135-143.

Kjaer, M., 1980. Variations of brain stem auditory potentials correlated to duration and severity of multiple sclerosis. Acta Neurol. Scand. 61:157-166.

Kjaer, M., 1983. Evoked potentials. With special reference to the diagnostic value in multiple sclerosis. Acta Neurol. Scand. 67:67-89.

Matthews, W.B., Small, D.G., Small, M., Pountnay, E., 1977. Pattern reversal evoked visual potential in the diagnosis of multiple sclerosis. J. Neurol. Neurosurg. Psychiat. 40:1009-1014.

Robinson, K., Rudge, P., 1977. Abnormalities of the auditory evoked potentials in patients with multiple sclerosis. Brain, 100:19-40.

Robinson, K., Rudge, P., 1980. The use of the auditory evoked potential in the diagnosis of multiple sclerosis. J. Neurol. Sci. 45:235-244.

Rudge, P., 1983. Clinical Neuro-otology, Churchill Livingstone, Edinburgh, p. 202.

Section II
Immunology

14

Multiple Sclerosis and Immunity: Facts, Fiction and Future Development

J. MERTIN

The current view of most workers in the field of multiple
sclerosis (MS) research is that the disease is a) autoimmune
in nature and b) causally related to a defect in immunoregulation. The latter belief has, in many laboratories, stimulated
a search for abnormalities in various arms of the immune response. Their quest has been successful, and a plethora of abnormalities in immune function in MS have been reported in the
literature. The question that must now be asked is which of
the defects detected are genuine manifestations of the disease
and which are byproducts of technical manipulation.

The field of MS research is very fertile, and has produced a host of reviews listing all the observed deviations in
immunoregulation. Indeed, many of us here have written such
reviews, all of us read them. They inevitably conclude that
whilst many details are known, there is still no unifying explanation for the role of the immune system in the aetiology
and pathogenesis of MS. On an occassion such as this, therefore, there is no need for yet another such review. As an
alternative let me instead briefly summarise the most important facts of about MS and immunity, with a few comments on
what I consider to be fiction. I will, thereafter, propose
some new approaches to the problem.

The facts about the putative autoimmune nature of MS are
listed on table 1.

Table 1: Multiple Sclerosis and the Immune Response

Facts   1) local immunoglobulin production
             in the central nervous system (CNS)

         2) oligoclonal bands in the cerebro-
             spinal fluid - pattern maintained
             throughout the course of the
             disease

         3) mononuclear cell infiltrates in
             the CNS

         4) disease susceptibility is influenced
             by genetic factors

         5) characteristics 1-4 are shared with an
             experimental autoimmune disease,
             chronic relapsing experimental allergic
             encephalomyelitis (CREAE)

         6) there is poor correlation in MS and
             CREAE between clinical signs of disease
             and the actual pathological activity
             within the CNS

What about the fiction? It is my belief that the fiction
in this field arises out of the idea that MS is a truly relapsing and remitting disease - at least in the majority of
cases. Indeed, in the past the finding by the pathologist of
"silent" lesions was considered to be exceptional, and clinical exacerbations followed by complete or partial remission
to be a true reflection of the activity of the disease process. Modern diagnostic methods such as evoked potentials,
computerised tomography, and nuclear magnetic resonance (NMR)
tomography have, however, confirmed Tourtelotte's proposition
that "MS never sleeps". Rather, the disease appears to be
chronicly progressive, being characterised by constantly emer-
ging and disappearing lesions which are often not clinically
manifest. It follows, therefore, that any premise which
attemps to link alterations in immunological parameters with
clinical changes such as relapses, is likely to be ficticious.
There are many examples of such observed changes shortly before or during relapses, including alterations in numbers

and/or activity of so-called suppressor T cells, of _in vitro_
lymphocyte responses to mitogens or antigens, of natural
killer cell activity and numbers, and in the concentrations of
components of the complement system. These observations are
frequently used to support the notion that MS is the result of
defective immunoregulation. Such a proposition is premature,
however, for whilst many details are known about the regulation of the normal immune response - regulation both "from
within" and "from without" - there is still no unifying concept of how the immune system functions. It would thus appear
rather speculative to assume a defect in the regulation of a
system as yet incompletely understood. In the future improved
diagnostic methods, and a better understanding of the regulation of the immune system, may provide us with an insight into
the immunopathology of MS. Greater knowledge of the immunological capacities of the central nervous system (CNS) itself
may, further, allow identification of those immunological
parameters which truly correlate with disease activity of MS.
Here I arrive at the point where I hope that MS research will
in future do better than it has to date.

When immunologists deal with autoaggressive conditions
they usually focus upon the immune system as the aggressor and
regard the target organ as an innocent victim, analogous, for
example, to target cells in an _in vitro_ cytotoxic assay.

This 'blinkered' view has meant that in the search for a
cause of MS attention has centred upon the immune response and
its postulated dysregulation. Such an approach has proved far
from successful, possibly because the target organ has not
been allowed its full share of responsibility. Perhaps one
should assign a more active role for the CNS in the pathogenic
process, for is it not possible that disturbances such as mentioned in table 2 may be instrumental in provoking a normal
immune system to attack a defective CNS, thereby causing inflammation, demyelination and/or failure to remyelinate?

Table 2:   The Target in MS

Observation:	Decrease in the concentrations of polyunsaturated fatty acids (PUFA) within the CNS (e.g. Thompson, 1975)
Consequence:	Decreased resistance of the CNS? (in experimental allergic encephalo-myelitis susceptibility to and clinical severity of the disease are increased following decrease of PUFA within the CNS when a) PUFA-deficient diet (Clausen and Moller, 1967), or b) treatment with phenylalanine (Mertin and Hunt, 1976) is given)
Observation:	Alteration of lipid-phase behaviour in the myelin of MS patients, with inability of MS myelin protein to organise/order the myelin bilayer (Chia et al., 1984)
Consequence:	Decreased resistance of the CNS?

The last point I wish to make may appear yet more speculative. There is increasing evidence that the CNS represents
the highest level of command for the overall regulation of
immune responses (table 3). One may suggest, therefore, that

Table 3:   Regulation of the Immune System by the CNS

Brain stem	- influence on humoral immune responses (Jankovic and Isakovic, 1973)
Cortex	- influence on cell-mediated immune responses (Renoux et al., 1984)
?	- intra-thecal route of antigen inoculation is most powerful in eliciting immune responses (Quirico Santos and Valdimarsson, 1982)

the real cause of MS is founded in a defect in the brain's own
regulatory controls of immune function. A disturbance in such
control circuits could lead to a lowering of defenses of the
CNS thereby provoking a normal immune system to attack.

Only by adopting a multidisciplinary approach, such as that we hope to initiate at this meeting, can we clarify the problems of MS and immunity upon which I have touched. As to the role neuroimmunology in this concerted action, I feel it would benefit us all greatly if neuroimmunologists laid more stress upon the "neuro" and ceased to be solely immuno-neurologists.

References

Chia, L.S., Thompson, J.E. and Moscarello, M.A., 1984, Alteration of lipid-phase behaviour in multiple sclerosis myelin revealed by wide-angle x-ray diffraction. Proc. Natl. Acad. Sci. (USA), 81: 1871-1874.

Clausen, J. and Moller, J., 1967, Allergic encephalomyelitis induced by brain antigen after deficiency in polyunsaturated fatty acids during myelination. Is multiple sclerosis a nutritive disorder? Acta Neurol. Scand., 43: 375-388.

Jankovic, B.D. and Isakovic, K., 1973, Neuro-endocrine correlates of immune response. I. Effects of brain lesions on antibody production, Arthus reactivity and delayed hypersensitivity in the rat. Int. Archs. Allergy appl. Immunol., 45: 360-372.

Mertin, J. and Hunt, R., 1976, Hyperphenylalaninaemia and experimental allergic encephalomyelitis. J. Neurol. Sci., 29: 351-357.

Quirico Santos, T. and Valdimarsson, H., 1982, T-dependent antigens are more immunogenic in the subarachnoid space than in other sites. J. Neuroimmunol., 2: 215-222.

Renoux, G., Biziere, K., Renoux, M. and Guillaumin, J.M., 1983, The production of T-cell-inducing factors in mice is by the brain neocortex. Scand. J. Immunol., 17: 45-50.

Thompson, R.H.S., 1975, Unsaturated fatty acids in multiple sclerosis. In: A.N. Davison, J.H. Humphrey, A.L. Liversedge, McDonald, W.I. and Porterfield, J.S. (Editors), Multiple Sclerosis Research, HMSO London, pp. 184-197.

15

The Spectrum of Experimental Allergic Encephalomyelitis

H. LASSMANN and K. VASS

Experimental allergic encephalomyelitis (EAE) is an autoimmune disease of the central nervous system (CNS), induced by active sensitization of susceptible animals with CNS tissue. The basic lesion in the brain of EAE animals is the perivenous inflammatory reaction, which appears to be essentially mediated by a cellular immune reaction directed against myelin basic protein (MBP), a component of myelin sheaths (Ben Nun et al., 1981). The clinical and pathohistological expression of the disease, however, can to a large extent be modified by other, including humoral immune reactions (Paterson, 1982; Schwerer et al., 1984). This modification seems to be partially responsible for the extensive diversity between different EAE models (Lassmann, 1983).

EAE not only mimicks multiple sclerosis (MS) but also all other inflammatory demyelinating diseases. In fact, all acute most passive transfer and some chronic EAE models rather reflect the lesions of acute perivenous or hemorrhagic leucoencephalomyelitis than MS itself. Even within chronic EAE models, which overall reflect MS pathology more closely than the acute ones, a large variety of structural changes in the lesions is noted. Chronic EAE lesions in Hartley or Strain 13 guinea pigs are very similar to MS plaques, regarding the extent and patterns of demyelination, gliosis and reparative phenomena or their topographical distribution

(Lassmann, 1983; Raine, 1984). However, even in this model the clinical course, the number and size of demyelinating lesions and the structural appearence of plaques is variable from animal to animal. Chronic EAE in SJL-mice (Lublin et al., 1981; Brown and McFarlin, 1981) is a predominately inflammatory disease with very little selective demyelination, even in animals with prolonged clinical disease course. Larger CNS lesions sometimes present in these animals, are generally accompanied by extensive destruction of other CNS elements and Wallerian degeneration. Chronic EAE in rats may lead to extensive demyelinated plaques, the morphology of the lesions, however, in many respect differs from that in guinea pigs and from MS patients (Lassmann, 1983).

Immunization with purified myelin proteins (MBP or proteolipid protein) instead of native CNS tissue resulted in acute or chronic inflammatory diseases of the CNS, without the formation of confluent, selectively demyelinated plaques (Rev: Lassmann, 1983; Cambi et al., 1983). With the addition of myelin lipids to MBP in the sensitization medium the extent of demyelination was augmented, although the numbers and size of demyelinated plaques invariably was smaller compared to those found after sensitization with native CNS tissue (Madrid et al., 1981; Raine et al., 1981).

All these above described models are useful to study certain aspects of the pathogenesis of inflammatory demyelinating diseases. However, the variability of acute and chronic EAE implies to carefully select from the wide range of models available the best suited for the answer of a specific question.

As mentioned above, the basic EAE lesion, the perivenous inflammatory infiltrate apparently is mediated by a cellular immune response. On a tissue level this can be best studied in passive transfer experiments, using monospecific MBP reactive T-cell lines (Wekerle, 1984). In this situation first inflammatory infiltrates in the CNS are predominately composed of T-cells, carrying the T-helper/inducer phenotype. A principially similar pattern of inflammatory reaction is also noted in rats and mice, actively sensitized for EAE (Hickey et al., 1983; Sriram et al., 1982). During recovery from the disease the majority of T-cells in the lesions express the T-suppressor/cytotoxic phenotype. In addition a large number of Ia-positive cells with structural features of monocytes and macrophages are present in active lesions, which according to immuneelectronmicroscopic studies appear to be the main effector cells in the demyelinating process. B-lymphocytes and plasma cells are generally numerous in the lesions of chronic EAE, regardless the animal species investigated.

There are at present not enough data available to evaluate, to what extent these fluctuations in the composition of inflammatory infiltrates allow conclusions regarding regulation of disease activity or structural expression of the lesions. Similar comparative studies in multiple different EAE models are required to determine possible general patterns of the inflammatory reaction in EAE and MS.

The second hallmark of inflammatory demyelination is the selective primary demyelination. Primary demyelination, like that found in MS does not just mean loss of myelin, but implies the selective destruction of myelin sheaths with preservation of axons, neurones and astrocytes. Thus the unselective tissue destruction, found in the lesions of some models of acute and chronic EAE (e.g. chronic EAE in monkeys and SJL-mice) cannot be regarded as suitable for the study of primary selective demyelination.

Recent evidence from chronic EAE in guinea pigs, the model which at present is accompanied by the most widespread and selective demyelination, suggests that antibodies against other antigens than MBP are additionally required for the demyelinating process. In this model extensive plaque like demyelination only appears in the chronic stage of the disease at a time point when high titres of antibodies against myelin are present in the sera of affected animals. Furthermore we found a significant correlation between anti myelin antibodies in the sera with the extent of demyelination in the central nervous system (Lassmann et al., 1984). Studies on the demyelinating activity of EAE sera in vitro and in vivo further support the view, that humoral immune response can be involved in the demyelinating process.

It is evident, that the target antigen for selective demyelination must be located on the surface of myelin sheaths and so be accessible for the immune system. Thus it is not surprising that antibodies against MBP failed to induce demyelination in vitro. Several studies suggest, that galacto cerebroside is one of the antigens, recognized in the demyelinating process (Dubois-Dalq et al., 1970; Saida et al., 1979). It is, however, interesting to note that in chronic EAE in guinea pigs a significant

number of animals do not show detectable antibodies against galactocerebroside, in spite of extensive active demyelination in the CNS and high
titrest of in <u>vivo</u> demyelinating activity of their sera (Schwerer <u>et al</u>.,
1984). Thus there appear to be multiple target antigens in the demyelinating process.

In conclusion the wide spectrum of changes found in different EAE
models covers not only the pathological alterations of MS, but also those
of other related hyman inflammatory demyelinating diseases. EAE thus
offers the change to study principle mechanisms related to the pathogenesis of inflammatory demyelination in the human brain. The variability of
EAE models and the complexity of the disease process, however, makes it
necessary to carefully select the right model for the specific question
asked. Furthermore it appears to be dangerous to draw generalized conclusions on the pathogenesis of inflammatory demyelination from observations
obtained in a single EAE model.

REFERENCES

Ben Nun, A., Wekerle, H. and Cohen, I.R., 1981. The rapid isolation of
    clonable antigen specific T lymphocyte lines capable of mediating auto-
    immune encephalomyelitis. Eur. J. Immunol., 11: 195.
Brown, A.M. and McFarlin, D.E., 1981. Relapsing experimental allergic
    encephalomyelitis in SJL mouse. Lab. Invest., 45: 278.
Cambi, F., Lees, M.B., Williams, R.M. and Macklin, W.B., 1983. Chronic
    EAE produced by bovine proteolipid apoprotein. Ann. Neurol., 13: 303.
Dubois-Dalq, M., Niediek, B. and Buyse, M., 1970. Action of anticerebro-
    side sera on myelinated nerves tissue culture. Path. Europ., 5: 331.
Hickey, W.F., Gonatas, N.K., Kimura, H and Wilson, D.B., 1983. Identifi-
    cation and quantitation of T lymphocyte subsets in the spinal cord of
    the Lewis rat during acute experimental allergic encephalomyelitis.
    J. Immunol., 131: 2805.
Lassmann, H., 1983. Comparative neuropathology of chronic experimental
    allergic encephalomyelitis and multiple sclerosis. Neurology Series
    vol. 25, Springer, Berlin, Heidelberg, New York, Tokyo.
Lassmann, H., Suchanek, G., Kitz, K., Stemberger, H., Schwerer, B. and
    Bernheimer, H., 1984. Antibodies in the pathogenesis of demyelination
    in chronic relapsing EAE (cr-EAE). In: E.C. Alvord, M.W. Kies, A.J.
    Suckling (Editors), Experimental allergic encephalomyelitis. Alan Liss
    Inc. New York, pp 165.
Lublin, F., Maurer, P.H., Berry, R.H. and Tippett, D., 1981. Delayed re-
    lapsing experimental allergic encephalomyelitis in mice. J. Immunol.,
    126: 819.
Madrid, R.E., Wisniewski, H.M., Igbal, K., Pullarkat, R.K. and Lassmann,
    H., 1981. Relapsing experimental allergic encephalomyelitis induced
    with isolated myelin and with myelin basic protein plus myelin lipids.
    J. Neurol. Sci., 50: 399.
Paterson, P.Y., 1982. Current perspective of neuroimmunologic disease:
    Multiple sclerosis and experimental allergic encephalomyelitis. Clin.

Immunol. Rev., 1: 581.

Raine, C.S., 1984. Biology of disease. Analysis of autoimmune demyelination: Its impact upon multiple sclerosis. Lab. Invest., 50: 608.

Raine, C.S., Tarugott, U., Farooq, M., Bornstein, M.B. and Norton, W.T., 1981. Augmentation of immune mediated demyelination by lipid haptens. Lab. Invest., 45: 174.

Saida, K., Saida, T., Brown, M.J. and Silberberg, D.H., 1979. In vivo demyelination induced by intraneural injection of anti galactocerebroside serum. Am. J. Path., 95: 99.

Schwerer, B., B., Kitz, K., Lassmann, H. and Bernheimer, H., 1984. Serum antibodies against glycosphingolipids in chronic relapsing experimental allergic encephalomyelitis. J. Neuroimmunol., 7: 107.

Sriram, S., Solomon, D., Rouse, R.V. and Steinman, L., 1982. Identification of T cell subsets and B lymphocytes in mouse brain experimental allergic encephalomyelitis lesions. J. Immunol., 129: 1649.

Wekerle, H., 1984. The lesion of acute experimental autoimmune encephalomyelitis. Lab. Invest., 51: 199.

16

T-cell Subsets in Multiple Sclerosis

M. A. BACH and E. TOURNIER-LASSERVE

INTRODUCTION

The attention has been recently focused on the possible involvement of T-cells in the pathophysiology of MS, since T-cells play a major role in regulating immune responses and maintaining self-tolerance, and also act as effector cells of immune damage in experimental models of demyelinating disease and in viral infections. The development of monoclonal antibodies directed against human T-cells has allowed to delineate two major T-cell subsets: one bearing the T4 marker, recognizing antigens associated with MHC class II molecules and expressing in most assays helper/inducer functions; the other bearing the T8 marker, recognizing antigens in the context of class I MHC molecules and preferentially exhibiting cytotoxic and suppressive activities (Reinherz et al., 1983). We have used these monoclonal antibodies to study T-cell subsets in MS, in parallel to in vitro T-cell dependent functions.

MATERIAL AND METHODS

Patients: Patients were followed at the Neurological Clinic of the Henri Mondor Hospital (Créteil, France) by Dr. J.D. Degos and Dr. C. Martin and J.-F. Eizenbaum, and were classified as definite MS according to Schumacher's criteria. None of them received corticoid or immunosuppressive therapy at the time of study. Healthy subjects or patients suffering other neurological diseases (OND) served as controls.

Lymphocyte isolation: Peripheral blood mononuclear cells (PBMC) were isolated from heparinized venous blood over a Ficoll-Hypaque gradient. Cerebrospinal fluid (CSF) samples were collected by lumbar puncture and immediately added with 10% foetal calf serum (FCS).

T-cell subset phenotyping: Monoclonal antibodies OKT3 (pan-T), OKT4 and OKT8 (Ortho Pharmaceuticals, Raritan, N.J., USA) were used as described elsewhere (Bach et al., 1980) in an indirect immunofluorescence assay to enumerate the corresponding T-cell subpopulations in blood and CSF.

PWM-Ig synthesis: IgG, IgM and IgA content of culture supernatants were measured as already described (Tjernlund et al., 1984) by immunoprecipitation with corresponding anti human Ig class specific antibodies using an automatic laser nephelometer (Hyland, Lessien, Belgium) after a 7 day culture in RPMI medium in the presence or absence of 0.1 µg/ml PWM (Gibco).

Con-A-induced suppression of MLR: The assay extensively described elsewhere (Tjernlund et al., 1984) consisted in stimulating PBMC with Con A (7.5 µg/ml) for 2 days and then adding after mitomycin C treatment Con A-stimulated and control unstimulated PBMC to mixed leucocyte cultures, where responder cells were autologous PBMC and stimulating cells were mitomycin C-treated allogeneic PBMC. ^{3}H-thymidine incorporation was measured on day 5. The suppression index was calculated as follows:

$$SI = 1 - \frac{\text{cpm in MLR plus Con A-stimulated cells}}{\text{cpm in MLR plus control cells}} \times 100$$

Xenogeneic cell-mediated lympholysis (CML) assay: The xenogeneic CML assay described by Carnaud et al. (1977) was used. In brief, 20 x 10^6 PMBC were suspended in 20 ml RPMI culture medium supplemented with 10% AB serum, together with 20 x 10^6 mitomycin C-treated DBA/2 mouse spleen cells. After 7 days of culture, the cells recovered were used as effector cells in a microcytotoxicity assay using DBA/2 P815 mastocytoma cells previously labelled with 51 Cr O$_4$Na$_2$ as target cells, at effector to target cell ratios grading from 10/1 to 200/1. The results were expressed as lytic units (LU 50) per culture as described by Cerottini et al., (1974).

RESULTS

Monoclonal-antibody defined T-cell subsets in blood: The results of our studies are summarized in Table 1 (Bach et al., 1980; Bach et al., 1984). Patients in remission showed normal T-cell subset number and distribution. Patients suffering from progressive MS exhibited significantly higher T4/T8 ratios than normal controls. Patients suffering from exacerbations presented with variable T-cell subset patterns, according to the time elapsed after the onset of acute attack: the highest values of T4/T8 ratios were recorded from 2 weeks before to one week after onset. During the second and third week, although some patients still showed abnormal T-cell subset distribution (T4/T8 ratio > 3.2) the mean difference between patients and controls did not reach statistical significance. Surprisingly, significantly high T4/T8 ratios were seen again in patients investigated later (from 3 weeks to 2 months after relapse).

In chronic progressive MS, as well as in exacerbating-remitting cases, elevated T4/T8 ratio resulted primarily from a decrease of T8+ cells percentage, associated to a minor increase (Which did not reach statistical significance) of T4+ cells.

Monoclonal antibody defined T-cell subsets in CSF (Table 1): As compared with patients suffering from other neurological diseases, MS patients showed a T-cell subset imbalance within CSF similar to that observed in blood with elevated T4/T8 ratios at the beginning of acute phase; conversely values recorded during the third week were found similar to that of OND controls (Cashman et al., 1982).

In vitro assays for T-cell functions: The amount of in vitro synthesized IgG (Table 2) after PWM stimulation, a helper T-cell dependent phenomenon, was found higher in rapidly progressive MS (with a Kurtzke index having increased of more than 1 within the 2 years preceding the study) than in slowly progressive cases or during remission. Similar data were obtained for IgM and IgA synthesis. No increase of spontaneous Ig synthesis was found for any Ig class in any group of patients.

Con-induced suppression of MLR (Table 3) was found significantly depressed among patients showing progressive MS, regardless of the recent evolution of the clinical status.

Table 1 : T-CELL SUBSETS IN BLOOD AND CSF

SUBJECTS	BLOOD			CSF	
	T4/T8 RATIO	% OVER NORMAL LEVEL		T4+T8 RATIO	% OVER NORMAL LEVEL (a)
MS PATIENTS					
Remission	1.7 ± 0.1^b (22)^c	5 % (1/22)		3.2 ± 0.4 (9)	11 % (1/9)
0-14 days before relapse	$\underline{3.5 \pm 0.6^d}$ (7)	43 % (3/7)	14 days before to 14 days after relapse	$\underline{4.8 \pm 1.3}$ (11)	64 % (7/11)
0-6 days	$\underline{3.3 \pm 0.4}$ (13)	62 % (8/13)			
7-13 days (after relapse)	2.2 ± 0.4 (3)	13 % (1/8)			
14-20 days	1.9 ± 0.3 (8)	13 % (1/8)	14-20 days	2.4 ± 0.5 (8)	13 % (1/8)
21-60 days	3.0 ± 0.4 (14)	43 % (6/14)	< 20 days	3.6 ± 0.4 (11)	10 % (1/11)
Chronic progression	$\underline{2.8 \pm 0.5}$ (29)	41 % (12/29)		-	-
HEALTHY CONTROLS	1.8 ± 0.1 (61)	5 % (3/61)		-	-
OND	2.0 ± 0.2 (15)	0 % (0/15)		2.6 ± 0.3 (15)	7 % (1/15)

a) values exceeding the 5 % confidence upper limit of healthy controls (for blood : 3.2, for CSF : 4.6)
b) Mean ± SEM   c) Number of subjects
d) Values significantly different from controls are underlined.

The generation of xenogeneic CML in mixed xenogeneic cultures was not found altered in MS patients suffering active disease (Table 4). A single stable patient was studied, who exhibited a normal CML value. A majority of patients tested for in vitro T-cell functions were also studied at the same time for T-cell subset markers. No individual correlation was noticed between the T4/T8 ratios and the data obtained from functional assays.

Table 2 : SPONTANEOUS AND PWM-DRIVEN IgG SYNTHESIS

	T4/T8 RATIO	SPONTANEOUS	PWM-DRIVEN
		Ig secretion (ng/ml)	
- Normal subjects (29)	1.8 ± 0.1^a	679 ± 76	1.666 ± 134
- M S			
Rapid progression (12)	$\underline{2.8 \pm 0.5}^b$	893 ± 129	$\underline{4.418 \pm 800}$
Slow progression (7)	$\underline{3.0 \pm 0.6}$	478 ± 59	1.981 ± 523
Remission (10)	2.0 ± 0.3	799 ± 125	1.891 ± 320

a) Mean $\pm$ SEM
b) Values significantly different from controls are underlined.

Table 3 : CON A-INDUCED SUPPRESSION OF MLR

	T4/T8 RATIO	% SUPPRESSION
Healthy controls (43)	1.8^a ± 0.1	61 ± 2
MS patients :		
Progressive form (16)	2.7^b $\pm \underline{0.4}$	49 $\pm \underline{6}$
Remission (8)	1.9 ± 0.2	68 ± 5

a) Mean $\pm$ SEM

b) Values signficantly different from controls are underlined

Table 4 : XENOGENEIC T-CELL MEDIATED CYTOTOXICITY

	T4/T8 RATIO	Anti mouse xenogeneic cytotoxocity (I U 50/culture)
Normal subjects	1.8 ± 0.1^{a} (61)	21 ± 6 (8)
MS patients		
Remission	1.0	25
Active disease	1.3	23
	2.0	25
	2.3	0
	$\underline{3.3}^{b}$	41
	$\underline{3.8}$	25

a) Mean $\pm$ SEM. Number of subjects is indicated in parenthesis.

b) Values exceeding the 5 % confidence upper limit of normal values are underlined.

DISCUSSION

A significant change of T4/T8 ratios in blood and CSF was found in active MS, due to decreased T8+ cell percentage. Although similar data were reported by others (Reinherz et al., 1980; Sanberg-Wollheim, 1983), some groups fail to evidence such an abnormality in exacerbating-remitting cases (Rice et al., 1984). The present work suggests that conflicting data might de explained by the peculiar kinetics of the T-cell subset disorder, which is transient, occurs early during the attack and may even precede it.

The reasons for such a rapid fluctuations of the T-cell subset balance are unclear. The selective migration of T8+ cells to CNS or lymphoid organs would be a likely hypothesis, but conflicting data have been reported about the composition of the cellular infiltrates of CNS in MS patients (Brinkman et al., 1982; Nyland et al., 1982). Another tentative hypothesis, the modulation of the T8 molecule by antilymphocyte auto-antibodies, has not yet been confirmed (Oger et al., 1982). We also observed abnormal regulatory T-cell functions in active MS patients with an increase of PWM-driven Ig synthesis and a decrease of

Con A triggered suppression of MLR, suggesting a failure of suppressor
T-cell function, in agreement with other authors (Goust et al., 1982).
Unexpectedly the deficit of suppressor T-cell function does not seem to
be directly related to the decreased number of T8+ cells. It must be
noted in that respect that regulatory T-cell function does not involve
the latter subset alone, but rather the cooperation between a subset of
T4+ suppressor-inducer cells and the T8+ suppressor effector cells.
Interestingly, the cytotoxic T-cell function, as explored by the generation of xenogeneic cytotoxic T-cells is not altered by the T-cell
balance disturbance.

Finally although active MS seem to be associated with marked abnormalities of regulatory T-cell subset distribution and functions, the
exact role of these disorders in the triggering mechanisms of relapses
remains unknown.

REFERENCES

Bach, M.A., Phan Dinh Tuy, F., Tournier, E., Chatenoud, L., Bach, J.F.,
    Martin, C. and Degos, J.D., 1980. Deficit of suppressor T-cells in
    active multiple sclerosis. Lancet, 2: 1221.
Bach, M.A., Martin, C., Cesaro, P., Eizenbaum, J.F. and Degos, J.D.
    T-cell subsets in multiple sclerosis: a longitudinal study of exa-
    cerbating remitting cases. J. Neuroimmunol. In press.
Brinkman, C.J.J., ter Laak, H.J., Hommes, O.R., Poppema, S. and Delmotte,
    P., 1982. T lymphocyte subpopulations in multiple sclerosis lesions.
    N. Eng. J. Med., 307: 1644.
Carnaud, C., Fadaï-Gotbi, M., Lesavre, P. and Bach, J.F., 1977. Educa-
    tion of human lymphocytes against mouse cells: specific recognition
    of H2 antigens. Eur. J. Immunol., 7: 81.
Cashman, N., Martin, C., Eizenbaum, J.F., Degos, J.D. and Bach, M.A.,
    1982. Monoclonal antibody defined immunoregulatory cells in multiple
    sclerosis cerebrospinal fluid. J. Clin. Invest., 70: 387.
Cerrotini, J.C., Euger, M.D., MacDonald H.R. and Brunner, K.T., 1974.
    Generation of cytotoxic T lymphocytes in vitro. I Response of normal
    and immune mouse spleen cells in mixed leucocyte cultures. J. Exp.
    Med., 140: 703.
Goust, J.M., Hogan, E.L. and Arnaud, P.A., 1982. Abnormal regulation of
    IgG production in multiple sclerosis. Neurology, 32: 228.
Nyland, H., Matre, R., Mork, S., Bjerke, J.R. and Noess, A., 1982. T
    lymphocyte subpopulations in multiple sclerosis lesions. N. Eng. J.
    Med., 307: 1643.
Oger, J., Jackevicius, S., Antel, J. Rosenkoetter, P. and Arnason, B.,
    1982. Multiple sclerosis: regeneration of T suppressor cell markers
    in culture. Ann. Neurol., 12: 81.
Reinherz, E.L., Weiner, H.L., Hauser, S.L., Cohen, J.A., Distaso, J.A.
    and Schlossman, S.F., 1980. Loss of suppressor T-cells in active
    multiple sclerosis. Analysis with monoclonal antibodies. N. Engl. J.
    Med., 303: 125.

Reinherz, E.L., Meuer, S.C. and Schlossman, S.F., 1983: The human T-cells receptor: analysis with cytotoxic T-cell clones. Immurol. Rev., 74: 83.

Rice, G.P.A., Finney, D.F., Brahemy, S.L., Knobler, R.L., Sipe, J.C. and Oldstone, M.B.A., 1984. Disease activity markers in multiple sclerosis. Another look at suppressor cells defined by monoclonal antibodies OKT4, OKT5 and OKT8. J. Neuroimmunology, 6: 75.

Sandberg-Wollheim, M., 1983. Lymphocyte populations in the cerebrospinal fluid and peripheral blood of patients with multiple sclerosis and optic neuritis. Scand. J. Immunol., 17: 575.

Tjernlund, U., Cesaro, P., Tournier, E., Degos, J.D., Bach, J.F. and Bach, M.A., 1984. T-cell subsets in multiple sclerosis: a comparative study between cell surface antigens and functions. Clin. Immunol. Immunopathol., 32: 185.

17

Functional Differences between Cerebrospinal Fluid and Peripheral Blood T-cells in Multiple Sclerosis

M. S. WOLLHEIM and E. C. DEFREITAS

INTRODUCTION

Available evidence implies an altered immune response in multiple sclerosis (MS) and suggests that immune reactions in the central nervous system take place in partial isolation from the rest of the immune system. This is suggested by the phenotypic examinations of B and T cell populations as well as by functional studies of these cells.

There is a significantly lower proportion of B cells in the cerebro-spinal fluid (CSF) than in the peripheral blood (PB) of patients with MS, irrespective of disease activity (Sandberg Wollheim, 1983). However, the number of cells with cytoplasmic immunoglobulin (Ig) is significantly higher in CSF than in PB in MS patients, and in CSF these cells are pre-dominantly of IgG-type and frequently show an altered k/l ratio (Sandberg Wollheim & Turesson, 1975). The local humoral immune reactivity is also evidenced by the demonstration of the spontaneous synthesis in vitro of IgG with restricted heterogeneity (Sandberg Wollheim, 1974) as well as specific antibody (to be publ.). Studies of sequential paired samples of MS CSF and serum revealed not only the presence of various antibodies in CSF at onset of disease, but also the appearance or disappearance of one or more antibody bands with no relation to clinical course (to be publ.).

It has also been shown that total CSF T cells are increased compared to PB T cells in MS patients (Cashman &al, 1982; Sandberg Wollheim, 1983). In disease activity, T suppressor cells decreased without significant changes in the T helper cell subpopulation.

Because of the central role of T helper cells in the immune response we wished to investigate its function in MS and to compare the CSF and PB T lymphocytes with respect to their ability to respond to antigen by proliferation and to deliver helper signals to autologous B cells.

PATIENT MATERIAL

CSF and PB were obtained from patients with definite MS as well as from a normal volunteer. One of the MS patients and the normal donor were booster immunized with tetanus toxoid prior to the experiment.

RESULTS

Proliferative response.   We have produced antigen-activated T cell lines from CSF and PB of several MS patients and from a normal donor. Freshly isolated CSF and PB lymphocytes were stimulated with several antigens as described in Fig 1. The growth curves of one MS patient are shown. The MS CSF T cells proliferated more rapidly than the PB T cells both in response to antigen and during subsequent growth in Interleukin 2 (Il 2). When equal numbers of CSF and PB T cells were restimulated with antigen, the CSF cells again grew faster. CSF T cells survived longer than PB T cells without Il 2 (data not shown). PB T cells were 90% non-viable after 3 days in Il 2-free medium compared to 7 days for CSF T cells, as demonstrated both with trypan blue and ^{3}H-TdR incorporation.

Identical experiments were carried out with CSF and PB cells from a normal donor. At first normal CSF T cells proliferated faster than PB T cells upon antigen stimulation and after addition of Il 2. But by day 16, the growth rate was the same for both cell populations, also after re-stimulation with antigen. The normal CSF and PB T cells showed no difference in Il 2 dependency, both cell populations dying by day 3 in Il 2-free medium.

CSF and PB T cell lines from one of the MS patients were tested for antigen-specific proliferation after 2 months in culture, when 98% of the cells phenotypically were T helper cells (Leu 1+3+2-). T cells from the lines were added to wells with various concentrations of tetanus antigen (TET). The response of the CSF T cell line was greater than that of the

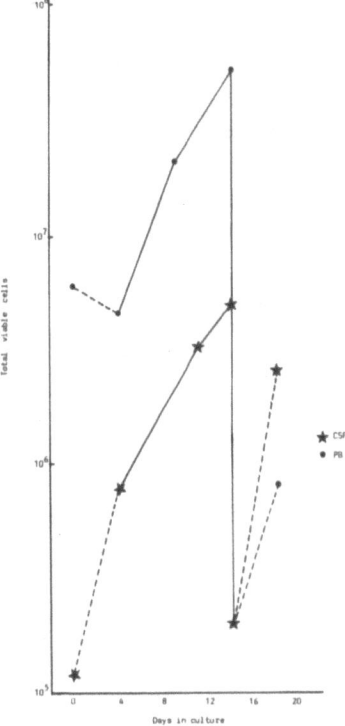

FIGURE 1.   Growth curve of TET-activated T cells derived from CSF (★)
or PB (●) of an MS patient. Cells were alternately stimulated with TET
(10 ug/ml) (-----) and expanded in Il 2 (———) as indicated.

METHOD. CSF cells were washed, resuspended in RPMI-1640 supplemented with
glutamin and 10% human AB serum, and seeded in 24-well cluster plates. As
accessory cells were added 4 x 10^6 gamma-irradiated autologous PB cells.
Non-irradiated PB lymphocytes were resuspended at 4 x10^6/ml and seeded in
parallel wells. As antigens were added: TET (tetanus toxoid; Connaught
Labs; 10 ug/ml), PPD (purified protein derivative; Connaught Labs), or
Reovirus-WW strain (Dr W. Gerhard, Wistar Inst; 10 infectious units/ml).
After 4 days in 5% CO_2 at $37^{o}C$ all cultures were supplemented with medium
with 5% lectin-free, human Il 2 (Cellular Products). New medium was added
twice a week. At intervals, the cells were washed, resuspended at 2 x10^5/
ml and restimulated with antigen in the presence of accessory cells.

PB-derived line at all antigen concentrations (Fig. 2). The CSF line
showed marked proliferation even at low antigen concentrations. The TET-
induced proliferation of both cell lines was dependent upon the presence
of autologous accessory cells. Other antigens than TET did not stimulate
the growth of the cells (data not shown).

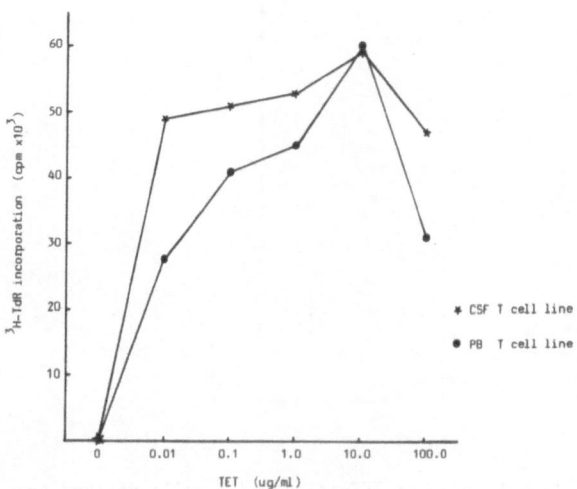

FIGURE 2.   Proliferative response to TET of $2x10^4$ cells from the T cell
lines derived from an MS patient's CSF (★) and PB (●).

METHOD.   After more than two months in culture, cells from the cell
lines were seeded in microtiter wells and stimulated with varying concentrations of TET (or other antigens) and accessory cells for 3 days. The
cultures were pulsed for the final 18 hr with 1 uCi/well ^{3}H-TdR. The response of both CSF and PB T cell lines to TET in the absence of accessory
cells was <400 cpm. Other antigens in the presence of accessory cells
gave responses <800 cpm.

Helper activity.   Cells from the CSF T cell line, titrated into
Mishell-Dutton cultures containing autologous PB-derived B cells and
monocytes, induced greater specific antibody synthesis per cell than did
cells from the PB T cell line. As few as 20 CSF T cells gave detectable
helper activity for 2×10^5 B cells and monocytes (Fig. 3). Optimal amounts
of antibody was induced by the CSF T cell line at a 100-fold lower
concentration of TET than by the PB T cell line (Fig. 4).

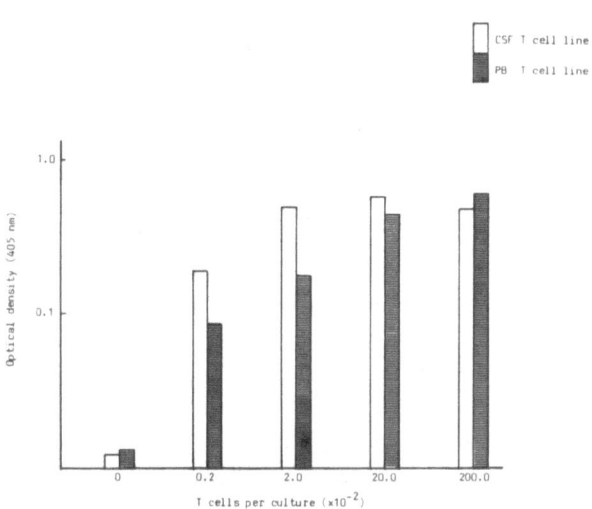

FIGURE 3.   Helper activity of TET-specific T cell lines derived from an
MS patient's CSF and PB. Cells from the CSF T cell line induced greater
specific antibody synthesis per cell than did cells from the PB T cell
line.

METHOD.   Varying numbers of T cells from the CSF and PB lines were added
to 2×10^5 autologous PB-derived B cells and monocytes in the presence of
10 ng/ml TET in Mishell-Dutton cultures (Mishell & Dutton, 1967). Supernatants were assayed for TET-specific IgG in a solid-phase ELISA.

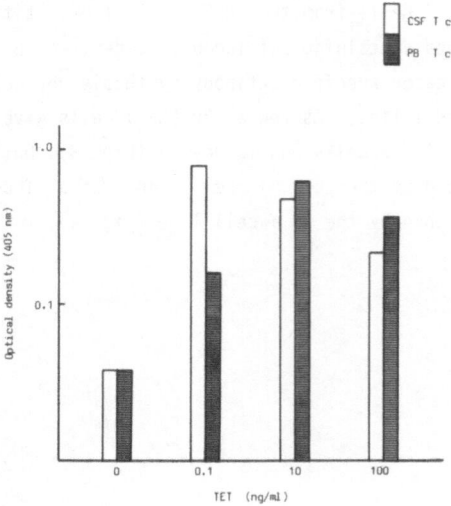

FIGURE 4.   Helper activity of TET-specific T cell lines derived from an MS patient's CSF and PB. Cells from the CSF T cell line induced optimal amounts of specific antibody synthesis at a 100-fold lower concentration of TET compared to cells from the PB T cell line.

METHOD. Equal numbers of cells ($2x10^4$/culture) from the CSF and PB T cell lines were added to $2x10^5$ autologous PB-derived B cells and monocytes and varying concentrations of TET in Mishell-Dutton cultures. Supernatants were assayed for TET-specific IgG in a solid-phase ELISA.

Frequency of antigen-reactive T cells in CSF- and PB- derived lines. Limiting dilution analysis of MS CSF and PB T cell lines was carried out by seeding twenty-four parallel microtiter wells with between 3 and 100 T cells and 4×10^5 gamma-irradiated autologous PB lymphocytes. The cells were stimulated with either 0.1 or 10.0 ug/ml TET. After 4 and 8 days, Il 2 (final conc. 10%) was added. After 16 days, wells were scored for viable colonies of cells with a phase contrast microscope. The frequency of TET-reactive cells was derived from the Poisson formula (inverse of cell concentration giving 67% responding cultures) (Elliott &al, 1984).

The frequency of T cells responding to high (10 ug/ml) TET concentration was the same for both cell populations, 1 in 12. In contrast, the frequency of cells reacting to low (0.1 ug/ml) TET concentration was three times higher in the CSF line than in the PB line, 1 in 14 compared to 1 in 45 (data not shown).

DISCUSSION

Our previous demonstration that MS CSF cells spontaneously produce oligoclonal IgG (Sandberg Wollheim, 1983) and specific antibody (unpubl.) indicates that the various cells required for Ig and antibody synthesis are present in the CSF. The central role of the T cell, notably the T helper cell, in regulating the immune response, prompted us to study the function of CSF T cells in comparison with PB T cells in MS patients.

In most patients insufficient CSF cell numbers are obtained for analysis of the helper function, since large numbers of pure T cells are required. We therefore generated antigen-specific T cell lines from the CSF and PB of MS patients and a normal donor.

Our studies demonstrated functional differences between MS CSF and PB T cells. CSF-derived T cells (1) proliferated more rapidly in response to tetanus toxoid and at lower concentrations; (2) required, but were less dependent upon exogeneous Il 2 for proliferation; (3) per cell induced greater specific antibody synthesis by autologous PB B cells at both high and low antigen concentrations; and (4) exhibited greater frequency of antigen-reactive cells at low antigen concentrations.

During the initial days of culture, the more rapid proliferation of MS CSF T cells could be due to the lower proportion of suppressor cells in CSF, but by day 14, the CSF and PB populations were phenotypically identical, and yet the CSF cells expanded more rapidly. The prolonged growth of CSF cells in Il 2 alone, may suggest that antigen-activated CSF T cells maintain Il 2 receptors longer. This could mean, that once stimulated by antigen CSF T helper cells persist in CSF in an "activated" state for a longer period of time.

The greater ability of the TET-specific CSF T cell line to provide help to B cells could result from both the higher frequency of antigen-specific cells in the cell line and a greater production of lymphokines essential for B cell proliferation and differentiation or the secretion of these factors for longer periods of time.

REFERENCES

Cashman, N., Martin, C., Eizenbaum, J.F., Degos, J.D. and Bach, M.A. 1982. Monoclonal antibody-defined immunoregulatory cells in multiple sclerosis cerebrospinal fluid. J. clin. Invest., 70:387.

Elliott, L., Brooks, W. and Roszman, T. 1984. Cytokinetic basis for the impaired activation of lymphocytes from patients with primary intra-cranial tumors. J. Immunol., 132:1208.

Mishell, R. and Dutton, R. 1967. Immunization of dissociated spleen cell cultures from normal mice. J. Exp. Med., 126:423.

Sandberg Wollheim, M. 1974. Immunoglobulin synthesis in vitro by cerebro-spinal fluid cells in patients with multiple sclerosis. Scand. J. Immunol., 3:717.

Sandberg Wollheim, M. and Turesson, I. 1975. Lymphocyte subpopulations in the cerebrospinal fluid and peripheral blood in patients with multiple sclerosis. Scand. J. Immunol., 4:831.

Sandberg Wollheim, M. 1983. Lymphocyte populations in the cerebrospinal fluid and peripheral blood of patients with multiple sclerosis and optic neuritis. Scand. J. Immunol., 17:575.

18

Characterization of T-cell Subsets and Macrophages in Active Demyelinating Multiple Sclerosis Lesions

H. NYLAND, S. MÖRK, R. MATRE and A. NAESS

INTRODUCTION

Active demyelinating lesions of multiple sclerosis (MS) is characterized by increased cellularity,presence of numerous macrophages and astrocytes,increased vascularity,and perivenous mononuclear cell infiltrates
(Adams,1977).The mononuclear cell infiltrates consist mainly of T lymphocytes (Nyland et al.,1982;Traugott et al.,1983),and a small number of B
lymphocytes/plasma cells (Esiri,1980).The macrophages in MS lesions
possess receptors for the Fc part of IgG,FcR (Nyland et al.,1980),and show
capping of surface IgG indicating that they may be engaged in immune mediated phagocytosis of myelin (Prineas & Graham,1981).

In this study we have further characterized the phenotype of the
mononuclear cells in active MS lesions by immunocytochemical identification of the T8,T4 and the Ia-like (HLA-DR) antigens.Macrophages were identified cytochemically by reactions for alpha-naphthyl acetate esterase.

MATERIALS AND METHODS

Patients.

4 patients with clinical definite MS were studied. Some selected
clinical data are presented in Table 1.

Table 1 Clinical data of the 4 patients with multiple sclerosis studied.

	Ages (years)	Sex	Duration of illness (years)	Disease course
Patient 1	45	F	8	Progressive
Patient 2	50	F	17	Progressive
Patient 3	46	F	1	Acute
Patient 4	53	F	15	Progressive

Tissue.

   Brain and spinal cord were obtained at autopsy.The macroscopic examination revealed lesions of various size and age.Specimens were taken
from grossly visible lesions and also surrounding normal-appearing white
matter,quick-frozen in liquid nitrogen and sectioned (4-6μm) in a cryostat.
The sections were picked up on coverslips and stained with haematoxylin
and eosin (H&E) and for myelin.Serial cryostat sections were examined for
comparison of the density of the cell infiltrates and positivity of the
reactions.

Antisera.

   The monoclonal antibodies OKT3,OKT4,OKT8 and OKIa1 (HLA-DR antigens)
were obtained from Ortho Pharmaceutical Corporation,Raritan,N.J.,USA.
Fluorescein isothiocyanata (FITC)-conjugated swine antimouse IgG was pur-
chased from Nordic Immunological Laboratories,Tilburg,Holland (code no.
12-380,protein concentration 10mg/ml,molar F/P ratio between 1 and 4).

Immunofluorescence staining.

   Cryostat sections (4-6μm) were incubated with an appropriate antibody
dilution for 30min.The adherent antibodies were labelled using FITC-conju-
gated swine anti-mouse IgG diluted in PBS.The preparations were examined
in a Zeiss Fluorescence microscope with an Osram HBO-200 mercury lamp.

Immunoperoxidase staining.

   Cryostat sections were incubated with the antibody dilutions followed
by incubation with rabbit anti-mouse IgG diluted 1:20,and then swine anti-
-rabbit serum 1:20.The peroxidase reaction was carried out with complexes
of peroxidase-antiperoxidase.

Demonstration of ANAE-activity.

   Frozen sections were examined for (ANAE)-activity according to Müller
et al., 1975.

RESULTS

Active multiple sclerosis lesions.

The active MS lesions showed increased cellularity with hypertrophic astrocytes and numerous macrophages throughout the demyelinating lesions (Fig.1a,b).Perivascular mononuclear cell infiltrates were localized to

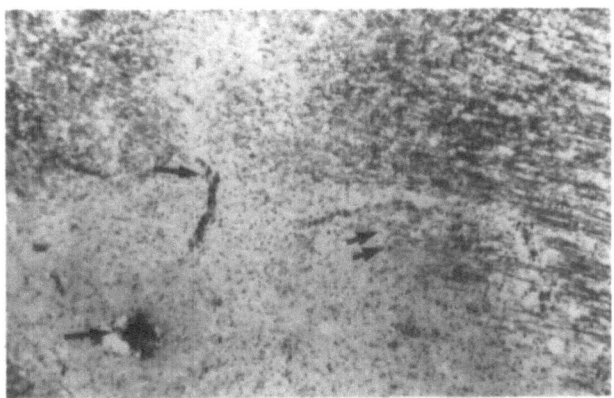

Figure 1a: Active demyelinating MS lesion in cerebral white matter. Central venule (single arrow), edge of demyelinating zone (double arrow)

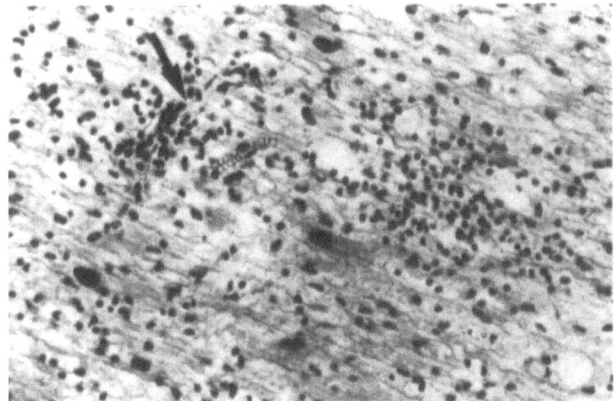

Figure 1b: The hypercellular margin of the lesion in the vicinity of a small venule (arrow). The astro-cytes and macrophages are identified by morphological criteria, while identification of the other cells present is difficult.

small and larger vessels within the lesions and in the adjacent normal myelinated tissue (Fig.2a,b).Staining of the active MS lesions with the

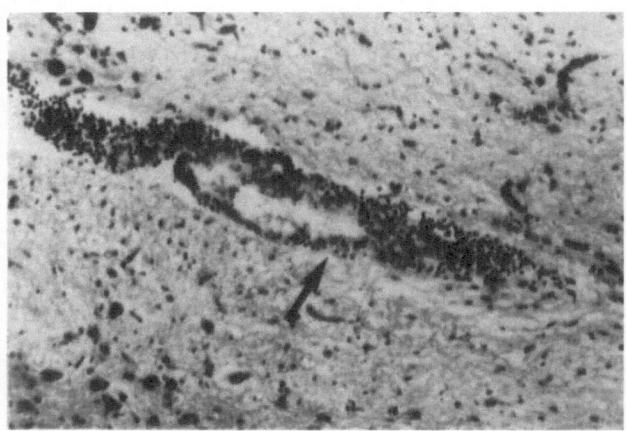

Figure 2a: A perivenous (arrow) infiltration of mono-nuclear cells in a demyelinated MS lesion.

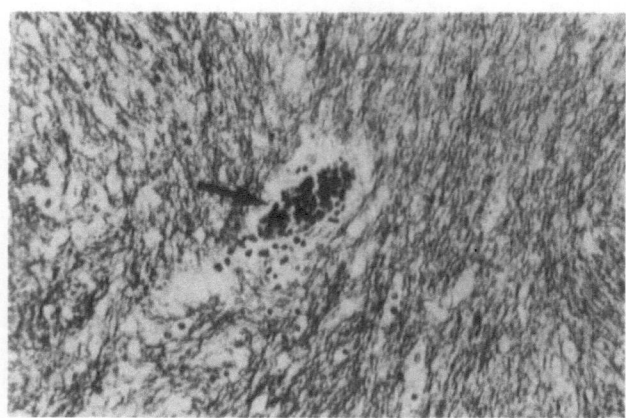

Figure 2b: Modest perivenous infiltration of lympho-cytes in apparently normal myelinated cerebral white matter.

OKT3 antibody showed that the majority of the perivascular mononuclear cells consisted of T lymphocytes (Fig.3).In addition,T lymphocytes

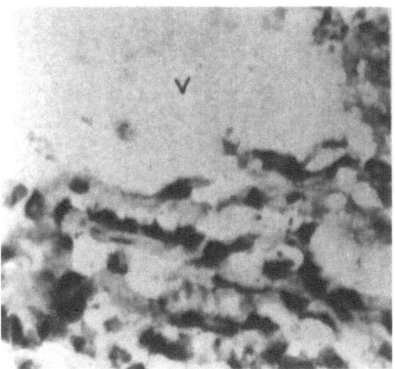

Figure 3:   Immunoperoxidase staining of an active MS lesion. Dense infiltrate of T3+ cells in a perivascular infiltrate of a venule (V)

occurred outside the perivascular spaces within the neural parenchyma.The perivascular mononuclear infiltrates consisted mainly of T4$^+$ T cells,while the number of T8$^+$ T cells varied,but were generally low,the overall proportion of T4$^+$/T8$^+$ T cells was 3:1 (Fig.4).The majority of the cells in

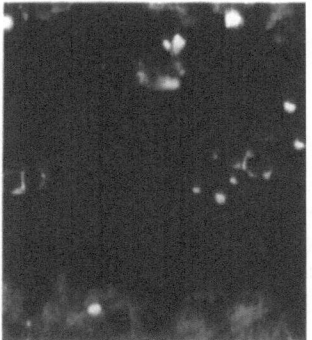

Figure 4:   Immunofluorescence staining of a few T8+ cells in a dense perivascular infiltrate of an active MS lesion.

the perivascular spaces were Ia-positive (Fig.5).In addition,strongly Ia-
-positive macrophages were seen in the perivascular infiltrates.

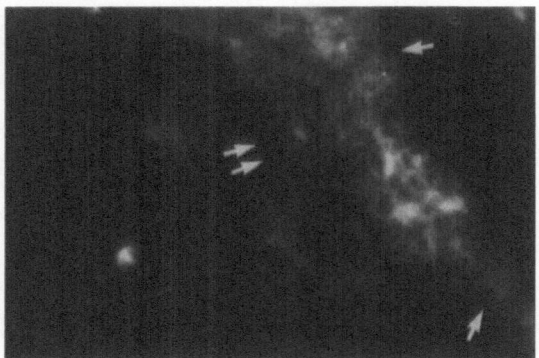

Figure 5: Immunofluorescence staining of a perivascular infiltrate with anti-Ia. Large numbers of
Ia$^+$ cells (singel arrows). The venule in the center
(double arrow).

T8$^+$ T cells were invading the neural parenchyma,often clustered together (Fig.6),both just outside and at a distance from the vessels.The

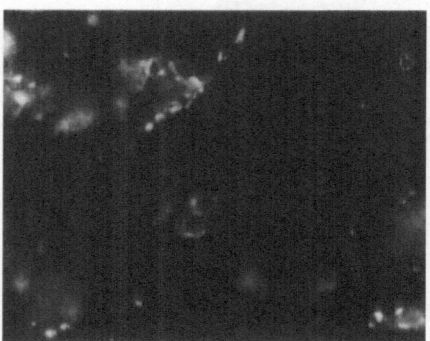

Figure 6: Immunofluorescence staining
of an active MS lesion with anti-T8.
small clusters of T8$^+$ cells in the parenchyma.

macrophages within the demyelinating areas,especially at the active edges,
were strongly Ia-positive (Fig.7).

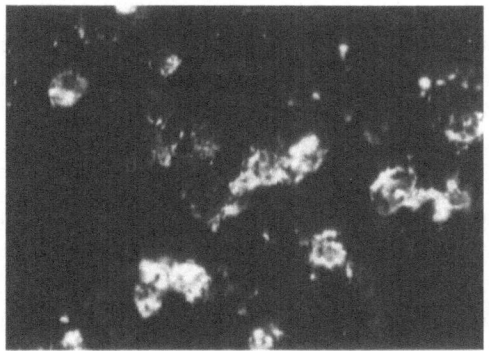

Figure 7:   Immunofluorescence staining of
Ia+ cells with the morphologic characteristics of macrophages at the edge of an active
demyelinating lesion.

DISCUSSION

The nature and significance of the inflammatory reactions in MS
brains are not understood to date. The present study confirms previous
observations that the inflammatory cell infiltration in MS brain lesions
consists essensially of T lymphocytes and macrophages (Nyland et al.,1982;
Traugott et al.,1983).The prominent perivascular accumulation of mononuclear cells in this material consisted mainly of Ia-positive,presumably
activated T4+T cells.A reduced number of T8+T cells were seen in the perivascular spaces, the distribution was similar to that reported both in
peripheral blood and cerebrospinal fluid (Arnason et al.,1982).The perivascular spaces of normal nervous tissue are the sites for inflammatory
reactions in different condition.The adventitial cells express macrophage-
-like properties and may participate in antigen processing and interaction
with T lymphocytes (Nyland and Nilsen,1982).

In zones of active demyelination,especially at the active edges,
strongly Ia-positive macrophages were numerous.The macrophages probably
are derived from microglial cells.The expression of FcR and Ia antigen

link them to the monocyte-macrophage cell linkeage and recent experimental
data show that normal brain contain an Ia-positive cell population which
probably have a bone marrow origin (Ting et al.,1983).In the brain parenchyma we also demonstrated T8[+] T cells,probably cytotoxic T cells, in
addition to few T4[+]T cells.Similar findings have been reported by Boss et
al. (1984),while Traugott et al. (1983) observed numerous T4[+]T cells in
the brain parenchyma.A smaller number of these mononuclear cells were also
Ia-positive.

The precise functional role of the inflammatory cells cannot be read
from the immunohistochemical examination.The macrophages may have cytotoxic, phagocytic and antigen-presenting properties. The T8[+]T cells may
have suppressive and cytotoxic functions. Our study suggest that myelin
damage may be mediated by cytotoxic T cell and macrophages.

REFERENCES

1. Adams,C.W.M.,1977. Pathology of multiple sclerosis:progression of the
   lesion. Br.Med.Bull.,33:15-20.
2. Arnason,G.G.W.,Oger,J.J.-F.,Antel,J.P.&Szuchet,S.,1982. Lymphocyte
   function in multiple sclerosis.Neurosciences 7:(Suppl.9).
3. Boss,J.,Esiri,M.,Tourtelotte,W. & Mason,Y.,1984.Quantitative study of
   T cells in the central nervous system in multiple sclerosis.Neuropath.
   Appl.Neurobiol.10:305 (Abstract).
4. Esiri,M.M.1980b. Multiple sclerosis: a quantitative and qualitative
   study of immunoglobulincontaining cells in the central nervous system.
   Neuropathol.appl.Neurobiol. 6:9-21.
5. Mueller,J.,Brun Del Re,G.,Buerki,H.-U.,Keller,H.U.,Hess,M.W.&Cottier,H.
   1975. Nonspecific esterase activity:a criterion for differentiation of
   T and B lymphocytes in mouse lymph nodes.Eur.J.Immunol.,5:270-274.
6. Nyland,H. & Nilsen,R.,1982. Localization of Fcγ receptors in the human
   central nervous system.Acta path.microbiol.immunol.scand.Sect.C,90:
   217-221.
7. Nyland,H.,Mörk,S. & Matre,R.,1982. In situ characterization of mononuclear cell infiltrates in lesions of multiple sclerosis. Neuropathol.
   appl.Neurol.8:403-411.

8. Prineas,J.W. & Graham,B.A.,1981. Multiple sclerosis:capping of surface immunoglobulin G or macrophages engaged in myelin breakdown.Ann. Neurol. 10:149-158.

9. Ting,J.P-Y.,Nixon,D.F.,Weiner,L.P. & Frelinger,J.A.,1983. Brain Ia antigens have a bone marrow origin.Immunogenetics,17:295-301.

10.Traugott,U.,Reinherz,E.L. & Raine,C.S.,1983. T cell subsets and Ia--positive macrophages in lesions of different ages.J.Neuroimmunol.4: 201-221.

19

Determination of Lymphocyte Subsets in Cerebrospinal Fluid (CSF)

W. M. NILLESEN and B. M. J. UITDEHAAG

We have developed a new indirect immune fluorescence micro method for the determination of lymphocytes in CSF.

In suspension the cells are first labelled with a mono- or polyclonal antibody followed by a second labelling with goat-anti-mouse FITC. After being labelled the cells are fixated in 1% paraformaldehyde and for nuclear staining ethidiumbromide is added. Then the cells are cytocentrifugated and embedded in 9 parts glycerol with 1 part PBS/NaN_3 and examined by fluorescence microscopy.

The advantages of this technique are:

1. it can be applied on CSF with < 1 cell/μl.
2. every mono- or polyclonal antibody can be used.
3. it is linear with the conventional method used in the blood.
4. it is relatively cheap.

CONCLUSION

By using the method we describe here it is possible to determine CSF lymphocyte-subsets in all patients, regardless of the cellnumber in the CSF. Therefore this method is suited to gain an insight into the subset-ratio in healthy persons or patients without pleiocytosis of the CSF. Furthermore the effect of immunosuppressant and/or cytotoxic drugs on lymphocyte-subsets can be studied.

In the table the results are shown of the patients we have examined so far. The numbers of patients in the different groups are as yet too small to draw any conclusions.

Some results in patients with multiple sclerosis (MS) and other neurological diseases (OND)

	Cells/µl Leuco's 10^9/l	% Lympho's	T4/T8	IgT	Ia
MS rapid progr. (n=4)					
CSF	11.0 (10.5)	90 (6)	3.41 (1.16)	6.5 (4.2)	13.5 (7.1)
Blood	6.0 (0.9)	35 (12)	2.19 (0.71)	13.0 (12.5)	3.5 (1.3)
MS slow progr. (n=5)					
CSF	5.2 (5.9)	88 (5)	2.08 (0.55)	10.8 (5.4)	21.0 (10.9)
Blood	8.4 (1.6)	35 (9)	2.80 (1.9)	5.6 (5.0)	3.2 (0.8)
OND (n=7)					
CSF	1.2 (0.8)	88 (6)	3.20 (1.83)	9.0 (4.3)	17.3 (9.9)
Blood	6.8 (1.7)	32 (11)	2.81 (1.66)	6.2 (4.9)	3.3 (2.1)

standard deviation between brackets

20

Ia-Presenting Cells in early Multiple Sclerosis Lesions and Adjacent Normal Looking White Matter; A Morphological Study

H. J. TER LAAK and O. R. HOMMES

INTRODUCTION

Till now it is still unknown which initial factors are involved in the demyelination process in MS. Recent and established lesions have been extensively described by various authors using histological and enzyme-histological methods (Adams, 1975, 1977; Friede and Arbor, 1961; Friede and Knoller, 1964).

New immunohistological methods will give a deeper understanding and especially the availability of monoclonal antibodies to hematopoietic cells (Berger et al., 1981) will much contribute to clarify the immune response in MS resulting in demyelination.

It has been proven that lymphocytes (especially T-helper/inducer cells and T suppressor/cytotoxic cells) and macrophage-like cells take part in the immune response as seen in fresh MS lesions (Nyland et al., 1982; Brinkman et al., 1982; Traugott et al., 1982, 1983). Many genes of the "human leukocyte antigen" system (HLA system) are thought to be closely concerned in the initiation and effector phase of immune responses (Schwartz, 1982); the products of class II HLA-genes (HLA-DR, DQ, DP and others, collectively referred to as Ia) play an important role in the induction of an immune response while the products of class I genes (HLA-A, B and C) are important as target molecules (Hancock, 1984; Appleyard et al., 1985).

From in vitro studies it has been proven that antigen recognation can only take place in cooperation with Ia presentation (Weinberger et al., 1982; DeFreitas et al., 1983); so, antigen presenting cells (APC's) can probably only elicit immune responses in vivo if they present both the antigen and Ia. At first a major role for combining both functions was attributed to macrophages (Unanue, 1972); later on the dendritic cell concept of Steiman added follicular dendritic cells and interdigitating reticulum cells of lymphoid tissues (Steinman, 1981) and also Langerhans cells of the skin and interstitial cells in the connective tissue, to the APC's. Furthermore, it was found that human endothelial cells and fibroblasts could be recognized by lymphocytes in vitro (Hirschberg et al., 1982; Pober et al., 1983). From lightmicroscopical examinations it appeared that in many normal human tissues Ia-positive cells may occur (Scott et al., 1980; Newman et al., 1980; Natalie et al., 1981; Morris and Ting, 1982), but Ia was undetectable in brain (Williams et al., 1980).

In this study the presence of Ia-positive cells in normal and MS brain tissue will be investigated in order to trace those locations where the putative antigen, if any, might be present.

MATERIALS AND METHODS

Cerebral white matter was obtained from a 59-year old woman about 3 hours after death; she was suffering from MS. The cerebrum from a 35-year old man who died from a traffic accident and the cerebrum from an 1-year old child with severe mental retardation served as controls. Both control brains showed lightmicroscopically no abnormalities. These brains were obtained within 3 and 12 hours after death respectively. Cerebral white and grey matter and cerebellum specimen were excised and immediately frozen in cooled isopenthane ($-40^{\circ}C$). Fresh serial sections (8 μm) were cut using a cryostate, air-dried, fixed in acetone during 10 minutes and dried again. The sections were incubated during 30 minutes with the monoclonal antibody OKIa1 (from Orthoclone) to detect Ia-positive elements in the tissue. Monoclonal antibody to glial fibrillary acid protein (GFA) was used to detect astrocytes. OKIa1 is known to detect monocytes and lymphocytes and is directed to the framework of class II molecules of the HLA system (Reinherz et al., 1979). Peroxidase conjugated rabbit-anti-mouse antibodies (1:20) were used as second step incubations; there after staining was achieved by incubating the sections in a solution with AEC (3-amino-9 ethylcarbazole) and H_2O_2; counterstaining took

place with haematoxilin. Second step solutions were diluted with 1%
normal human serum. Control sections were obtained by incubating the
sections with phosphate buffered saline (PBS) instead of OKIa1 or anti-
GFA.

RESULTS

Normal cerebral white matter

All the sections incubated with OKIa1 were characterized by an almost complete absence of positive elements; only sporadically scattered-
Ia-positive elements were found in the cerebral white matter; the smaller and larger veins were mostly negative but sometimes there was a
slight partial positivity of the inner layer representing the endothelium cells. Sporadically a positive cell adjacent to a vein was found.
Both the cerebral white matter of the child and the adult contained
about a small Ia-positive spots or cells per 40 mm^2.

Other normal central nervous tissues

The adjacent cerebral grey matter contained about equal or less Ia-
positive elements with respect to the above mentioned white matter. However, in the adhering meningeal tissue many positive elements were seen
and sometimes positive blood vessels were also present. The child's cerebellum showed occasionally positive endothelial cells; the total number
did not outrange the number in the cerebral white matter.

MS-tissue

From the cerebral white matter of the MS patient a small waxy trans-
parant looking area was excised. This area appeared to contain a small
(2 mm) recent lesion which contained many cells: the inner part of the
brain was devoid of myelin. After staining with OKIa1 there was a remarkable positivity in the section.
- The central part of the lesion was filled with many heavily stained
  large rounded cells. Ia-positivity was present both at the surface and
  in the cytoplasm of these cells. These cells were found around the
  veins and in the already demyelinated tissue; they were often found in
  close contact with lymphocytes (OKT8 positive) and these large cells
  showed a clear Sudan Black B-positivity; apparently these cells represent cells of the macrophage lineage. The veins in the lesion were

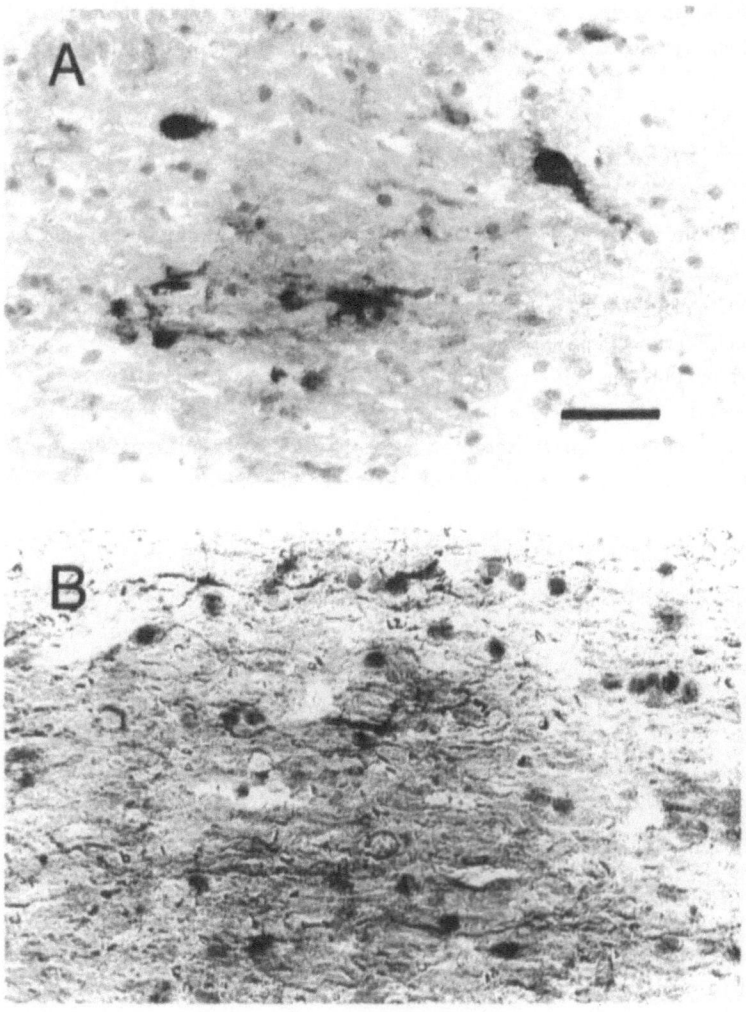

Fig. 1: Serial sections of a longitudinal tract in the cerebral "normal-
        looking" white matter of a MS patient. Ia-antibodies (OKIa1)
stain rounded cells and cells with a dendritic shape (Figure A); in
Figure B the longitudinal arranged processes of astroglial cells have
been stained (antibodies to GFA).
Bar: 100 μm.

negative for Ia. GFA antibodies clearly stained cells in this region
which were quite different from the macrophage-like cells.
A small zone adjacent to the lesion - this zone may extend to about
2 mm - with normal looking white matter (as seen by the Sudan Black B
stain) appeared to contain many Ia-positive cells; the density of these
cells decreased from the edge of the lesion. These cells had a "dendritic" shape, but became more and more rounded as they were located
closer to the lesion. Apparently these cells represent precursors of
the macrophage-like cells in the lesion. The veins did not show any Ia-
positivity of the endothelium, but positive cells could be frequently
seen between these small veins and the surrounding limiting membrane
consisting of astroglial feet; these cells were often quite large and
looked like the macrophage-like cells, but also smaller rounded cells
and sometimes very small cells (pericytes?) were observed. Cells clearly positive for GFA antibodies could not be observed in this region.
In the remaining white matter present in the sections there were
regions without Ia-positive cells (like the controls), but also regions,
even several millimeters apart from the lesion, containing cells with
a dendritic appearance. Serial sections of a longitudinal tract in
such a region which was stained on the presence of astroglial cells
(with GFA antibodies) and Ia-positive cells (with OKIa1), revealed
that the "dendritic" Ia-positive cells were quite different from the
astroglial cells with their long processes; these processes could not
be observed in the sections stained with OKIa1 (Fig. 1). In the remaining white matter two capillaries or post-capillary venules were
seen which showed a clear Ia-positivity of the endothelium cells (Fig.
2); one of these capillaries was in close contact with an Ia-positive
large rounded cell.

DISCUSSION

In this study the data of Williams et al. (1980) were confirmed, viz.
that in human brain tissue only very small amounts or no Ia occur. We
showed that only some cells were positive; the kind of these cells is
not always clear, but at least some of these cells were endothelium cells
and some were possibly resting macrophages. However, it is possible that
in vivo more Ia might be present because of the long period of at least

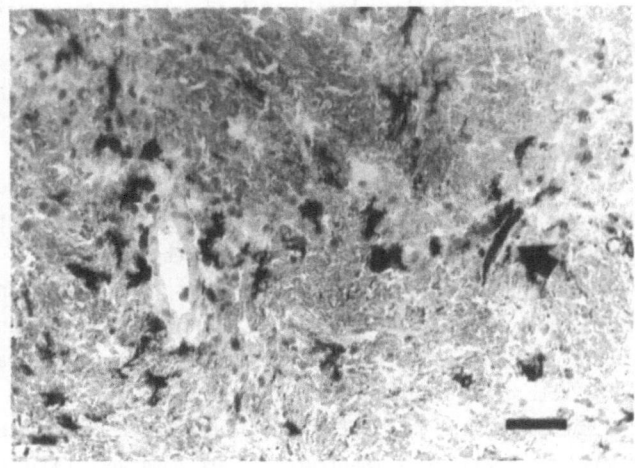

Fig. 2:   Several Ia-positive cells are present in the cerebral
           "normal-looking" white matter of a MS patient. Note
the negative endothelium of a larger vein (left) and the positive endothelium of a capillary or small vein (right; arrow).
Bar: 100 μm.

3 hours before the tissues could be frozen. Nevertheless there is a re-
markable difference in Ia-content of the normal tissue and the MS tissue.
Increase of Ia-content in a diseased condition was also described by
Volc-Platzer et al. (1984) for human keratinocytes in cutaneous T-cell
lymphoma and for thyroid epithelial cells in Hashimoto thyroiditis
(Aichinger et al., 1985).

The occurrence of many Ia-positive cells in the lesion area and
directly adjacent to the lesion area and the occurrence of many transitional forms strongly suggests that we are dealing with the same kind of
cell. Both the findings in the described longitudinal tract and in the
lesion area exclude in all probability that these cells are astrocytes.
The capability of these cells to phagocytize myelin further excludes the
possibility that these cells are oligodendroglial cells. So, it might be
possible that these cells are activated microglial cells or activated
monocytes from the blood or both. However, cell counts indicate that
there is no elevated total cell number in the adjacent myelinated area
although many cells show Ia-positivity. So, it is likely that for the

greater part these Ia-positive cells represent activated microglial cells.

The question remains by which humoral or cellular factor these cells were activated. The circular arrangement of the positive cells around the lesion suggest a soluble factor from the lesion (from leaking veins or from cells in the lesion); this might be important for the perpetuation of the demyelination. But in this study we were especially interested in the location of those sites where possibly induction of the immune response could or can take place. It might be possible that the Ia-positive small veins or capillaries represent these locations.

Expression of HLA-DR is of great functional importance for the induction of an immune response (McDevitt, 1980; Unanue, 1981) and in this context the clear positivity of endothelium cells of some smaller vessels is an intriguing observation. What factors cause these cells to be Ia-positive? Are they cells and do they originate from the peripheral blood (sensitized lymphocytes and/or their lymphokines) or from the central nervous system (viz. astroglial cells)? Ia-expression of human endothelial cells (Pober et al., 1983) and rat astrocytes (Fierz et al., 1984) can be induced by y-interferon; astrocytes can produce interleukin-1 (Fontana et al., 1982). The putative antigen, whatever it may be and if there is an antigen, in MS may originates from abnormal myelin breakdown products transported by astroglial cells to the veins.

Many questions remain to be solved; from this study it will be clear that our attention in future have to be focussed not only on the lesions in MS patients, but also on the normal looking myelin of MS patients.

REFERENCES

Adams, C.W.M., 1975. The onset and progression of the lesion in multiple sclerosis. J. Neurol. Sci., 25: 165-182.
Adams, C.W.M., 1977. Pathology of multiple sclerosis: progression of the lesion. Br. Med. Bull., 33: 15-20.
Aichiger, G., Fill, H. and Wick, G., 1985. In situ immune complexes, lymphocyte subpopulations, and HLA-DR-positive epithelial cells in Hashimoto thyroiditis. Lab. Invest., 52: 132-140.
Appleyard, S.T., Dubowitz, V., Dunn, M.J. and Rose M.L., 1985. Increased expression of HLA ABC class I antigens by muscle fibres in Duchenne muscular dystrophy, inflammatory myopathy, and other neuromuscular disorders. Lancet, 361-363.

Berger, C.L., Kung, P., Goldstein, G., Depietro, W., Takezaki, S., Chu, A., Fithian, E. and Edelson, R.L., 1981. Use of orthoclone monoclonal antibodies in the study of selected dermatologic conditions. Int. J. Immunopharmacol., 3: 275-282.

Brinkman, C.J.J., Laak ter, H.J., Hommes, O.R., Poppema, S. and Delmotte, P., 1982. T-lymphocyte subpopulations in multiple sclerosis lesions. N. Engl. J. Med., 307: 1644-1645.

De Freitas, E.C., Chesnut, R.W., Grey, H.M. and Chiller, J.M., 1983. Macrophage-dependent activation of antigen-specific T cells requires antigen and a soluble monokine. J. Immunol., 131: 23-29.

Fierz, W., Endler, B., Wekerle, H. and Fontana, A., 1984. Immune-specific interaction between astrocytes and T-lymphocytes: regulation of Ia-antigen expression on astrocytes by immune-interferon (IFN-y) and its effects on antigen presentation. In: Annual report of the Max-Planck-Society, Clinical Research Unit for multiple sclerosis, pp 70-76.

Fontana, A., Kristensen, F., Dubs, R., Gemsa, D. and Weber, E., 1982. Production of prostaglandin E and an interleukin-1 like factor by cultured astrocytes and C6 glioma cells. J. Immunol., 129: 2413-2419.

Friede, R.L. and Arbor, A., 1961. Enzyme histochemical studies in multiple sclerosis. Arch. Neurol., 5: 433-443.

Friede, R.L. and Knoller, M., 1964. Quantitative enzyme profiles of plaques of multiple sclerosis. Experientia, 20: 130-132.

Hancock, W.W., 1984. Analysis of intragraft effector mechanisms associated with human renal allograft rejection: immunohistological studies with monoclonal antibodies. Immunol. Rev., 77: 61-84.

Hirschberg, H., Braathen, L.R. and Thorsby, E., 1982. Antigen presentation by vascular endothelial cells and epidermal Langerhans cells: the role of HLA-DR. Immunol. Rev., 66: 57-77.

McDevitt, H.O., 1980. Regulation of the immune respons by the major histocompatibility system. N. Engl. J. Med., 303: 1514-1517.

Morris, P.J. and Ting, A., 1982. Studies of HLA-DR with relevance to renal transplantation. Immunol. Rev., 66: 103-131.

Natali, P.G., DeMartino, C., Quaranta, V., Nicotra, M.R., Frezza, F., Pellegrino, M.A. and Ferrone, S., 1981. Expression of Ia like antigens in normal human non-lymphoid tissue. Transplant., 31: 75-78.

Newman, R.A., Ormerod, M.G. and Greaves, M.F., 1980. The presence of HLA-DR antigens on lactating human breast epithelium and milk fat globale membranes. Clin. exp. Immunol., 41: 478-486.

Nyland, H., Matre, R., Mørk, S., Bjerke, J.-R. Bjerke, and Naess, A., 1982. T-lymphocyte subpopulations in multiple sclerosis lesions. N. Engl. J. Med., 307: 1643-1644.

Pober, J.S., Collins, T., Gimbrone, M.A., Corran, R.S., Gitlin, J.D., Fiers, W., Clayberger, C., Krensky, A.M., Burakoff, S.J. and Reiss, C.S. 1983. Lymphocytes recognize human vascular endothelial and dermal fibroblast Ia antigens induced by recombinant immune interferon. Nature, 305: 726-729.

Reinherz, E.L., Kung, P.C., Pesando, J.M., Ritz, J., Goldstein, G. and Schlossman, S.F., 1979. Ia determinants on human T-cell subsets defined by monoclonal antibodies. J. Exp. Med., 150: 1472-1482.

Schwartz, B., 1982. The human major histocompatibility HLA complex. In: Stites et al., (Ed.) Basic and clinical immunology, Lange Medical Publications, Los Altos, California, 4th edition, p. 60.

Scott, H., Solheim, B.G., Brandtzaeg, P. and Thorsby, E., 1980. HLA-DR-like antigens in the epithelium of the human small intestine. Scand. J. Immunol., 12: 77-82.

Steinman, R.M., 1981. Dendritic cells. Transplant., 31: 151-155.
Traugott, U., Reinherz, E.L. and Raine, C.S., 1982. Multiple sclerosis: distribution of T cell subsets within active chronic lesions. Science, 219: 308-310.
Traugott, U., Reinherz, E.L. and Raine, C.S., 1983. Multiple sclerosis. Distribution of T cells, T cell subsets and Ia-positive macrophages in lesions of different ages. J. Neuroimmunol., 4: 201-221.
Unanue, E.R., 1972. The regulatory role of macrophages in antigenic stimulation. Adv. Immunol., 15: 95-165.
Unanue, E.R., 1981. The regulatory role of macrophages in antigenic stimulation. II Symbiotic relationship between lymphocytes and macrophages. Adv. Immunol., 31: 1-136.
Volc-Platzer, B., Majdic, O., Knapp, W., Wolff, K., Hinterberger, W., Lechner, K. and Stingl, G., 1984. Evidence of HLA-DR antigen biosynthesis by human keratinocytes in disease. J. Exp. Med., 159: 1784-1789.
Weinberger, O., Germain, R.N., Springer, T. and Burakoff, S.J., 1982. Role of syngeneic Ia+ accessory cells in the generation of allospecific CTL responses. J. Immunol., 129: 694-697.
Williams, K.A., Hart, D.N., Fabre, J.W. and Morris, P.J., 1980. Distribution and quantitation of HLA-ABC and DR (Ia) antigens on human kidney and other tissue. Transplant., 29: 274-279.

21

Developmental Aspects of Oligodendrocyte Structure and Function

M. SCHACHNER

An understanding of the development and function of oligodendrocytes is a central issue in assessing the contribution of these cells to the pathology of multiple sclerosis. In particular, repair processes, especially those which relate to neuron-glia and possibly also to astrocyte-oligodendrocyte interactions, have to be considered in terms of developmental plasticity. In addition, the characterization of oligodendrocyte-specific cell surface antigens is expected to elucidate the possible antigenic targets of immune mechanisms leading to the elimination of oligodendrocytes in the disease. We have started to characterize cell surface markers recognized by monoclonal antibodies to define developmental stage- and subclass-specific oligodendrocyte populations and probe for their relation to oligodendrocyte differentiation and interactions with other neural cell types. Furthermore, we have investigated the membrane properties of cultured oligodendrocytes using electrophysiological methods and have compared these to the other macroglial population, the astrocyte.

After initial attempts to characterize markers of oligodendrocytes by polyclonal antibodies (Berg and Schachner, 1982; Schachner, 1974; Schachner and Willinger, 1979), we succeeded in isolating monoclonal antibodies to cell surface markers of oligodendrocytes characteristic of different developmental stages (Kuhlmann-Krieg et al., 1985; Nieke et al., 1985; Schachner et al., 1981; Schnitzer and Schachner, 1982; Sommer et al. 1985; Sommer and Schachner, 1981, 1982). Immunoselection of live oligodendrocytes was achieved using antibodies coupled to magnetic beads

153

(Meier et al., 1982; Meier and Schachner, 1982), thus providing the basis for the controlled investigation of pure oligodendrocytes in culture.

Of the twelve monoclonal antibodies designated O1 through O12 and which have been characterized so far, O3, O4, O5 and O6 have been shown to react with sulfatide. Galactocerebroside is recognized by antibodies O1, O2 and O7. Antigens O8, O9 and O11 are yet unidentified glycolipids. Antigen O10 is no longer detectable on trypsin-treated live cells and is therefore most likely a protein or glycoprotein. During development this group of antibodies is the first to react in the intact brain tissue in prospective white matter tracts and in vitro with the cell surface of live cultured cells. The group of antigens to appear subsequently within the population of O4 antigen-positive cells consists of antigens O7, O1 and O2. Antibodies O8 through O11 recognize subsets of O4-positive oligo-dendrocytes at differentiative stages advancing with increasing O number. Antigens O11 and O12 are the latest to become recognizable within the set of O4 antigen-positive cells. Interestingly, O11 antigen-positive cells are not completely comprised within the O10 antigen-positive cell popula-tion, since O11 antigen-positive cells can be recognized that are not O10 antigen-positive. Similarly, not all O8 antigen-positive cells appear to be comprised within the O4 antigen-positive cell population. Antigens O11 and O12 are recognized predominantly on a morphologically distinct cell type of "hairy eyeball" morphology with large, sometimes bipolar cell bodies (up to 30 μm) surrounded by high amounts of membranous material de-void of cytoplasm. These observations suggest that the monoclonal anti-bodies recognize not only different developmental stages, but also diffe-rent subclasses of oligodendrocytes.

Antigen O10 is expressed in the central, but not peripheral nervous system and in the hypomyelinating mouse mutants quaking, shiverer and Trembler, but not in jimpy nor the rat mutant myelin deficient (md). Since antigens O11 and O12 are detectable in jimpy and myelin deficient animals, the absence in expression of O10 antigen points to a specific defect rather than to a more general abnormality in oligodendrocyte differentiation. All antigens are expressed in addition to mouse and rat also in rabbit, lamb, chicken and human.

Astrocytes support the differentiation of oligodendrocytes in culture, but under our culture onditions not all signals are present to induce complete differentiation of these cells (Meier et al., 1985; Schachner et al., 1983).

Membrane properties of cultured oligodendrocytes, such as membrane potential, input resistance and K^+ pump activity are not modified by O antibodies over a time period of several hours (Kettenmann et al., 1985b; see also Gilbert et al., 1984; Kettenmann et al., 1982; Kettenmann et al., 1983a, b; Kettenmann et al., 1984b, c, d; Kettenmann et al., 1985a). Also, some O antibodies seem to affect the capacity of oligodendrocytes to myelinate in organotypic cultures of mouse spinal cord (Kuhlmann-Krieg and Schachner, unpubl. observations).

Further support for a heterogeneity in oligodendrocyte populations comes from the observation that γ-aminobutyric acid (GABA) depolarizes in a dose-dependent manner approximately one-third of all immunologically identified oligodendrocytes in heterogeneous cultures of mouse spinal cord. Measurements of $\left[K^+\right]_o$ indicate that the response to GABA is not due to K^+ released from active neurons. The depolarization is not accompanied by a change in cell input resistance. Replacement of sodium in the bathing solution abolishes the entire response, whereas ouabain only inhibits the repolarization phase. Bicuculline and picrotoxin, but not nipecotic acid reduce the GABA effect. Pentobarbital and chlordiazepoxid also reduce the GABA-induced depolarization. Muscimol produces a depolarization similar to that of GABA. These pharmacological investigations suggest that the receptor mechanism has some similarity to the neuronal $GABA_A$ receptor. Further, heterogeneity in oligodendrocyte populations is also indicated by the observation that some cells respond to both GABA and glutamate, while others respond only to one and some are not responsive to either. A similar heterogeneity in response to the neurotransmitters GABA and glutamate has so far not beenfound in cultured astrocytes (Kettenmann et al., 1984a).

Our study supports the notion that oligodendrocyte differentiation is revealed by changes in the pattern of cell surface antigen expression and that oligodendrocyte populations in culture are heterogeneous with respect to expression of cell surface markers and to functional cell surface properties, such as the receptor mechanisms for direct membrane responses to GABA. Furthermore, abnormalities in cell surface properties specific for one particular antigen could be detected in the particular case of two hypomyelination mutants, jimpy and myelin, but not in others, suggesting that a specific gene detect may result in a specific loss of a central nervous system marker of myelinating cells rather than a more general loss or retardation of oligodendrocyte differentiation. In addition, the observation that the myelin associated glycoprotein (MAG) shares a functionally relevant carbohydrate epitope (Keilhauer and Schachner, 1985) with the cell surface glycoproteins L1 and N-CAM involved in cell adhesion and recognition among neural cells (Kruse et al., 1984) opens the possibility to investigate oligodendrocyte cell surfaces in the context of cell adhesion mechanisms. Since this carbohydrate epitope is also recognized by HNK-1, a monoclonal antibody directed against lymphocyte subpopulations including natural killer cells, a search for the functional relevance of this epitope and the cells expressing it seems warranted, particularly with regard to disorders of the immune system affecting the nervous system.

ACKNOWLEDGEMENTS

Support by Gemeinnützige Hertie-Stiftung und Hermann and Lilly Schilling-Stiftung for Multiple Sclerosis Research is gratefully acknowledged.

REFERENCES

Berg, G. and Schachner, M., 1982. Immunoelectron microscopic characterization of galactocerebroside and nervous system antigen-1 (NS-1) positive oligodendrocytes in culture. Neuroscience Letters, 28: 75-80.
Gilbert, P., Kettenmann, H. and Schachner, M.,1984. GABA directly depolarizes cultured oligodendrocytes. J. Neurosci., 4: 561-569.
Keilhauer, G. and Schachner, M., 1985. Differential inhibition of neuron-neuron, neuron-astrocyte and astrocyte-astrocyte adhesion by L1, L2 and N-CAM antibodies. Submitted for publication.
Kettenmann, H., Backus, K.H. and Schachner, M., 1984a. Aspartate, glutamate and GABA depolarize cultured astrocytes. Neuroscience Letters, 52: 25-29.
Kettenmann, H., Gilbert, P. and Schachner, M., 1984b. Depolarization of cultured oligodendrocytes by glutamate and GABA. Neuroscience Letters, 47: 271-276.
Kettenmann, H., Orkand, R.K. and Lux, H.D., 1984c. Some properties of single potassium channels in cultured oligodendrocytes. Pflügers Arch. 400: 215-221.
Kettenmann, H., Orkand, R.K., Lux, H.D. and Schachner, M., 1982. Single potassium channel currents in cultured oligodendrocytes. Neuroscience Letters, 32: 41-46.

Kettenmann, H., Orkand, R.K. and Schachner, M., 1983a. Coupling among identified cells in mammalian nervous system cultures. J. Neurosci., 3: 506-516.

Kettenmann, H., Orkand, R.K. and Schachner, M. Potassium uptake mechanisms of cultured oligodendrocytes studied with ion-sensitive electrodes. Submitted for publication.

Kettenmann, H., Sommer, I. and Schachner, M., 1985b. Monoclonal cell surface antibodies do not affect short-term electrical properties of oligodendrocytes in culture. Neuroscience Letters, in press.

Kettenmann, H., Sonnhof, U., Camerer, H., Orkand, R.K., Kuhlmann, S. and Schachner, M., 1984a. Electrical properties of oligodendrocytes in culture. Pflügers Arch., 401: 324-332.

Kettenmann, H., Sonnhof, U. and Schachner, M., 1983b. Exclusive potassium dependence of the membrane potential in cultured mouse oligodendrocytes. J. Neurosci., 3: 500-505.

Kruse, J., Mailhammer, R., Wernecke, H., Faissner, A., Sommer, I., Goridis, C. and Schachner, M., 1984. Neural cell adhesion molecules and myelin associated glycoprotein share a common, developmentally early carbohydrate moeity recognized by monoclonal antibodies L2 and HNK-1. Nature, 311: 153-155.

Kuhlmann-Krieg, S., Sommer, I. and Schachner, M., 1985. Ultrastructural features of cultured oligodendrocytes expressing stage-specific cell surface antigens. Submitted for publication.

Meier, D.H., Keilhauer, G., Kuhlmann, S., Nieke, J. and Schachner, M., 1985. Astrocytes support incomplete differentiation of an oligodendrocyte precusor cell. Submitted for publication.

Meier, D.H., Lagenaur, C. and Schachner, M., 1982. Immunoselection of oligodendrocytes by magnetic beads. I. Determination of antibody coupling parameters and cell binding conditions. J. Neurosci. Res., 7: 119-134.

Meier, D.H. and Schachner, M., 1982. Immunoselection of oligodendrocytes by magnetic beads. II. In vitro maintenance of immunoselected oligodendrocytes. J. Neurosci. Res., 7: 135-145.

Nieke, J., Sommer, I. and Schachner, M., 1985. Stage-specific cell surface antigens of oligodendrocytes in the peripheral nervous system. Expression during development and regeneration and in myelin-deficient mutants. Submitted for publication.

Schachner, M., 1974. NS-1 (nervous system antigen-1), a glial cell specific antigenic component of the surface membrane. Proc. Nat. Acad. Sci. (USA), 7: 1795-1799.

Schachner, M. and Willinger, M., 1979. Developmental expression of oligodendrocyte-specific cell surface markers: NS-1 (nervous system antigen-1), cerebroside, and basic protein of myelin. In: P.A. Miescher, L. Bolis, S. Gorine, T.A. Lambo, G.J.V. Nossal, G. Torrigiani (Editors), The menarini Series on Immunopathology, Schwabe, Basel/ Stuttgart, 2: 37-60.

Schachner, M., Faissner, A., Kruse, J., Lindner, D., Meier, D.H., Rathjen, F.G. and Wernecek, H., 1983. Cell type-specificity and developmental expression of neural cell surface components involved in cell interactions and of structurally related molecules. Cold Spring Harbor Symp. Quant. Biol., 48: 557-568.

Schachner, M., Kim, S.U. and Zehnle, R., 1981. Developmental expression in central and peripheral nervous system of oligodendrocyte cell surface antigens (O antigens) recognized by monoclonal antibodies. Develop. Biol., 83: 328-338.

Schnitzer, J. and Schachner, M., 1982. Cell type specificity of neural cell surface antigen recognized by monoclonal antibody A2 B5. Cell and Tissue Research, 224: 625-636.

Sommer, I., Kuhlmann-Krieg, S. and Schachner, M., 1985. Expression of stage specific cell surface antigens of oligodendrocytes in normal and myelin-deficient mutant mice. Submitted for publication

Sommer, I. and Schachner, M. 1981. Monoclonal antibodies (O1 to O4) to oligodendrocyte cell surfaces: an immunocytological study in the central nervous system. Develop. Biol., 83: 311-327.

Sommer, I. and Schachner, M., 1982. Cells that are O4 antigen-positive and O1 antigen-negative differentiate into O1 antigen-positive oligodendrocytes. Neuroscience Letters, 29: 183-188.

22

Monoclonal Antibodies Against Oligodendrocytes;
A Morphological Study

H. J. TER LAAK, M. SCHACHNER and O. R. HOMMES

INTRODUCTION

Recently various monoclonal antibodies against oligodendrocytes (so-
called O-antibodies) were developed by Schachner and her co-workers
(Sommer and Schachner, 1981; Sommer et al., 1985). It is generally accepted that in MS demyelination of central nervous tissue is responsible for
the clinical abnormalities in the long run. This demyelination means that
the oligodendrocytes, which make the myelin, are concerned and it also
means that these cells at least lose their cell processes which cover the
axons. In spite of this demyelination there are various reports dealing
with some kind of remyelination (Hommes, 1980). Till now treatment of MS
is not always very successful and policies must be centered on inhibiting
this demyelination and on stimulating remyelination, if possible, via
direct or indirect ways. Therefore, accurate knowledge of de- and remyelination processes is necessary.

In principle Schachner's O-antibodies can inform us whether there is
remyelination or not, because these antibodies can recognize myelin in
distinct stages of differentiation. So, the monoclonal antibodies 03, 04,
05 and 06, which recognize sulfatide, are the first to react in intact
brain tissue in prospective white matter tracts; subsequently, antigenic
determinants of galacto-cerebroside (07, 01 and 02) are recognized and
finally the antibodies 08 through 011 recognize oligodendrocytes at further differentiative stages advancing with increasing O-number; the latter
antibodies are directed to unidentified glycolipids with the exception of
010 which represents a protein or glycoprotein.

In this study seven O-antibodies (designated O5 through O11) were tested on their capacity to detect oligodendrocytes and myelin in the central nervous system.

MATERIALS AND METHODS

Monoclonal antibodies against oligodendrocytes (O5 through O10) were obtained from hybridoma clones from mice injected with bovin corpus callosum (O5, O6 and O8 to O10) and with a preparation of synaptosomes (O7); monoclonal antibodies against the antigen O11 were obtained from a hybridoma clone from a rat injected with a membrane preparation of mouse cerebellum (Sommer et al., 1985). Polyclonal antibodies against glial fibrillary acid protein (GFA) were used to detect the presence of astrocytes.

Tissue specimens from normal human cerebrum and cerebellum, from the pons of a MS patient and from the myelum of a rat were frozen in cooled isopenthane and cut with a cryostate microtome (6 μm thickness); the sections were air-dried and prior to incubation fixed in acetone during 10 minutes; in another set of sections no acetone-fixation was applied. In a separate experiment deparaffinized sections (4 μm) from formaldehyde-fixed normal human cerebrum and cerebellum and from the medulla oblongata of a MS patient were also used to detect the efficiency of these monoclonal antibodies.

Immunostaining was achieved by incubating the cryostate sections with antibodies using the indirect peroxidase method and the deparaffinized sections with antibodies using the PAP-technique. The O-antibodies were used at a dilution of 1:10 or 1:20 during 30 minutes at room temperature (cryostate sections) and 18 hours at 4°C (deparaffinized sections). In the indirect method peroxidase-labeled rabbit-anti-mouse Ig (Dako) at a dilution of 1:10 was used and in the PAP-technique rabbit-anti-mouse IgG (1:20; Dako) and mouse-PAP (1:100; Pelfreez) were applied as the second and third step during 30 minutes at room temperature.

Immunostaining of astrocytes was achieved by using the following antibodies at appropriate dilutions: antibodies against GFA (Dako), peroxidase labeled goat-anti-rabbit (Nordic), swine-anti-rabbit IgG (Fc) from Nordic and rabbit-PAP (Nordic).

Specify was tested by using phosphate buffered saline (PBS) in the first step instead of O- or GFA-antibodies.

RESULTS

Formaldehyde-fixed tissues from normal human cerebrum and cerebellum and from the medulla oblongata of a MS patient appeared to be completely negative after immunostaining with the oligodendrocyte antibodies except for O10, which was only positive for the astroglial cells. These cells were also clearly stained after incubation with GFA-antibodies. Especially the sections from the medulla oblongata of a MS patient showed a remarkable resemblance of the plaque area after staining with O10- and GFA-antibodies.

The cryostate sections fixed for 10 minutes in acetone did show a clearly visible diffuse myelin positivity after being incubated with O7, O8, O9, O10 or O11; this was true for all human tissues examined in this investigation; however, the cell bodies of the oligodendrocytes could not be observed; O10 did stain the astroglial cells as seen by their processes and their astroglial feet around the blood vessels; antibodies against GFA also stained the latter elements, but with O10 the positivity was even better, especially in the transitional region between the grey and white matter in the normal human cerebrum. The molecular layer and the Purkinje cells in the cerebellum also appeared to be clearly positive after incubation with O10-antibodies, the positivity had a dotted aspect lightmicroscopically.

From longitudinal rat myelum sections it was observed that the white matter of the myelum itself was positive and that the peripheral white matter from the roots was negative both with O10- and O11-antibodies. The cryostate sections which were fixed with acetone and which were incubated with O5- or O6-antibodies did not show any positivity of the myelin.

However, if acetone fixation was omitted O5- and O6-antibodies did stain the myelin which was observed in normal human cerebrum and cerebellum and in the myelin containing areas outside the plaques in the pons.

DISCUSSION AND CONCLUSIONS

From the above mentioned results it will be clear that mature myelin of the central nervous system can be stained by using the O-antibodies. The cell bodies of the oligodendrocytes cannot be discerned in histological sections. It is also clear that unfixed tissues have to be used and

that even mild acetone-fixation ought to be omitted (especially for 05-
and 06 antibodies). Cross reactivity of 010-antibodies with astroglial
cells and Purkinje cells was observed in the experiments. From earlier
experiments (Sommer et al., 1981) it was already known that fixation of
cerebellum cultures leads to immunolabelling of astrocytes by 0-antibodies
which was due to intracellularly localized cross-reactive components in
these cells (Schachner, 1983); so, the specificity of the 0-antibodies for
oligodendroglial cells is only guaranteed for intact cells.

REFERENCES

Hommes, O.R., 1980. Remyelination in human CNS lesions. In: P.S. McConnell,
    G.J. Boer, H.J. Romijn, N.E. van de Poll and M.A. Corner (Editors),
    Adaptive capabilities of the nervous system. Progress in Brain
    Research, volume 53: 39-63.
    Elsevier/North-Holland Biomedical Press, Amsterdam-New York.
Schachner, M., 1983. Immunohistochemistry and immunocytochemistry of
    neural cell types in vitro and in situ. In: A.C. Cuello (Editor),
    Immunohistochemistry, 399-429.
Sommer, I., Kuhlmann-Krieg, S and Schachner, M., 1985. Expression of stage
    specific cell surface antigens of oligodendrocytes in normal and
    myelin deficient mutant mice. Submitted for publication.
Sommer, I. and Schachner, M., 1981. Monoclonal antibodies (01 to 04) to
    oligodendrocyte cell surfaces: an immunological study in the central
    nervous system. Develop. Biol., 83: 311-327.

23

The Relationship of Immunological and Histological Abnormalities in Multiple Sclerosis

I. V. ALLEN

It is well known that immunoglobulins generally and viral antibodies particularly have elevated levels in the cerebrospinal fluid (CSF) in multiple sclerosis. At least part of the IgG has a constant oligoclonal isofocusing (IEF) spectrum. The pathogenic significance of this finding is unknown though it is often assumed that the CSF IgG is produced, at least in part, by plasma cells in inflammatory cell infiltrates within recent plaques and may be directed against a primary antigen of pathogenetic significance. Several workers have succeeded in eluting IgG from plaques and from apparently normal white matter in the brain in MS. IgG of plaque origin has an oligoclonal IEF pattern which has not to date been compared with the CSF pattern in the same patient. By contrast, apparently normal white matter has a polyclonal pattern resembling that of serum (Glynn et al., 1982). Various detailed pathological studies have demonstrated the presence of plasma cells and lymphoid cells in active lesions in MS and immunohistochemistry has confirmed the positivity of these cells for IgG, supporting the view that they are the source of plaque IgG. It is recognised however that very early demyelinated lesions do not invariably contain inflammatory cells and further anomaly is Tavolta's (1975) finding that old plaques, when stained by immunofluorescent techniques, apparently contain more IgG than recent plaques. Because of the practical implications of the cellular source of IgG in the interpretation of immunochemical studies in MS and because of the possible basic pathogenetic significance of the IgG abnormalities in this disease, we have attempted to answer this question by

a detailed histological-immunochemical study of samples of postmortem
brain in which the cellular composition has been related to IgG content,
both in amount and IEF pattern.

MATERIAL AND METHODS

Postmortem brain samples were obtained from 5 cases of classical MS.
The brains were frozen slowly before sectioning to -20°C and stored at
-70°C. Partially thawed samples of plaque, periplaque, apparently normal
white matter and grey matter were dissected for biochemical and histological assessment according to a standard protocol (Table 1). Control

TABLE 1

THE RELATIONSHIP BETWEEN PLAQUE HISTOLOGY AND IgG STUDIES IN MS

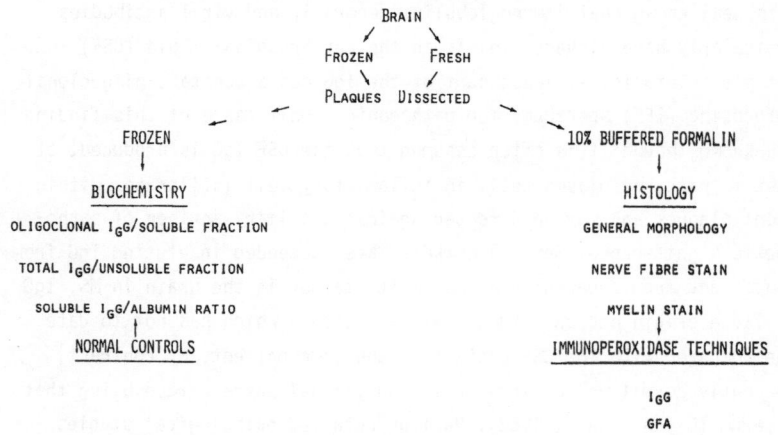

material for the biochemical study was obtained from 3 cases of subacute
sclerosing panencephalitis (SSPE) brain and from 9 normal brains. Control
material for the immunohistochemical study was obtained from one normal
brain, one case of SSPE and various samples of human glioma.

Methods for homogenising brain tissue, determinations of soluble and
particulate-bound IgG and albumin, and IEF with immunoperoxidase staining for IgG have been described previously (Glynn et al., 1982). All
formalin fixed samples were embedded in paraffin; sections were stained
by haematoxylin-eosin (H&E) and luxol fast blue (LFB) techniques. All
samples were also stained using a direct immunoperoxidase technique for

human IgG and for glial fibrillary acid protein. Control staining was done on selected sections: the various controls are given in Table 2.

TABLE 2

THE RELATIONSHIP BETWEEN PLAQUE HISTOLOGY AND IgG STUDIES IN MS

IgG CONTROLS

NEGATIVE	POSITIVE
NORMAL SWINE SERUM	LYMPHOID TISSUE - TONSIL
NON-IMMUNE NORMAL RABBIT SERUM	
IgG	
IgM	
MUMPS VIRUS	
INFLUENZA VIRUS	
CANINE DISTEMPER VIRUS	
FIBRONECTIN	

POST-MORTEM ABSORPTION OF IgG BY
ASTROCYTE CYTOPLASMIC RECEPTORS

Samples were assessed histologically without knowledge of the IgG results. The histological findings were recorded on a standard protocol and plaques were designated "recent", "active" or "inactive" according to the criteria given in Table 3. Many samples showed at least two

TABLE 3

THE RELATIONSHIP BETWEEN PLAQUE HISTOLOGY AND I_gG STUDIES IN MS

PLAQUE CATEGORISATION

"RECENT"	CELLULARITY	↑
	FREE LIPIDS	
	INFLAMMATION	
"ACTIVE"	CELLULARITY N OR ↓	
	FREE LIPIDS	
	INFLAMMATION	
"INACTIVE"	CELLULARITY	↓
	NO FREE LIPIDS	
	NO INFLAMMATION	

GRADINGS

+ → +++	SUBJECTIVE
±	"OF NO SIGNIFICANCE"

phases of demyelination and were included in a combined category. 33 Plaques were assessed. Of these none was categorised as "recent". There were 12 active, 6 showing both active and inactive features and 15 inactive plaques. Histological preservation and histochemical staining was good. There was no significant difference in IgG levels in active and inactive plaques.

SUMMARY AND CONCLUSIONS

The significant finding in this study was the lack of correlation between plaque activity, inflammation and plaque IgG content. Some previous studies have demonstrated immunocompetent cells with the MS plaque and others have shown that IgG can be eluted from plaques. The has led to a false conclusion that the source of IgG within plaques must inevitably be immune-competent cells.

The present study indicates that, while in recent or active lesions, immune-competent cells may make some contribution to the IgG content, in all plaques the astrocytes contain IgG and may be a significant source of the IgG eluted from plaques. The interpretation of these findings will be discussed.

24

Towards Cloning of Lymphoid Cells from Cerebrospinal Fluid

F. ROTTEVEEL, E. BRAAKMAN and C. J. LUCAS

INTRODUCTION

There is little doubt that T cells occur within the sites of inflammatory reactions seen in the central nervous system (CNS) of MS patients. Most probably, there is a relation between lesions of the CNS and the composition of CSF. Indeed, the evidence for involvement of the immune system in the etiology of MS stems from findings on the CSF: the CSF of MS patients has been found to contain IgG of restricted heterogeneity, most of which is synthesized within the CSF (Link, 1967). Moreover, the CSF of MS patients contains lymphoid cells. Many of the T cells present appear to be activated (Noronha et al., 1980).

Analysis of lymphoid cells in the CSF has led to conflicting results. Panitch and Francis (1982) reported that among T cells in the CSF, the proportion of $T8^+$ cells is relatively decreased. Sandberg-Wollheim (1983) also reported decreased $T8^+$ cell numbers but the differences were not significant. Cashman et al. (1982) observed low numbers of $T8^+$ cells only during exacerbations whereas Hauser et al. (1983) observed a normal proportion of $T8^+$ cells among T cells in the CSF. Finally, Hommes and Brinkman (1984) reported that a low proportion of $T8^+$ cells in the CSF is correlated with a high total CSF cell number. Although this finding needs to be confirmed it would lend support to the notion that a low level of suppressor cells (supposedly contained within the $T8^+$ subpopulation of human

T lymphocytes) can be held responsible for both the elevated IgG concentrations and the elevated cell numbers in the CSF.

The data from Hauser et al. (1983) and Weiner et al. (1984) suggest a relation between low T8[+] cell numbers in peripheral blood and a high number of total T lymphocytes in CNS. Such a correlation was not found by Steck and de Flaugergues (1984) and was not mentioned by Hommes and Brinkman (1984).

The study of lymphoid cells in compartmentalized areas (such as the CNS) has been hampered by the extremely small numbers of cells available for study. However, recent advances have made it possible to clone and expand T lymphocytes in the presence of interleukin 2 (Il-2), a T-cell growth factor (MacDonald et al., 1982; Moretta et al., 1983).

The following approaches to grow CSF T cells are possible:

1) Polyclonal activation of 'bulk' cultures (Clark et al., 1984).
2) Selective activation of 'bulk' cultures using specific antigens (Richert et al., 1983; Burns et al., 1984).
3) Culture of lymphocytes at limiting cell numbers in the presence of a polyclonal activator (Fleisher and Bogdahn, 1983).
4) Culture of cells at limiting numbers in the presence of specific antigens.

Recently two studies were reported where CSF cells were first grown in bulk cultures and subsequently cloned (Birnbaum et al., 1984; Santoli et al., 1984). Due to the small amount of published data and the differences in the methods of selection employed, it is not possible at this stage to present even a preliminary description of the types and specificities of T-cell lines or clones derived from MS CSF samples. However, it has already been demonstrated that clonal expansion of T cells from CSF is feasible.

Only few studies have been reported on the analysis of B lymphocytes in the CSF of MS patients. It has been observed that lymphocytes in the CSF contain lower proportions of B cells as compared to peripheral blood (Sandberg-Wollheim, 1974 & 1975; Kam-Hansen, 1980). CSF B lymphocytes can synthesize Ig in vitro (Sandberg-Wollheim, 1975; Henriksson et al., 1981). From the data of Hendriksson et al. (1981) it appears that B cells from CSF contain an increased proportion of cells which are actively synthesizing Ig. Based on the occurrence of oligoclonal IgG, the composition of which is apparently constant over prolonged periods of time, it is assumed that B lymphocytes in the CNS are of limited heterogeneity (Sandberg-Wollheim, 1974). There are indications that distinct heterogeneity patterns occur within each plaque (Mattson et al., 1980). To further elucidate this, it seems worthwhile to try to establish long-term cultures of CSF B lymphocytes.

Potentially the expansion of cloned CSF cells provides a powerful tool to study the immunologically relevant cells in the CSF. We have set out to study the cellular content of the CSF in a way which would allow characterization of a representative sample of the cells. A prerequisite is the availability of a culture method that allows the growth of virtually every single T cell. It would also be necessary to know the conditions to maintain functional activities of cell lines and clones. Currently available cloning procedures tend to favour outgrowth of T4$^+$, helper-type, proliferating cells rather than the T8$^+$ cytotoxic subpopulation.

MATERIALS AND METHODS

Isolation of lymphocytes from CSF. CSF lymphocytes from MS or other patients were obtained by diagnostic lumbar puncture. Approximately 7 ml of CSF was collected in a tube that contained 1 ml of foetal calf serum (FCS). The CSF-FCS mixture was immediately centrifuged. The supernatant (used for further analysis) was removed and the cells were resuspended in RPMI supplemented with 10% FCS. PBL from the same donors were also obtained. PBL were generally obtained by leucophoresis. Mononuclear cells were isolated by flotation on Ficoll/hypaque. All CSF lymphocytes and PBL were cryopreserved. CSF lymphocytes were stored in aliquots of 10^3-10^4 cells. Recovery after thawing was 80-90% and the viability was always greater than 95%.

Cloning of T lymphocytes. Lymphocytes were seeded in wells of Terasaki microtest plates at 1 cell/well in the presence of 10^4 irradiated, autologous PBL in 20 μl of RPMI-1640 medium supplemented with 20% pooled human serum and 15% of an Il-2 containing conditioned medium. To induce polyclonal activation 1% phytohaemagglutinin (PHA) was added. Wells were checked for growth every three days. Growing colonies were transferred to larger wells. From then on the medium was partially replaced every 3 to 4 days. Every 7-10 days irradiated autologous PBL were added as feeder cells.

Using specific stimulation in a similar protocol (omitting the PHA) we obtained specific T cell clones from antigen exposed bulk cultures. The autologous feeder cells are antigen-pulsed, virus-infected (measles virus or influenza virus) or virus-transformed.

RESULTS

Efficiency of polyclonal activation of single cell culture. Peripheral
blood lymphocytes from several donors were cultured at 1 cell/well (average) in the presence of 1% PHA and 15% Con-A supernatant as a source of
Il-2. A representative experiment is shown in Table 1. When taking into
account that the PBL sample contains approximately 70% T cells, the cloning efficiency can be estimated (using Poissons formula) to be around 50%.
When stained with anti-T4 or -T8 monoclonal antibodies the majority of the
clones proved to be T4$^+$.

TABLE 1.   CLONING EFFICIENCY WITH PHA and Il-2
          Number of wells with cell growth in a total of 240 wells*

Donor	D10	D11	D12	P11
	56	70	46	47

*PBL were plated at 1 cell/well (average)

Establishment and maintenance of cloned T cell lines. Although clones of
functional T lymphocytes can readily be grown, the maintenance of functionally active T cell clones is not always successful. We have been able
to prepare several antigen-specific proliferating cells which can serve as
positive controls in CSF T cell cloning studies. It has proved more difficult to establish and maintain specific cytotoxic cells. The time and time
interval of antigen presentation, the dose of antigen and the time of addition and the amount of Il-2 added, all appear to affect growth patterns
and functional cytotoxic activities. We found that re-exposure to the relevant antigen or addition of Il-2 can prolong cytolytic activities (Table
2A). Furthermore, we have observed that during a second cycle of antigen
presentation and addition of growth factor optimal results are obtained if
the addition of Il-2 is postponed 48 hours after addition of antigen
(Table 2B) which might be explained by increases in the level of Il-2
receptor expression. Using a protocol based on these findings we have suc-
cessfully prepared measles virus, influenza virus and Epstein Barr virus
specific cloned cytotoxic T cell lines.

TABLE 2.

A. MAINTENANCE OF CYTOTOXIC ACTIVITIES IN VITRO. EFFECT OF
   RE-EXPOSURE TO ANTIGEN-PULSED CELLS OR Il-2.

	Day of assay	LU/culture
restimulated day 7	14	<1
Il-2 day 7	14	82
restimulated day 10	14	10
Il-2 day 10	14	950

B. ADDITION OF Il-2 AFTER ANTIGEN RE-EXPOSURE APPEARS TO
   RESULT IN OPTIMAL RESTIMULATION

Ag	Il-2	Day of assay	LU/culture
10	8	11	0
10	10	13	16
10	12	15 .	129

Analysis of cells in CSF of an SSPE patient. CSF cells from an SSPE patient were stored in liquid nitrogen. After thawing cells were plated at
1 and 5 cells per well in the presence of PHA and Il-2. In addition, cells
were plated at 3 cells/well in the presence of measles virus-infected autologous antigen presenting cells. The remainder of the CSF cells were
cultured with measles virus-infected cells. No clones were obtained from
the cultures with measles virus. Approximately 150 clones were obtained
from the cultures which were stimulated with PHA. None could be shown to
proliferate in response to measles virus antigens and none of the clones
could kill measles virus-infected autologous target cells.

DISCUSSION

Only few studies have dealt with long-term growth of CSF T cells.
Clark et al. (1984), who made no attempts to clone, obtained several cell
lines, most of which had the $T3^+,T4^+$ phenotype. Birnbaum et al. (1984) and
Santoli et al. (1984) grew CSF cells in bulk culture and obtained a number
of clones from these bulk cultures that displayed alloreactivity or natural killer activity. Richert et al. (1983) obtained MBP-specific and
measles-specific T cell lines from the CSF of MS patients. However, the

fact that Burns et al. (1984) succeeded to obtain a tetanus-specific T cell line from CSF lymphocytes, indicates that mere selection of an antigen-specific T cell should be considered with caution. As far as we know the approach used by Fleisher and Bogdahn (1983) to use polyclonal activation of single cell cultures has not yet been exploited for MS-CSF cell study. Clearly, it is easier to follow such an approach with a CSF sample from a meningitis patient where the antigens of the responsible pathogen are known. We have shown that such an approach is feasible and that a large number of clones can be generated. We obtained $T4^+$ and $T8^+$ cytotoxic cell lines. So far we have not yet succeeded in obtaining an MBP-specific clone with cells from two different CSF samples from MS patients. Unfortunately such a comprehensive analysis of CSF cells cannot be done with more than a few CSF samples. Also it remains to be shown that at the level of a cloning efficiency of 50%, as we currently achieve, the growing cells are indeed representative.

Although the development of long-term growth of T cell clones using interleukin-2 will undoubtedly broaden our insight into the nature of lymphoid cells in CSF, one should realize the limitations. At the moment we can only hope that the use of this technique will help to identify the specific antigens involved in the etiology and pathogenesis of multiple sclerosis. It seems likely that cloning efficiency and growth patterns will vary from patient to patient and for a given patient will vary in time. The expected differences between patients necessitates population studies which have to be done in multicentre cooperation, by which exchange of control cell lines would facilitate analysis of the cell lines obtained.

ACKNOWLEDGEMENT: This study was supported by a grant from FUNGO (no. 13-40-05) to Francien Rotteveel and by a grant from the Princess Beatrix Fund to Eric Braakman.

REFERENCES
Birnbaum, G., Kotilinek, L., Schwartz, M. and Sternad, M., 1984. Spinal fluid lymphocytes responsive to autologous and allogenic cells in multiple sclerosis and control individuals. J. Clin. Invest., 74: 1307-1317.
Burns, J., Zwerman, B. and Lisak, R., 1984. Tetanus toxoid reactive T lym-

phocytes in the cerebrospinal fluid of multiple sclerosis patients. Immunol. Commun., 13: 361-369.

Cashman, N., Martin, C., Eizenbaum, J-F., Degos, J-D. and Bach, M-A., 1982. Monoclonal antibody-defined immunoregulatory cells in multiple sclerosis cerebrospinal fluid. J. Clin. Invest., 70: 387-392.

Clark, R.B., Dore-Duffy, P., Donaldson, J.O., Pollard, M.K. and Muirhead, S.P., 1984. Generation of phenotypic helper/inducer and suppressor/ cytotoxic T-cell lines from cerebrospinal fluid in multiple sclerosis. Cell. Immunol., 84: 409-414.

Fleisher, B. and Bogdahn, U., 1983. Growth of antigen specific, HLA restricted T lymphocyte clones from cerebrospinal fluid. Clin. Exp. Immunol., 52: 38-44.

Hauser, S.L., Reinherz, E.L., Hoban, C.J., Schlossman, S.F. and Weiner, H.L., 1983. CSF cells in multiple sclerosis: monoclonal antibody analysis and relationship to peripheral blood T-cell subsets. Neurology, 33: 575-579.

Henriksson, A., Kam-Hansen, S. and Andersson, R., 1981. Immunoglobulin-producing cells in CSF and blood from patients with multiple sclerosis and other inflammatory neurological diseases enumerated by protein-A plaque assay. J. Neuroimmunol., 1: 299-309.

Hommes, O.R. and Brinkman, C.J.J., 1984. T-cell subsets in spinal fluid of multiple sclerosis patients. J. Neuroimmunol., 6: 123-130.

Kam-Hansen, S., 1980. Distribution of lymphocytes from the cerebrospinal fluid and blood in patients with multiple sclerosis. Acta Neurol. Scand., 62: suppl. 75.

Link, H., 1967. Immunoglobulin G and low molecular weight proteins in human cerebrospinal fluid - chemical and immunological characterization with special reference to multiple sclerosis. Acta Neurol. Scand., 43: suppl. 28.

Mattson, D.H., Roos, R.P. and Arnason, B.G.W., 1980. Isoelectric focusing of IgG eluted from multiple sclerosis and subacute sclerosing panencephalitis brains. Nature, 287: 335-337.

MacDonald, H.R., Sekaly, R.P., Kanagawa, O., Thiernesse, N., Taswell, C., Cerottini, J-C., Weiss, A., Glasebrook, A.L., Engers, H.D., Kelso, A., Brunner, K.T. and Bron, C., 1982. Cytolytic T lymphocyte clones. Immunobiol., 161: 84-106.

Moretta, A., Pantaleo, G., Moretta, L., Cerottini, J-C. and Mingari, M.C., 1983. Direct demonstration of the clonogenic potential of every human peripheral blood T cell. J. Exp. Med., 157: 743-754.

Noronha, A.B.C., Richman, D.P. and Arnason, B.G.W., 1980. Detection of in vivo stimulated cerebrospinal fluid lymphocytes by flow cytometry in patients with multiple sclerosis. New Engl. J. Med., 303: 713-717.

Paniteh, H.S. and Francis, G.S., 1982. T-lymphocyte subsets in cerebrospinal fluid in multiple sclerosis. New Engl. J. Med., 307: 560-561.

Richert, J.R., McFarlin, E.E., Rose, J.W., McFarland, H.F. and Greenstein, J.I., 1983. Expansion of antigen-specific T cells from cerebrospinal fluid of patients with multiple sclerosis. J. Neuroimmunol., 5: 317-324.

Sandberg-Wollheim, M., 1974. Immunoglobulin synthesis in vitro by cerebrospinal fluid cells in patients with multiple sclerosis. Scand. J. Immunol., 3: 717-730.

Sandberg-Wollheim, M. and Turesson, I., 1975. Lymphocyte subpopulations in the cerebrospinal fluid and peripheral blood in patients with multiple sclerosis. Scand. J. Immunol., 4: 831-836.

Sandberg-Wollheim, M., 1983. Lymphocyte populations in the cerebrospinal fluid and peripheral blood of patients with multiple sclerosis and optic neuritis. Scand. J. Immunol., 17: 575-581.

Santoli, D. Defreitas, E.C., Sandberg-Wollheim, M., Francis, M.K. and Koprowski, H., 1984. Phenotypic and functional characterization of T cell clones derived from the cerebrospinal fluid of multiple sclerosis patients. J. Immunol., 132: 2386-2392.

Steck, A.J. and de Flaugergues, J-C., 1984. Local and systemic immune response in multiple sclerosis: analysis of CSF inflammatory changes and peripheral blood T-cell subsets. J. Neurol., 231: 126-129.

Werner, H.L., Hafler, D.A., Fallis, R.J., Johnson, D., Ault, K.A. and Hauser, S.L., 1984. Altered blood T-cell subsets in patients with multiple sclerosis. J. Neuroimmunol., 6: 115-121.

25

Activation of Natural Cytotoxic Activity *In Vitro* with Lymphocytes from Patients with Multiple Sclerosis

E. BRAAKMAN, A. VAN TUNEN and C. J. LUCAS

INTRODUCTION

Natural killer (NK) cells are defined as lymphocytes with the capacity to lyse certain tumor cells and virus-infected cells without prior
immunization (Herbermann and Holden, 1978). These cells constitute a heterogeneous subset of the lymphoid cell population. It has been demonstrated
that interferon (IFN) plays an important role in the regulation of NK activity (Ortaldo et al., 1983). Recently, it has been demonstrated that
interleukin-2 (Il-2) can also enhance NK cell activity (Grimm et al., 1983;
Devos et al., 1984). Furthermore Il-2 has an important role in the regulation of IFNγ production (Kawase et al., 1983). This was confirmed with
pure recombinant Il-2 by Svedersky et al., 1984 and by ourselves. Although
the role of the endogenously produced IFNγ in the augmentation of NK activity by Il-2 has been a controversial issue, there is increasing evidence
that the enhancement of NK activity by Il-2 is only partly mediated by
IFNγ (Svedersky et al., 1984; Braakman et al., manuscript in preparation).
Although the precise mechanisms by which NK activity are regulated remain
to be established it is attractive to hypothesize that NK cells play a
significant role in the natural resistance against virus infections. Among
the immunoregulatory abnormalities in MS patients it has been reported
that NK activity is decreased (Benczur et al., 1980; Hauser et al., 1981;

Uchida et al., 1982, and Neighbour et al., 1982) and that IFN production
is impaired (Neighbour and Bloom, 1979, and Benczur et al., 1980).

In this report we have studied the endogenous NK activity and the NK
activity augmented by recombinant Il-2 and recombinant IFNγ in lymphoid
cells from 40 MS patients in comparison with 40 age and sex matched healthy controls. Possible mechanisms of dysregulation of NK activity in MS
patients will be discussed.

PATIENTS AND METHODS

Patients and healthy donors. Patients came from three neurological clinics.
The cooperation of Drs van Walbeek, Koetsier and Sanders from respectively:
Onze Lieve Vrouwengasthuis, The Free University Hospital, both in Amsterdam, and the Academic Hospital Leiden, is gratefully acknowledged. In all
patients a definite diagnosis of MS was established. The median age of the
patients was 41, the youngest being 23, the oldest 62. The group includes
23 females and 17 males. Twenty-three patients had the chronic progressive
form of the disease. At the time of study none of the patients were treated with corticosteroids or other immunosuppressive agents. Fourty healthy blood donors matched for age and sex were used as controls.

Culture conditions and NK assay. All experiments were performed with peripheral blood lymphocytes (PBL) that had been stored in liquid nitrogen.
Cells were cultured in RPMI 1640 supplemented with 2 mM L glutamine, 100
U/ml penicillin, 100 µg/ml streptomycin and 6% pooled human plasma at a
concentration of $2-10^6$ cells/ml in a volume of 2 ml. Endogenous NK activity was measured on the next day. K562 cells were used as target cells in
a 5-hr chromium release assay.

Treatment with rec Il-2 and rec IFNγ. Recombinant human interferon-γ was
a gift from Boehringer. Recominant human Il-2 (Batch 37 B, Biogen S.A.,
Geneva, Switzerland) was a generous gift from Dr. W. Friers, Ghent,
through Dr. H. Schellekens, Primate center TNO, Rijswijk, The Netherlands.
At the onset of culture 50 U/ml rec Il-2 or 50 U/ml rec IFNγ was added.
The NK activity was then measured on day 4.

Statistics. The nonparametric method of Mann Whitney was applied to perform the statistical analysis. Significance was accepted throughout at the
P<0.05 level.

RESULTS

Endogenous NK activity. PBL from 40 MS patients and 40 age and sex matched healthy controls were tested for endogenous or spontaneous NK activity on K562 target cells. The endogenous NK activity of each individual patient or control donor at an effector to target (E/T) ratio of 40:1 is shown in Figure 1. It can be seen that extensive variation in the level of endogenous NK activity exists between individual patients as well as between individual controls. Statistical analysis reveals that the group of MS patients have a significantly lower (p=0.03) endogenous NK activity than the healthy control group.

Fig. 1. Endogenous, Il-2- and IFNγ augmented NK activity of MS patients and healthy controls.

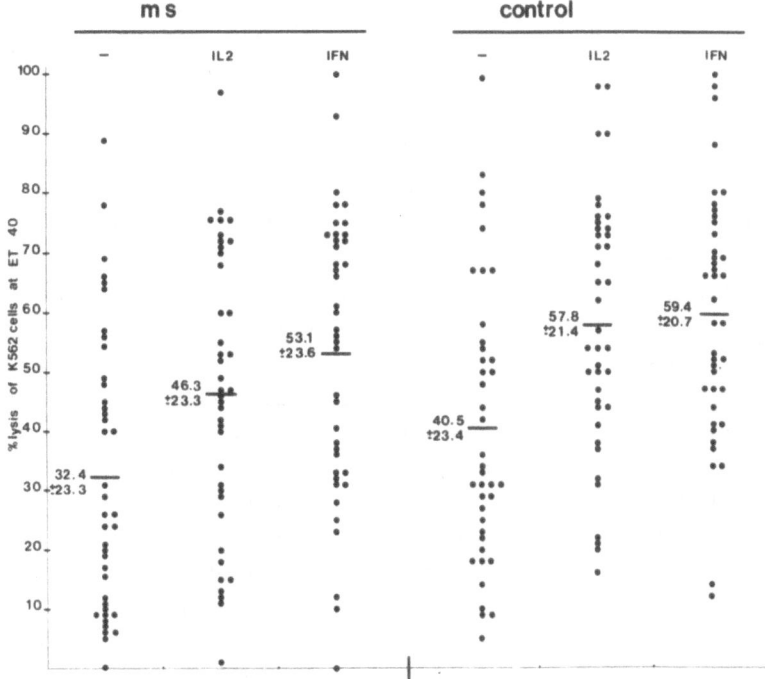

Each dot represents the endogenous, Il-2- or IFNγ augmented NK activity of one MS patient or healthy donor. Data are given as percentage lysis of K562 at an E/T ratio of 40:1.

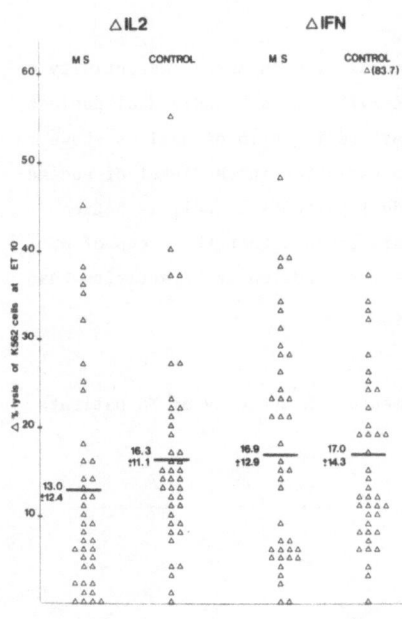

Fig. 2. Augmentation of NK activity induced by Il-2 and IFN in MS patients and healthy controls

Increment is given at an E/T ratio of 10:1. Each triangle represents the difference between the augmented NK activity and the endogenous NK activity on day 4.

NK activity augmented by Il-2 and IFNγ. Previous studies from this laboratory showed that Il-2 and IFNγ can enhance NK activity in cultures of lymphoid cells of healthy blood donors. Part of the enhancing effect of Il-2 on NK activity is mediated by the endogenously produced IFNγ and part is direct activation of NK precursor cells by Il-2 in an IFNγ-independent way. The NK activity of MS patients can also be enhanced by Il-2 and IFNγ (Fig. 1). The NK activity enhanced by Il-2 is significantly lower in MS patients than in controls (p=0.03). In contrast, the NK activity generated after 4 days of culture in the presence of IFNγ did not significantly differ between patients and controls (p=0.13). Figure 2 shows the increase by Il-2 and by IFNγ for each individual. Each triangle represents the difference between the NK activity after culture in the presence of Il-2 or IFNγ and the endogenous NK activity on day 4 of one given cell sample from a patient or a control individual. Since in a number of cultures the cytotoxic activity at a 40:1 E/T ratio could be at or near the plateau level, we have calculated the increment seen with Il-2 or IFNγ for the data obtained at an E/T ratio of 10:1. NK activity of nearly all patients and controls can be enhanced by both Il-2 and IFNγ. It can be seen that there are more low responders to Il-2 in the MS group compared to the healthy control group. This results in a significantly smaller increase of NK activity due to Il-2 treatment in the group of MS patients than in the controls (p= 0.02). However, there is no difference in the increase of NK activity by IFNγ between MS patients and controls (p=0.48).

An association of low NK activity with the presence of HLA DR2 has been suggested by Benczur et al., 1980. This could not be confirmed by Hauser et al., 1981. We have compared DR2[+] MS patients with DR2[-] MS patients. No differences were observed between these two groups with respect to endogenous NK activity or NK activity enhanced by Il-2 (Table I). Merrill et al., 1982, reported an association of low NK activity with the active and chronic form of MS whereas stable MS patients were similar to the control group. In our group of 40 MS patients, no differences were observed between chronic progressive and stable MS patients with respect to endogenous NK activity or NK activity enhanced by Il-2 (Table I).

TABLE I. NK activity in different patient groups.

Group	No. of Patients	Endogenous NK	Il-2 augmented NK
Dr2[-]	15	35.1 ± 22.4	41.7 ± 23.2
Dr2[+]	18	32.6 ± 17.3	42.0 ± 22.0
Chronic			
progressive	22	34.4 ± 20.5	43.1 ± 19.7
Remission	16	35.0 ± 24.0	45.5 ± 27.3

NK activities of lymphocytes from several groups MS patients before and after stimulation with Il-2. Data are presented as percentage lysis of K562 cells at an E/T ratio of 40:1. Analysis of data at 10:1 E/T gave similar results.

DISCUSSION

Our data confirm that endogenous NK activity of PBL of MS patients is significantly lower than that of healthy controls. In addition, we have shown that PBL of MS patients are poor responders to Il-2. Or, perhaps more to the point, a greater number of MS patients respond poorly to Il-2 than controls do. The low endogenous NK cell function and the diminished enhancement after Il-2 exposure may be ascribed to a defective response to Il-2 which could lead to defective IFNγ production. Alternatively, it is possible that addition of Il-2 results in adequate amounts of newly syn-

thesized IFNγ but that the response of the cells to IFNγ with regard to NK
induction is impaired in PBL from MS patients. A poor response to IFNγ
seems unlikely since PBL of MS patients can respond equally well to exogenous IFNγ as controls (Fig. 2). Hence, we would favour the notion that
leukocytes from MS patients have a low direct response to IL-2 both in
terms of produced IFNγ as well as in terms of induction of NK activity. In
agreement with the hypothesis of a decreased direct response to Il-2 in MS
patients is a recent report of Merrill et al., 1984, who showed a reduced
proliferative response to Il-2 in PBL of MS patients. At least three explanations, not mutually exclusive, can be given for the diminished responsiveness to Il-2. First, the number of actually responding cells to
Il-2 can be lower. There seems to be, however, no difference in the percentage of Il-2 receptor bearing cells among PBL of MS patients compared
to controls (Merrill et al., 1984). Nearly all functional human NK cells
are IgG Fc receptor positive (Santoli et al., 1978) and part of the NK
precursor cells sensitive for Il-2 are FcR$^+$ (Braakman et al., manuscript
in preparation). Literature data on the percentage FcR$^+$ cells in MS patients are inconclusive. We did not observe a significantly lower number
of FcR$^+$ cells in peripheral blood of MS patients (data not shown). Nevertheless, the endogenous and the Il-2 augmented NK activity is lower in MS
patients as a group. A second possibility is that in MS patients certain
inhibitory factors such as prostaglandin E (PGE) are produced in higher
quantities both in vivo and in vitro and/or NK cells and T cells from MS
patients could be more sensitive to the effects of PGE (Merrill et al.,
1983a,b). Also higher concentrations of immune complexes in serum of MS
patients could interfere with the activation or lytic activity of NK cells
by binding to FcR$^+$ cells. A third possibility to explain the low responsiveness of PBL from MS patients to Il-2 with respect to the augmentation
of NK activity is that MS patients have more NK cell specific suppressor
cells, as described by Zöller and Wigzell, 1982, than healthy controls. As
far as we know, no data are available on these suppressor cells in MS
patients.

It was suggested that IFN production by PBL of MS patients is decreased. Most data concern the production of IFNα. Neighbour and Bloom,
1979, described lower IFN production in response to measles virus and
Benczur et al., 1980, described lower IFN production in response to poly
IC. Santoli et al., 1981, reported normal IFN production in response to a

variety of viruses. Preliminary data from the 40 MS patients we studied, suggest a lower IFNγ production in response to exogenous recombinant human Il-2 (data not shown), which in itself supports the hypothesis that leucocytes from MS patients respond poorly to Il-2; in other words, the low IFN production is only a secondary result of low reactivity to Il-2 (Merrill et al., 1984; this paper).

In conclusion, a primary low response of PBL from MS patients to Il-2 results in low Il-2 augmented NK activity. A similar mechanism could be the cause of the low endogenous reactivity. The lower Il-2 induced NK activity can result from a defect at two different levels, the IFNγ dependent and the IFNγ independent induction pathways. These conclusions are based solely on analysis of a group of patients and controls both of which show extensive variation between individuals. Whether therefore these conclusions still hold for individual MS patients remains to be established. Currently we are investigating the relative contribution to augmentation of NK activity of the IFNγ dependent and the IFNγ independent pathways of activation in individual patients. It could be that the relative contributions are distorted in MS patients.

One of the prominent hypotheses on the etiology of MS is a persistent virus infection. An important role in the in vivo resistance against virus infections has been contributed to NK cell function (Rager-Zisman and Bloom, 1980). Therefore, it could be that low NK cel function and diminished IFN production play a role in the etiology of MS as one of the predisposing factors making an individual susceptible to MS.

ACKNOWLEDGEMENTS: The authors thank Drs van Walbeek, Koetsier and Sanders for providing us with blood samples from MS patients. This study was supported by the Princes Beatrix Fonds.

REFERENCES

Benczur, M., Petrányi, G.Gy., Palffy, Gy., Varga, M., Talas, M., Kotsy, B., Foldes, I. and Holden, S.R., 1980. Dysfunction of natural killer cells in multiple sclerosis: a possible pathogenic factor. Clin. Exp. Immunol., 39: 657-662.

Devos, R., Plaetinck, G. and Fiers, W., 1984. Induction of cytolytic cells by pure recombinant human interleukin 2. Eur. J. Immunol., 14: 1057-1060.

Grimm, E.A., Robb, R.J., Roth, J.A., Neckers, L.M., Lachmann, L.B., Wilson, D.J. and Rosenberg, S.A., 1983. Lymphokine activated killer cell phenomenon. III. Evidence that Il-2 is sufficient for direct activation of peripheral blood lymphocytes into lymphokine-activated killer cells. J. Exp. Med., 158: 1356-1361.

Hauser, S.L., Ault, K.A., Levin, M.J., Garovoy, M.R. and Weiner, H.L., 1981. Natural killer cell activity in multiple sclerosis. J. Immunol., 127: 1114-1117.

Herbermann, R.B. and Holden, H.T., 1978. Natural cell mediated immunity. Adv. Cancer Res., 27: 305.

Kawase, I., Brooks, C.G., Kuribayashi, K., Olabuenaga, S., Newman, W., Gillis, S. and Henney, C.S., 1983. Interleukin 2 induces γ interferon production: participation of macrophages and NK-like cells. J. Immunol., 131: 288-292.

Merrill, J.E., Jondal, M., Seeley, J., Ullberg, M. and Sidén, A., 1982. Decreased NK killing in patients with multiple sclerosis: An analysis on the level of the single effector cell in peripheral blood and cerebrospinal fluid in relation to the activity of the disease. Clin. Exp. Immunol., 47: 419-430.

Merrill, J.E., Myers, L.W. and Ellison, W., 1983a. Regulation of natural killer cell cytotoxicity by prostaglandin E in the peripheral blood and cerebrospinal fluid of patients with multiple sclerosis and other neurological diseases. Part 2. Effect of exogenous PGE_1 on spontaneous and interferon induced natural killer. J. Neuroimmunol., 4: 239-251.

Merrill, J.E., Gerner, R.H., Myers, L.W. and Ellison, G.W., 1983b. Regulation of natural killer cell cytotoxicity by prostaglandin E in the peripheral blood and cerebrospinal fluid of patients with multiple sclerosis and other neurological diseases. Part 1. Association between amount of prostaglandin produced, natural killer, and endogenous interferon. J. Neuroimmunol., 4: 223-237.

Merrill, J.E., Mohlstrom, C., Uittenbogaart, C., Kermaniarab, V., Ellison, G.W. and Myers, L.W., 1984. Response to and production of interleukin 2 by peripheral blood and cerebrospinal fluid lymphocytes of patients with multiple sclerosis. J. Immunol., 133: 1931-1937.

Neighbour, P.A. and Bloom, B.R., 1979. Absence of virus induced lymphocyte suppression and interferon production in multiple sclerosis. Proc. Natl. Acad. Sci. USA, 76: 476-480.

Neighbour, P.A., Graynel, A.I. and Miller, A.E., 1982. Endogenous and interferon-augmented natural killer cell activity of human peripheral blood mononuclear cells in vitro. Studies of patients with multiple sclerosis, systemic lupus erythematosus or rheumatoid arthritis. Clin. Exp. Immunol., 49: 11-21.

Ortaldo, J.R., Mantovani, A., Hobbs, D., Rubinstein, M., Pestka, S. and Herbermann, R.B., 1983. Effects of several species of human leukocyte interferon on cytotoxic activity of NK cells and monocytes. Int. J. Cancer, 31: 285-289.

Rager-Zisman, B. and Bloom, B.R., 1980. Natural killer cells in resistance to virus-infected cells. Springer Sem. Immunopathol., 4: 397-414.

Santoli, D., Trinchieri, G., Moretta, L., Zmijewski, C.M. and Koprowski, H., 1978. Spontaneous cell-mediated cytotoxicity in humans. Distribution and characterization of the effector cell. Clin. Exp. Immunol., 33: 309-318.

Santoli, D., Hall, W., Kastrukoff, L., Lisak, R.P., Perussia, B., Trinchieri, G. and Koprowski, H., 1981. Cytotoxic activity and interferon production by lymphocytes from patients with multiple sclerosis. J. Immunol., 126: 1274-1278.

Svedersky, L.P., Shepard, H.M., Spencer, S.A., Shalaby, M.R. and Palladine, M.A., 1984. Augmentation of human natural cell mediated cytotoxicity by recombinant human interleukin 2. J. Immunol., 133: 714-718.

Uchida, A., Maida, E.M., Lenzhofer, R. and Micksche, M., 1982. Natural killer cell activity in patients with multiple sclerosis: Interferon and plasmaphoresis. Immunobiol., 160: 392-402.

Zöller, M. and Wigzell, H., 1982. Normally occurring inhibitory cells for natural killer cell activity. II. Characterization of the inhibitory cell. Cell. Immunol., 74: 27-39.

26

Molecular and Cellular Basis of Autoimmune Encephalitogenesis

H. WEKERLE

Many distinct lines of evidence suggest that immunopathological mechanisms are involved in onset und course of multiple sclerosis (MS). As examples, abnormally distributed immunoglobulins in the cerebrospinal fluid, shifts in T lymphocyte subset equilibria, and abnormalities in natural killer functions are commonly cited (McFarlin & McFarland, 1982; Waksman, 1983; Weiner & Hauser, 1982). Perhaps the most impressing argument in favor of an immunopathogenesis is, however, the morphological appearance of the MS lesion within the CNS white matter. Focal round cell infiltrations mainly around postcapillary venules, activation of astrocytes, and destruction of myelin are the key features. A practically identical lesion pattern is inducible by immunizing experimental animals with autologous white matter (Lassmann, 1983). The similarity between the inducible experimental autoimmune diesease and MS are so far the most compelling evidence for autoimmune mechanisms in the pathogenesis of MS.

In an attempt to learn more about the structural requirements of CNS autoimmunity, and, more generally, about the cellular organisation of the physiological immune responsiveness within the CNS, we made use of a transfer model of acute rat EAE. In this model, highly defined permanent T lymphocyte lines specific for circumscript molecular portions of myelin basic proteins are used as highly pathogenic encephalitogens, and as probes to study the cascade of events leading to CNS autoimmune disease.

MBP Specific T Lymphocyte Lines

Permanent T lymphocyte lines recognizing MBP or other protein antigens were first isolated from in vivo primed inbred rats by Ben-Nun et al. (1981). This method relies on strong positive selection pressures required to single out oligo-and monoclonal T cell populations from the natural repertoire. A first enrichment of antigen positive cells is reached by in vivo priming. In a second step, the primed lymph nodes are dissociated, and the cells exposed in vitro to the relevant antigen. Only specific T cells transform to activated blasts, and these can be selected by density gradient centrifugation. The third selection step makes use of the fact that activated rat T cells express much higher densities of receptors for interleukin-2 (Il-2)than inactive T lymphocytes (Osawa & Diamantstein, 1983). Freshly isolated T cells are incubated in IL-2 containing propagation medium, which leads to continous proliferation of the activated cells, and an out-dilution of the nonactivated ones. Stabile, specific T populations are established by repeated cycles of antigen-dependent restimulation of the T populations interchanging with IL-2 driven propagation in the absence of antigen or antigen presenter cells.

Genetic Control of Potentially Autoimmune T Lymphocytes within the T Lymphocyte Repertoire.

It has been known for many years that among all rat strains tested, only very few are susceptible to induction of EAE by active immunization. It is further known, that susceptibility and resistance to EAE is genetically controlled and that control is exerted by genes situated within the Major Histocompatibility Complex (MHC), Ir genes, as well as genes located in the non-MHC genetic "background". Both types of genes cooperate to render rats of strain Lewis highly susceptible, and BN rats resistant to active indcution of EAE (Gasser et al., 1975; Günther et al., 1978).

Attempts to select MBP-specific, encephalitogenic T cell lines from immunized BN rats failed in most laboratories (Ben-Nun & Cohen, 1982). The cells selected were able to recognize certain MBP structures, but were unable to mediate disease. This apparent absence of encephalitogenic T clones in immunized BN rats could be the result of active suppression by suppressor T cells during the immune response. More recent work, focussed on in vitro selection of MBP specific T lines from completely normal, unprimed BN rat lymph nodes, was, however, equally unable to produce MBP specific T lines transferring EAE. There is the possibility that the natural T cell repertoire of BN rats, in contrast to Lewis rats, has only a very small proportion of potentially autoaggressive MBP-specific T clones, and that the relative content of encephalitogenic clones is subject to genetic control (Schlüsener & Wekerle, submitted).

This notion is further supported by the functional properties of T lymphocyte lines selected from (Lewis x BN)F1 hybrid animals. F1-derived T lines recognize their antigen as all other T lymphocyte populations only if presented by presenter cells sharing at least one set of MHC antigens. Thus, F1 T lines recognizing tuberculin can be activated by syngeneic F1 presenter cells, but also by both types of parental presenters. In contrast, MBP-specific F1 T line cells recognize MBP only if presented by either F1 or by Lewis presenters. MBP on BN presenter cells is not recognized.

When the antigen fine specificity of these clones is tested using defined peptide fragments of the MBP molecule, it becomes clear that the F1 and Lewis T lines recognizing MBP on F1 or Lewis presenter cells all are specific for the same molecular epitope, the encephalitogenic peptide for Lewis rats defined by amino acid positions 68-88. All these T lines are efficient mediators of EAE. The few BN lines responding to MBP, recognize distinct epitopes on MBP; they all are unable to transfer EAE.

These results suggest that a) normal immune systems may include substantial numbers of potentially encephalitogenic cells in the physiological state; b) since a normal rat does not undergo spontaneous EAE, the potentially autoreactive cells must be controlled by regulatory mechanisms; c) different individuals may have varying proportions of potentially autoaggressive T clones in their T repertoire, and this distribution seems to be regulated by genes of the MHC.

Homing of Autoaggressive T Cells to their Target Organs.

In the T line transfer models of EAE, the pathogenic cells are activated in vitro, injected intravenously, and cause overt disease usually within 3-4 days. There must be mechanisms, enabling the circulating T cells to specifically retrieve their relevant target tissues, since the homing specificity is remarkable. As described, MBP-specific T lines almost exclusively cause lesions within the CNS, but normally spare the PNS. In contrast, T lines, which were recently selected for reactivity to the peripheral nerve myelin protein P2 (Linington et al., 1984; Izumo et al., in press), exclusively migrate to and destroy peripheral nerves.

It appears that elements of the blood brain barrier (BBB) are actively involved in target retrieval by autoaggressive T lymphocytes. The essential role of the BBB was demonstrated recently, when equal doses of encephalitogenic T line cells were injected either into the cerebrospinal fluid space, or into the blood circulation. Surprisingly, only those animals developed EAE, which were injected i.v. The intrathecally injected animals failed to develop any demonstrable clinical symptoms. A histological analysis revealed that i. th. injected cells did not directly invade the brain parenchyme, but rather entered the meningeal blood vessels. Having circulated through the blood stream, these cells seemed to reenter the CNS via the "front door", the BBB. Their number or their state of activation may have become insufficient to cause transfer-EAE, as did the directly i.v. injected cells (Lassmann & Wekerle, in preparation).

If the BBB is essential for target retrieval of encephalitogenic cells, where is the signal of specificity localized? The first cellular candidate is the endothelial surface directly lining the cerebral blood vessels. Indeed, it has been reported that under certain conditions, endothelial cells can be induced to express Ia determinants and to immunogenically present antigen to T cells (Hirschberg et al., 1980; Pober et al., 1983). In the normal brain myelin products could be expressed along with Ia determinants on endothelial cells, and could be thus specifically guide the circulating cells into the white matter. So far, however, no traces of Ia have been demonstrable on endothelium either of normal or of EAE rat brains (Wekerle, 1984). Ia determinants, where, however, densely expressed on pericytic elements of EAE lesions (Vass et al., submitted). Second, only activated, but not resting T line cells are able to penetrate the BBB and to retrieve the white matter (Naparstek et al., 1983). If MBP/Ia recognition were the signal of entry, resting cells should recognize the antigen complex as well as activated blasts.

Recent work has, however, established that activated T blasts have unusual enzymatic activities, which enable them to cross endothelial layers with high efficiency. When cultured with xenogeneic endothelial monolayers, rat and mouse activated T lymphocytes have the tendency to attach to the endothelial surfaces, and to cross the monolayers (Savion et al., 1984; Naparstek et al., 1984). It is possible that proteolytic enzymes are involved in temporarily opening intercellular tight junctions, which are of particular importance in the BBB. In addition activated T blasts produce glycosidases which can locally digest basal laminas. It is possible that activated T blasts behave in a similar manner in the CNS as well, and that their passage through the endothelial part of the BBB is nonspecific.

The Pivotal Role of the Astrocyte in T Cell Homing and Symptom Generation.

A possible clue for the localization of the tissue specific signal comes from studies from our laboratory, where pure monolayer cultures of Lewis rat astrocytes were tested for their capacity to present antigen to syngeneic T line cells. These studies were based on preceding observations by Fontana, that T cells and astrocytes can interact in a bidirectional way. Astrocytes on the one hand can secrete interleukin-1 which is a mediator participating in T cell activation (Fontana et al., 1981), and conversely, activated T cells release mediators activating astrocytes (Fontana et al., 1982). For example, T cell-derived interferon-γ induces Ia antigens on astrocytes, which normally are negative (Hirsch et al., 1983; Wong et al., 1984).

T line cells which are incubated on syngeneic astrocytes in the absence of specific antigen, loosely attach to the astrocyte surfaces and seem to migrate on top of the monolayers. After addition of antigen, the T cells become immediately firmly attached, and within 24 hrs., they are fully activated to morphological transformation and proliferation. Antigen presentation obeys all rules of T cell recognition: it is antigen dose dependent and MHC-restricted, and contact dependent. It was found that during antigen presentation, Ia antigens were induced on the membranes of astrocytes. It is at present not yet clear, whether resting astrocytes have low doses of membrane Ia undetectable by conventional immunocytochemical techniques, or whether they are completely negative (Fierz et al., in press).

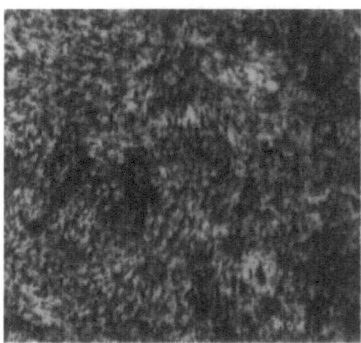 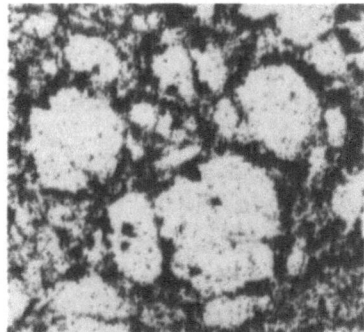

Fig. 1

Lysis of MBP-presenting astrocytes by syngeneic encephalitogenic T line cells in vitro. Brain-derived astrocytes from newborn Lewis rats were induced to express Ia by immune interferon containing medium were cultured with syngeneic MBP-specific, encephalitogenic T line cells in absence (left) and presence of soluble MBP (5μg/ml; right).

A more profound role of antigen presenting astrocytes in the generation the EAE symptoms was revealed by very recent experiments by D. Sun, which were based on the morphological observation that during antigen recognition, astrocytes are radically lysed by the recognizing MBP-specific, encephalitogenic T line cells (Fig. 1). Applying a conventional isotope release test , it was found that astrocyte lysis was exquisitely antigen-dependent, and Ia-restricted. The most surprising finding was, however, that only encephalitogenic T line cells lyse the antigen presenting astrocytes. T line cells recognizing other proteins, such as ovalbumin or tuberculin, fully activated by the antigen presenting astrocytes, but fail completely to lyse the presenter cells (Sun & Wekerle, submitted).

It is tempting to speculate about the possibly dual role of the astrocytes in the pathogenesis of CNS autoimmune disease. On the one hand, as in vitro, astrocytes could be the antigen presenting cells in the CNS as well. This is especially probable, as they can be expected to express on their surface metabolic products of myelin turn over, including MBP. An activated MBP-specific T cell having passed the endothelial part of the BBB could therefore be confronted with its specific antigen, MBP, expressed in a potentially immunogenic fashion on an astrocyte process, which is known to form the third layer of the BBB cycle leading to local accumulating of proliferating and recruited lymphoid and mononuclear cells.

As the in vitro interaction with MBP-specific T cells with antigen presenting astrocytes in vitro leads to astrocyte death, similar, though possibly milder, astrocyte damage could occur in situ as well. Even, if sublethal, interactions with I cells could paralyse the function of astrocytes, and, considering the central role of astroglia in the CNS tissues, functional deterioration of local brain function would be the result. It should be noted that astrocytes are thought to warrant correct neuronal function by creating subtle microenvironmental compartments, and by establishing stable electrolyte and mediator equilibria (Kimelberg, 1983). Both functions could be impaired after T cell action, and the resulting defects of neuronal function could be at least one factor contributing to the acute early symptoms of EAE.

Conclusion

We have outlined experimental data which have been recently obtained in a transfer model of T line mediated EAE, and which have lead to some new insights into the pathogenesis of CNS autoaggression. In particular, they seem to be helpful in

TABLE I: Critical Requirements for a Protein Antigen to Act as an Encephalitogen

1. Sufficient representation of complementary T lymphocyte clones within the normal immune repertoire; (genetic control by MHC)

2. activation on complementary T clone cells outside of the nervous system; (by the antigen itsef or a cross-reacting molecule)

3. immunogenic expression of the determinant within the CNS; (preferentially on astrocyte membranes)

4. induction of presenter cell lysis during intra-CNS recognition of the antigen; (leads to astrocyte defects)

defining the structural requirements for a protein structure to become an encephalitogen. It appears that the first prerequisite is a sufficient number of complementary T lymphocyte clones within the natural repertoire of the immune system. This is genetically controlled, most probably including MHC-linked Ir genes. HLA DR-linkage of human disease might act on this level. The second requirement would be activation of the potentially encephalitogenic T clones outside the CNS, perhaps by crossreacting determinants. Virus antigens crossreacting with myelin components were discussed as precedent of molelular mimicry. The third requirement is the expression of the critical determinant on the CNS astrocytes. Finally, only such a determinant leading to astrocyte lysis after recognition by specific activated T cells could lead to damage within the white matter, and thus to clinical EAE.

ACKNOWLEDGEMENT

The Unit is supported by funds of the Hermann-and-Lilly-Schilling-Stiftung. Thanks are due to Mrs. B. Goebel for writing this manuscript, and to my colleagues who rendered available unpublished data.

LITERATURE

Ben-Nun, A., Eisenstein S., and Cohen, I.R. 1982. Experimental autoimmune encephalomyelitis (EAE) in genetically resistant rats: PVG rats resist active induction of EAE but are susceptible to and can generate EAE effector T cell lines. J. Immunol. 129: 918-919.

Ben-Nun, A., Wekerle, H., and Cohen, I.R. 1981. The rapid isolation of clonable, antigen-specific T lymphocyte lines capable of mediating autoimmune encephalomyelitis. Eur. J. Immunol. 13: 195-199.

Fierz, W., Endler, B., Reske, K., Wekerle, H., and Fontana, A. 1985. Astrocytes as antigen-presenting cells. I. Induction of Ia-antigen expression on astrocytes by T cells via immune-interferon, and its effect on antigen-presentation. J. Immunol. in press.

Fontana, A., Dubs, R., Merchant, R. Balsiger, S., and Grob, P.J. 1981. Glia cell stimulation factor (GSF): A new lymphokine. 1. Cellular sources and partial purification of murine GSF. role of cytoskeleton and protein synthesis in its production. J. Neuroimmunol., 2: 55-71.

Fontana, A., Kristensen, F., Dubs, R., Gemsa, D., and Weber, E. 1982. Production of prostaglandin E and an interleukin-1 like factor by astrocytes and C6 glioma cells. J. Immunol., 129: 2413-2419.

Gasser, D.L., Palm, J., and Gonatas, N. K. 1975. Genetic control of susceptiblity to experimental allergic encephalomyelitis and the AgB locus of rats. J. Immunol. 115: 431-433.

Günther, E., Odenthal, H., and Wechsler, W. 1978. Association between susceptibility to experimental allergic encephalomyelitis and the major histocompatibility system in congenic rat strains. Clin. Exp. Immunol. 32: 429-434.

Hirsch, M.-A., Wietzerbin, J., Pierres, M., and Goridis, C. 1983. Expression of Ia antigens by cultured astrocytes treated with gamma-interferon. Neurosci. Lett., 41: 199-204.

Hirschberg, H., Bergh, O.J., and Thorsby, E. 1980. Antigen-presenting properties of human vascular endothelial cells. J. Exp. Med., 152: 249-255.

Izumo, S., Linington, C., Wekerle, H., and R. Meyermann. 1985. A morphological study on experimental allergic neuritis mediated by T-cell line specific for bovine B$_2$ protein in Lewis rat. Lab.Invest., in press.

Kimelberg, H.K. 1983. Primary astrocyte cultures - a key to astrocyte function. Cell.Mol.Neurobiol. 3: 1-16.

Lassmann, H. 1983. Comparative neuropathology of chronic experimental allergic encephalomyelitis and multiple sclerosis. Springer Verl., Berlin

Linington, C., Izumo, S., Suzuki, M., Uyemura, K., Meyermann, R., and Wekerle, H. 1984. A permanent rat T cell line that mediates Experimental Allergic Neuritis in the Lewis rat in vivo. J. Immunol. 133: 1946-1950.

McFarlin, D.E., and McFarland, H.F. 1982. Multiple Sclerosis. N.E.J.M., 307: 1183-1188; 1246-1251.

Naparstek, Y., Ben-Nun, A., Holoshitz, J., Reshef, T., Frenkel, A., Rosenberg, M. and Cohen I.R. 1983. T lymphocyte lines producing or vaccinating against autoimmune encephalomyelitis (EAE). Functional aactivation induces peanut agglutinin receptors and accumulation in the rain and thymus of line cells. Eur. J. Immunol. 13: 418-423.

Naparstek, Y., Cohen, I. R., Fuks, Z., and Vlodavsky, I. 1984. Activated I lymphocytes produce a matrix-degrading heparan sulphate endoglycosidase. Nature, 310: 241-244.

Osawa, H., and Diamantstein, T. 1983. The characteristics of a monoclonal antibody that binds specifically to rat T lymphoblasts and inhibits IL-2 receptor functions. J. Immunol., 130: 51-55.

Poper, J.S., Gimbrone, M.A., Cotran, R.S., Reiss, C.S., Bukaroff, S.J., Fierz, W., and Ault, K.A. 1983. Ia expression by vascular endothelium is inducible by activated T cells and by human y-interferon. J. Exp. Med. 157: 1339-1353.

Savion, N., Vlodavsky, I., and Fuks, Z. 1984. Interaction of T lymphocytes and macrophages with cultured vascular endothelial cells: Attachment, invasion and subsequent degradation of the subendothelial extracellular matrix.J.Cell.Physiol. 118: 169-178.

Sun, D., and Wekerle, H. 1985. Antigen-specific, Ia-restricted lysis of rat brain astrocytes by syngeneic encephalitogenic T lymphocyte line cells. Epitope dependency of killing function? Submitted.

Vass, K., Lassmann, H., Wekerle, H., and Wisniewski, H.M. 1985. The distribution of Ia-antigen in the lesions of rat acute experimental allergic encephalomyelitis. Submitted.

Waksman, B.H. 1983. Immunity and the nervous system: Basic Tenets. Ann. Neurol., 13: 587-591.

Weiner, H.L., and Hauser, S.L. 1982. Neuroimmunology I: Immunoregulation in neurological disease. Ann. Neurol., 11: 437-449.

Wekerle, H. 1984. The lesion of acute Experimental autoimmune encephalomyelitis. Lab.Invest., 51: 199-205.

Wekerle, H., and Schlüsener, H.J. 1985. Autoaggressive T lymphocyte lines recognizing the encephalitogenic region of myelin basic protein: in vitro selection from unprimed rat T lymphocyte populations. Submitted.

Wong, G.H.M., Bartlett, P.F., Clark-Lewis, I., Battye, F., and Schrader, J.W. 1984. Inducible expression of H-2 and Ia antigens on brain cells. Nature, 310: 688-691.

27

Cytotoxic Antibodies in Multiple Sclerosis

L. RUMBACH, J. M. WARTER, M. M. TONGIO, C. MARESCAUX, S. MAYER and M. COLLARD

INTRODUCTION

　　Terasaki et al., (1970) demonstrated lymphocytotoxic antibodies (LCA) or lymphocytotoxins detectable at 15°C in the serum of systemic lupus erythematosus (SLE). Since then, cold LCA have been reported in many diseases including rheumatoid arthritis, various neurological diseases including Guillain-Barre syndrome, myasthenia gravis (Lisak et al., 1979) and multiple sclerosis (MS) (Kuwert and Bertrams, 1972). The present study was undertaken to further define the cold and warm LCA as well as the cold and warm monocytotoxic antibodies in MS sera and cerebrospinal fluid (CSF), and to investigate possible correlations between these cytotoxic activities and various clinical and biological parameters (Rumbach et al., 1982).

MATERIALS AND METHODS

　　Twenty-one patients were studied, 17 women and 4 men, average age 28 years. All had the "clinically definite" form of MS (criteria of Mac Alpine). For controls, the serum of 32 healthy blood donors and the serum and CSF of 6 patients with diseases other than MS were studied under the same conditions. The serum and CSF of each patient were tested at 15°C and 37°C with the autocells : total lymphocytes (TL), B lymphocytes (BL) and monocytes (M), and then with fresh allocells (TL, BL, M) of the same eight healthy blood donors. Tests were performed before and after absorption on platelets. Antibodies in the serum and CSF were detected by the microlymphocytotoxic technique of Terasaki and Mc Clelland (1964) as modified by Rumbach et al., (1982).

RESULTS

Serum of MS patients (Table 1)

In 9 patients all tests were negative at 15°C and 37°C. The sera of the other 12 MS reacted positively at 15°C, but there were differences at 37°C. Four of the 12 reacted negatively with TL, BL and M, 3 reacted negatively with TL and BL but positively with M, 4 reacted negatively with TL but positively with BL and M, and one reacted positively with TL, BL and M. After platelet absorption, the number of positive reactions was reduced. Autocellular cytotoxic activity tests showed that only 6 of the 21 MS sera reacted positively.

Table 1

Cytotoxic activity in sera of MS patients

+ = positive ;   -- = negative reactions

Tested in the presence of allocells

	15°C			37°C		
	TL	BL	M	TL	BL	M
n = 9	-	-	-	-	-	-
4	+	+	+	-	-	-
3	+	+	+	-	-	+
4	+	+	+	-	+	+
1	+	+	+	+	+	+

CSF of MS patients

Results differed from the previous ones. Reactions were positive against autocells and allocells in all the samples tested, before platelet absorption, at 15°C and 37°C. After platelet absorption, the number of positive reactions was reduced when allocells were tested, and mostly disappeared when autocells were tested.

Healthy controls

Only 5 of the 32 sera tested were positive with allocells.

Non-MS patients

No cytotoxic activity was detected in 5 of the 6 sera. However, the CSF cytotoxic activity before platelet absorption was strongly positive with allo- and autocells in all 6 patients.

No relation was found between cytotoxic activity and various clinical and biological parameters : age at onset of MS ; duration of disease development ; the patient's condition, remission or relapse ; or CSF albumin and immunoglobulin levels.

DISCUSSION

Cold LCA have been detected in the serum of 30 to 67 % of MS patients (Schocket et al., 1977), a finding we confirm. In our study, the cytotoxic activity was directed not only against TL and BL but also, and predominantly, against monocytes. Some of those antibodies were detected not only at 15°C but also at 37°C. All CSF reactions were strongly positive in MS and non-MS patients. The lysis of monocytes in absence of complement suggests that M lysis with CSF may not necessarily be linked to a classical immunological mechanism. The fewer positive reactions after absorption on platelets argues in favor that this phenomenon is perhaps not attribuable to an aspecific cytotoxic activity. Tests with autocells were positive in certain MS patients. The antibodies seem to "recognize" an antigenic determinant common to auto- and allocells. No correlation was found between cytotoxic activity and disease activity.

The role and significance of cytotoxic antibodies are unknown (Mayer and Tongio, 1984). They exist in some normal subjects without, apparently, any pathogenic effects. They could possibly have a beneficial effect on transplant survival. Cytotoxic antibodies are, however, more often found in various pathological conditions. In certain diseases, such as lupus, their pathogenic effect could be through action on certain lymphocyte populations or subsets, mainly during the active disease phase. This pattern of action has not yet been demonstrated for MS, partly due to the paucity of investigations and to the contradictory results on cellular populations reported (Scott and Spitler, 1983).

ACKNOWLEDGMENT

Text translated from the French by Sarah Dejours.

REFERENCES

Kuwert, E. and Bertrams, J., 1972. Leukocyte iso- and auto-antibodies in multiple sclerosis (MS) with special regard to complement-dependent cold-reacting autolymphocytotoxins (CoCoCy). Europ. Neurol., 7 : 65-73.

Lisak, R.P., Mercado, F. and Zweiman, B., 1979. Cold reactive antilympho-cyte antibodies in neurologic diseases. J. Neurol. Neurosurg. Psychiatry, 42 : 1054-1057.

Mayer, S. and Tongio, M.M., 1984. Autoimmunity against lymphocytes. In : C.P. Engelfriet, J.J. van Loghem and A.E.G.K. von dem Borne (Editors), Immunohematology. Elsevier, Amsterdam, pp. 275-283.

Rumbach, L., Tongio, M.M., Warter, J.M., Marescaux, C., Mayer, S. and Rohmer, F., 1982. Lymphocytotoxic and monocytotoxic antibodies in the serum and cerebrospinal fluid of multiple sclerosis patients. J. Neuroimmunol., 3 : 263-273.

Schocket, A.L., Weiner, H.L., Walker, J., Mc Intosh, K. and Kohler, P., 1977. Lymphocytotoxic antibodies in multiple sclerosis. Clin. Immunol Immunopathol., 7 : 15-23.

Terasaki, P.I. and Mc Clelland, J.D., 1964. Microdroplet assay of human serum cytotoxins. Nature (Lond.), 204 : 998-1000.

Terasaki, P.L., Mottironi, V.D. and Barnett, E.V., 1970. Autocytotoxins in lupus. N. Engl. J. Med., 283 : 724-728.

28

An Immunological Function for Astrocytes

W. FIERZ and A. FONTANA

The induction of a successfull immune reaction within the CNS is dependent
on several prerequisites: After initial contact with endothelial cells, T-
cells must penetrate the blood-brain-barrier (BBB), they must find their
antigen together with the Ia-antigens of the major histocompatibility complex (MHC) on the surface of antigen-presenting cells (APC) within the CNS-
tissue and they must be costimulated by Il-1. As astrocytes are spreading
their processes on the CNS-surface of the basal membrane of the BBB, they
are the first cells to be encountered by intruding T-cells. Therefore, a
physical contact between astrocytes and T-cells seems inevitable and could
be a major step in the activation of T-cells in the CNS. First functional
clues came from experiments by Fontana et al. (1982) which demonstrated
the production of an Il-1 like factor by astrocytes in vitro. Such experiments became possible because of the relative ease to grow pure astrocytic
monolayers from neonatal brain cells and because of the possibility to
identify astrocytes with antibodies against the glial fibrillary acidic
protein (GFAP) of the astrocytic intermediate filaments. Thus Il-1 was
produced in such mouse astrocyte cultures after stimulation with lipopoly-
saccharide (LPS) or spontaneously by rat astrocytes and by rat and human
glioblastoma cells. The glioblastoma cell derived Il-1 like factor has
been shown to be neutralized by an antiserum against human endogenous pyrogen (EP) and to bind to anti-EP immunoadsorbent columns. Apart from
Il-1, astrocytes also produced an Il-3 like factor which induced proliferation of Il-3 dependent cell lines and enhanced the expression of 20α-
hydroxysteroid dehydrogenase on spleen cells of nude mice. (Frei et al.

1984). In view of recent findings of Il-3 induced growth of macrophages
and haematopoietic stem cells, the production of Il-3 by astrocytes may
be important for the survival and expansion of inflammatory blood cells
invading the CNS.

To test whether, furthermore, astrocytes could function as antigen-
presenting cells (APC) we analyzed their interaction with T-cells which
were grown as myelin-basic-protein (MBP) - specific T-cell lines (Ben-Nun
et al. 1981). These pure T-cell lines must be regularly restimulated with
MBP on APC in the context of Ia-antigens of the MHC. In these experiments
we found that the normally used APC, like macrophages, could be replaced
by astrocytes (Fontana et al., 1984a). In cocultures of the T-cell lines
with astrocytes we observed 12 hours after addition of the antigen MBP,
an aggregation of the T-cells around astrocytes (Fig.1) and subsequently
the T-cells transformed into big blast-cells and started to proliferate

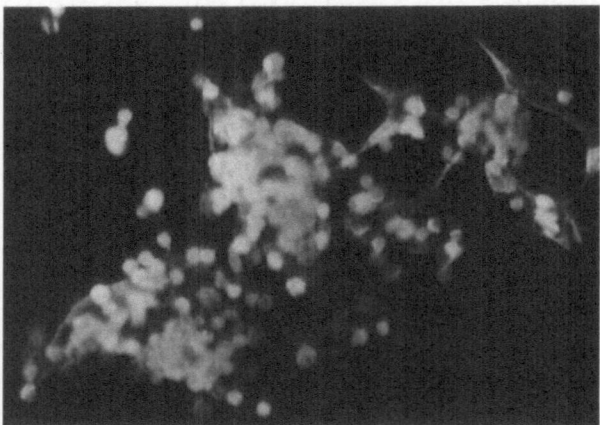

Figure 1
Antigen-presentation by astrocytes. Protoplasmic astrocytes interact
immuno-specifically with MBP-specific T-line cells in the presence of
MBP. Astrocytes are identified by immuno-cytochemical staining of the
GFAP-containing intermediate filaments. Cell nuclei are stained with
propidium iodide.

vigorously. This astrocyte mediated T-cell activation is antigen-specific
and MHC-restricted. i.e. MBP is presented by the astrocytes to the T-cells

in the context of Ia-antigens of the MHC. This reflects the rules of antigen-presentation but is somewhat surprising as astrocytes are Ia-negative
in vivo and in normal in vitro cultures. We found, however, that after the
interaction with the T-cells the astrocytes became Ia-positive. Independently, it was published by Hirsch et al. (1983) that Ia-antigens could be
induced on astrocytes in vitro by incubation with supernatants of stimulated spleen cells which contained immune-interferon (IFN-y), a product of
activated T-cells. In a subsequent series of experiments we have demonstrated that also pure recombinant IFN-y is able to induce Ia-antigens on
astrocytes (Fig.2). These Ia-antigens were functionally active: IFN-y

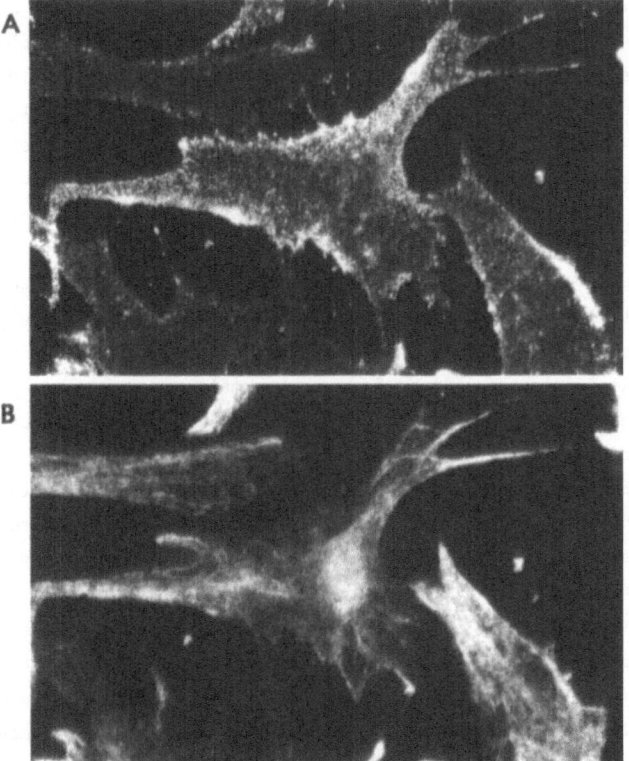

Figure 2
Astrocytes incubated with recombinant IFN-y show membrane immunofluo-
resent staining for Ia (A) and are identified as astrocytes with staining
for intracellular GFAP (B).

treated astrocytes were aggregating with T-cells already 2 hours after
addition of the antigen MBP and stimulated the T-cells to a much higher
degree than untreated, initially Ia-negative astrocytes (Fierz et al.,
subm.). Blocking studies with anti-Ia monoclonal antibodies showed that
initially Ia-negative astrocytes are only recognized by the T-cells
after about 12 hours, i.e. after Ia-expression has been induced on
the astrocytes by an activating signal (probably IFN-y) from the
T-cells. In conclusion, the immunospecific interaction of astrocytes and
T-cells is a mutually activating process.

Recent experiments have shown that activated T-cells are able to penetrate basal membranes (Naparstek et al. 1984). Such active T-cells would
then be able to induce Ia-antigens on astrocytes and, therefore, fulfill
the prerequisite for their own reactivation with CNS-antigens like MBP.
This suggested sequence of events is well supported in the EAE by the fact
that the MBP-specific T-line cells used in our experiments are encephalitogenic, after being transferred into naive recipients, but only when the
T-cells have been freshly activated before the transfer and have not been
irradiated. Such a pathogenetical model, however, implies primary activation of the T-cells outside the CNS. On the other hand, it is also conceivable that some abnormal stimulus, like e.g. virus infection, could induce Ia-antigens on astrocytes and, consequently, an interaction with
resting T-cells could take place. Such an abnormal induction of Ia-antigens by some stimulus could enable the astrocytes to present antigens
which are normally not immunogenic and this could be the basis for the
development of autoimmune disease in the CNS. However, also negative regulatory mechanisms have to be considered. It is known e.g. that prostaglandin E has an inhibitory effect on the expression of Ia-antigens by
macrophages (Snyder et al. 1982) and it could well be that such an inhibition of Ia-expression is also operating in the CNS leading to the observed lack of Ia-antigens on astrocytes in the normal CNS. In this context it is important to know that astrocytes themselves are able to produce prostaglandin E (Fontana et al. 1982) and that prostaglandin precursors have a marked suppressive effect on the development of EAE (Mertin
et al. 1978). Furthermore, a factor which suppresses the Il-2 induced T-
cell proliferation has been described to be produced by glioblastoma cells
(Fontana et al. 1984b). The partially purified factor (G-TsF) has a molecular weight of around 95.000 and an isoelectric point of 4.6(Schwyzer et

al., in press). Whether such a factor plays also a role in the normal CNS
for the negative regulation of astrocyte-T-cell interaction remains to be
seen.

The initially mentioned Il-1 production by astrocytes is not only important for the activation of T-cells but might have more general effects
on the development of inflammatory processes in the CNS. It is known, that
Il-1 is identical with the endogenous pyrogen, has chemotactic activity,
induces acute phase reactants and stimulates muscle protein degradation
(for review see Dinarello 1984). It was, therefore, very interesting to
find that astrocytes produce Il-1 not only in vitro but also possibly in
vivo, as Il-1 could be measured in intracellular brain extracts of LPS-
treated mice. (Fontana et al., 1984c). In further experiments we studied
the in vivo production and effects of Il-1 in animals with EAE induced
by adoptive transfer of MBP-specific T-cell lines. Il-1 was found in brain
extracts of rats already at the time of the very first paralytical symptoms
on day 3 to 4 after T-cell transfer (Fig 3). In contrast, no Il-1 activity

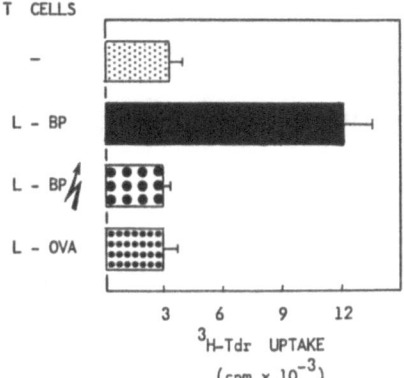

Figure 3
Il-1 activity in brain of rats after adoptive transfer of encephalitogenic T-cells. Il-1 is measured as the proliferative response of PHA-
stimulated thymocytes after addition of intracellular brain extracts
from rats which were injected intravenously with MBP-specific, activated
T-line cells. (L-BP). Control extracts were from normal rats (-) or
rats injected with irradiated cells (L-BP∦) or ovalbumin-specific T-
line cells (L-OVA).

could be measured in extracts of spleen, lung, liver and lymphnodes of such
animals. Parallel to the onset of Il-1 production in the CNS, a fever reaction was observed with a peak on day 4 which was followed by a hypothermia
24 hours later, when the animals had developed severe EAE (table 1). Furthermore, a rapid loss of about 10% of the body weight was observed at the

Table 1

Loss of body weight and fever reaction in rats after intravenous injection
of encephalitogenic T-line cells.

Rat	T-cells	Weight (g)			Temperature (^{o}C)				Clinic
		day 1	day 5	$\triangle$5-1	day 1	day 4	day 5	$\triangle$4-1	
1	L-BP	323	288	-35	37.2	37.6	26.4	+0.4	EAE
2	L-BP	324	284	-40	37.3	38.2	27.4	+0.9	EAE
3	L-BP	346	304	-42	37,2	38.3	30.5	+1.1	EAE
4	L-BP ⚡	320	328	+ 8	37.4	37.5	37.2	+0.1	normal
5	L-BP	356	317	-39	37.1	38.2	36.8	+1.1	EAE
6	L-BP ⚡	349	346	- 3	37.1	37.3	37.3	+0.2	normal

L-BP MBP-specific encephalitogenic T-line cells, freshly activated,
$\quad$ 5×10^{6} per animal
⚡ $\quad$ irradiated with 3000 rad
$\triangle$ $\quad$ difference between indicated days

same time. The mechanisms underlying the fever reaction are not clear so
far. One could speculate that Il-1 is produced locally in the CNS, possibly
by astrocytes, and reacts directly with the thermoregulatory centres in
the hypothalamus. Apart from its effect on body temperature, Il-1 may also
change other brain functions such as sleep. There is evidence that macrophage derived Il-1 has the capacity to increase slow-wave sleep (SWS) in
rabbits (Krueger et al.). In recent studies in rats, Il-1 like factors
prepared from supernatants of cultured astrocytes had also somnogenic effects (Tobler et al. 1984). However, despite of intracerebral Il-1 production in rats with EAE, we could not find an increase in SWS activity. In
fact the opposite became true, a marked decrease of SWS was observed which
developed before visible signs of EAE.

It is well known from morphological experience that astrocytes somehow take part in the pathological process inside the CNS-lesions of MS-
patients. Usually they are described in active plaques as "reactive" astrocytes and in old plaques as "scarring tissue". The new immune-functional
data on astrocytes may put them well into the centre of the pathological
events in the MS-lesion. It remains, however, to be seen whether the in
vitro observed immunological functions of astrocytes like antigen-presentation, Ia-expression an Il-1 production can also be identified in the in
vivo situation of the MS-plaque.

Acknowledgment

Part of the work was done at the Max-Planck-Society, Clinical Research
Unit for Multiple Sclerosis (Head: Prof. H. Wekerle), Würzburg, FRG.
This unit is supported by funds from the Hermann - and Lilly - Schilling
Foundation. Part of the work was supported by the Swiss National Foun-
dation (project no. 3.967-1.84) and the Swiss Multiple Sclerosis Society.

References

Ben-Nun, A., Wekerle, H. and Cohen, I.R., 1981. The rapid isolation of
    clonable, antigen-specific T lymphocyte lines capable of mediating
    autoimmune encephalomyelitis. Eur. J. Immunol., 11: 195-199.
Dinarello, Ch.A., 1984. Interleukin-1 and the pathogenesis of the acute-
    phase response. N, Engl. J. Med. , 311: 1413-1418.
Fontana, A., Kristensen, F., Dubs, R., Gemsa, D. and Weber, E., 1982.
    Production of prostaglandin E and interleukin-1 like factors by cul-
    tured astrocytes and C-6 glioma cells. J. Immunol., 129: 2413-2419.
Fontana, A., Fierz, W. and Wekerle, H., 1984a. Astrocytes present myelin
    basic protein to encephalitogenic T cell lines. Nature, 307:
    273-276.
Fontana, A., Hengartner, H., de Tribolet, N., and Weber, E., 1984 b.
    Glioblastoma cells release both interleukin-1 and factors inhibiting
    interleukin-2 mediated effects. J.Immunol., 132: 1837-1844.
Fontana , A., Weber , t. and Dayer J.M., 1984c. Synthesis of interleukin-1/
    endogenons pyrogen in the brain of endotoxin treated mice: a step in
    fever induction? J. Immunol., 133: 1696-1698.
Frei, K., Stadler, B. and Fontana, A., 1984. Astrocyte-derived interleukin-
    3 like factors. Lymphokine Res., 3: 243 (Abstr.).
Hirsch, M.R., Wietzerbin, J., Pierres M. and Goridis, C., 1983. Expression
    of Ia-antigens by cultered astrocytes treated with gamma-interferon.
    Neuroscience letters, 41: 199-204.
Krueger, J.M., Walter, J., Dinarello, C.A., Wolff, S.M. and Chedid, L.,
    1984. Sleep-promoting effects of endogenons pyrogen (interleukin-1).
    Am.J. Pysiol., 246: R 994- R 999.

Mertin, J. and Stackpoole, A., 1978. Suppression by essential fatty acids of experimental allergic encephalomyelitis is abolished by indomethacin. Prostaglandins and Medicin, 1: 283-291.

Naparstek, J., Cohen, I.R., Fuks, Z. and Vlodavsky I., Activated T lymphocytes produce a matrix-degrading heparan sulphate endoglycosidase. Nature, 310: 241-244.

Schwyzer, M. and Fontana A., in press. Partial purification and biochemical characterization of a T-cell suppressor factor produced by human glioblastoma cells. J. Immunol., in press.

Snyder, D.S., Beller, D.I. and Unanue, E.R., 1982. Prostaglandins modulate macrophage Ia expression. Nature, 299: 163-165.

Tobler, I., Borbely, A.A., Schwyzer, M. and Fontana A., in press. Interleukin-1 derived from astrocytes enhances slow-wave activity in sleep EEG of the rat. Eur. J. Pharmakol., in press.

Section III
Biochemistry, Neurobiology, Myelin

29

The Biochemistry of Myelin

J. M. MATTHIEU

Introduction

During the last twenty years our knowledge about myelin has improved
tremendously. Myelin has been purified, its chemical composition determined
and the metabolism of specific myelin constituents studied. By the use of
physicochemical, immunocytochemical and subfractionation techniques, our
understanding of myelin organization and assembly is progressing. Cell cultures provide a useful tool to study the differentiation of oligodendroglia, axon-glia interactions and the influence of growth factors on myelination. Some of the mechanisms involved in immune-mediated demyelination
have been investigated. Nevertheless, in spite of all the efforts and progress recently made, we are still ignorant of how an oligodendrocyte can
recognize the many axons it will myelinate, how the membrane wraps around
the axon and what changes cause layer upon layer of membrane to compact together to produce the mature myelin sheath. Similarly, the cause and pathogenesis of one of the more common diseases of the central nervous system
(CNS), multiple sclerosis (MS), remains unknown. In this brief review, I
would like to present some of the biochemical facts which could be relevant
for future research on MS.

Myelin lipids in the CNS

By dry weight analysis, the lipids represent 70% of the myelin sheath.
Phospholipids are predominant in myelin, but, in contrast to other plasma
membranes, it contains also high levels of cerebrosides (Table 1). Lipids
in myelin, as in other membranes, are distributed asymmetrically across the
bilayer (for a review, see Braun, 1984). Cholesterol is concentrated in the
inner leaflet of the bilayer. On the other hand, cerebrosides are predominantly localized toward the intraperiod line. Most phospholipids and particularly phosphatidylethanolamine are located in the inner half of the myelin bilayer. The carbohydrate portion of glycolipids in myelin (cerebrosides, sulfatides, gangliosides) can play an important role in antigen-
antibody reactions. For instance, cerebroside is probably the antigen recognized by some experimental allergic encephalomyelitis (EAE) antisera and
is that with which they react to cause demyelination.

TABLE I. LIPID COMPOSITION OF ADULT HUMAN MYELIN

	C N S	P N S
	(IN % OF DRY WEIGHT)	
PROTEIN	30	29
LIPID	70	7I
	(IN % OF LIPID WEIGHT)	
CHOLESTEROL	27.7	23.0
TOTAL GALACTOLIPID	27.5	22.I
TOTAL PHOSPHOLIPID	43.I	54.9
GANGLIOSIDE (G_{MI}...)	0.2	
GALACTOLIPIDS - CEREBROSIDES	22.7	
- SULFATIDES	3.8	
PHOSPHOLIPIDS - P-ETHANOLAMINE	15.6	19.2
P-CHOLINE	II.2	7.8
SPHINGOMYELIN	7.9	18.6
P-SERINE	4.8	9.3
P-INOSITOL	0.6	

P-, PHOSPHATIDYL. [A] DATA FROM W.T. NORTON, 1981. [B] DATA FROM SPRITZ ET AL., 1973.

Myelin proteins in the CNS

Proteolipid protein (PLP) is an integral myelin protein of 25 kilo-daltons (Kd) molecular weight (M_r) (Table 2, Fig. 1) present only in CNS myelin where it accounts for 20% of the protein content. It is synthesized on membrane-bound ribosomes and processed through the Golgi apparatus. PLP contains 276 residues; half the amino acids are nonpolar and a sharp seg-

TABLE 2. MAJOR PROTEINS OF HUMAN MYELIN

	C N S	P N S	M_R [A]
MAG	+	+	I00 - II0 KD [B]
WOLFGRAM	+	0 ?	46, 48 KD
P_0	0	+++	30 KD
PLP	++	0	25 KD
I OR DM-20	+	0	20 KD
MBP (P_I)	++	+	I8 KD
P_2	0	++	I2 KD

[A] APPARENT MOLECULAR WEIGHTS ARE EXPRESSED IN KILODALTONS

THE RELATIVE CONCENTRATIONS OF MYELIN IN A GIVEN SYSTEM ARE INDICATED BY PLUS(ES) SIGNS.

regation exists between hydrophobic and hydrophilic domains of the molecule. Three moles fatty acids/mole protein are covalently bound. A confor-
mation model suggests that the molecule spans the bilayer and interacts at
the external face with the adjacent bilayer to bring together apposed la-
mellar membranes (Laursen et al., 1983). In this location PLP could play an
important role in stabilizing the molecular structure of myelin. Furthermore, the segments of the molecule exposed at the external face of the membrane could be involved in pathological processes as receptors or antigenic
sites. The intermediate protein or DM-20 shows immunological cross-reactiv-
ity with PLP. It is not clear if the difference between both polypeptides
is due to internal sequence deletions, charge heterogeneity, posttransla-
tional modifications etc. (Lees and Brostoff, 1984).

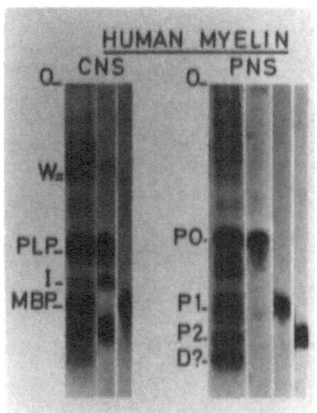

Figure 1. Human myelin proteins separated by electrophoresis. First lane of
CNS and PNS: Fast Green stained gel. All others: immunoblot analysis using
specific antisera. From left to right, CNS: PLP, MBP; PNS: P$_0$, P$_1$, P$_2$.
O, origin. W, Wolfgram protein or CNP. I, intermediate or DM-20 protein.
D, degradation product.

Myelin basic protein (MBP) is an extrinsic protein synthesized on free
ribosomes. A mRNA fraction seems to be located in the paranodal tongue processes and could be responsible for a peripheral synthesis of MBP. MBP consists of a family of polypeptides with different molecular weights but sharing for the major part of their molecules identical amino acid sequences.
The major MBP component in man is 170 amino acids long and has a molecular
weight of approximately 18 Kd. It contains a high percentage of basic residues. MBP is methylated and phosphorylated. MBP has been extensively studied in relation to MS since the discovery that it could elicit EAE, which
is so far the best experimental model for MS studies. Nevertheless, other
myelin constituents (e.g. cerebrosides) seem to play a role in certain forms
of EAE. MBP is localized on the cytoplasmic surfaces of the myelin bilayers
where it is involved in the formation of the major dense line and stabi-
lizes the multilayered structure (for a review see Matthieu and Omlin, 1984).

Myelin associated glycoprotein (MAG) is a quantitatively minor component of isolated myelin of about 110 Kd (Fig. 2). It contains 30% carbo-
hydrates and a relatively high content of nonpolar amino acids. Immunocytochemical studies indicate that MAG is restricted to myelin forming oligodendrocytes in the CNS, and particularly enriched in the periaxonal regions.
In this location it is believed to play an important role in axon-glial interactions and in maintaining the periaxonal space of myelinated axons
(Quarles, 1985). Glycoproteins are known to be cell surface antigens and
receptors for some viruses. Therefore, MAG could be involved in autoimmune
or viral aspects of MS and other demyelinating diseases (Quarles, 1985). In
MS plaques, the decrease in MAG immunostaining is one of the earliest biochemical events (Itoyama et al., 1980). This is probably not specific to MS
and was observed in demyelination following wallerian degeneration (Reigner
et al., 1981). The carbohydrate portion of glycoproteins can play an important role in antigen-antibody reactions by masking certain polypeptide
sites and, at the same time, directing the immune response, acting as immune decoys (Alexander and Elder, 1984). An interesting observation has
shown that a carbohydrate determinant in human MAG and other PNS myelin
glycoproteins can be recognized by human paraproteins associated with neuropathy and HNK-1, a monoclonal antibody used to identify human lymphocytes
with natural killer and suppressor functions (for a review, see Quarles,
1985). This carbohydrate epitope present on lymphocytes and myelin could be
of significance with regard to autoimmune demyelinating diseases. Murray
and Steck (1984) hypothesized that the presence of this epitope outside of
the nervous system could be involved in the initial sensitization to this
antigen.

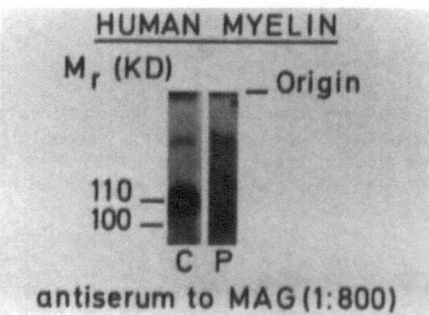

Figure 2. Immunoblot analysis of MAG in CNS myelin (C) and PNS myelin (P).
MAG in human CNS has an apparent molecular weight approximately 10 Kd
larger than in the PNS.

Myelin enzymes

Approximately 20 enzymes have been found in myelin indicating that
transport, synthesis and degradation take place in myelin. Among these enzymes, only two are specific to myelin: 2',3'-cyclic-nucleotide-3'-phospho-
hydrolase (CNP) and cholesterol ester hydrolase. The physiological function

of CNP is still unknown and that of cholesterol ester hydrolase is not clear since cholesterol esters are normally absent from the brain. CNP is closely associated with oligodendroglial plasma membranes and paranodal tongue processes.

Comparison between CNS and PNS myelin

Since the PNS is spared in MS, the comparison of CNS myelin with PNS myelin could lead to some novel ideas, especially when we argue that the similarities between the two myelins should tell us something about the fundamental processes of myelin formation, whereas the differences should reflect special susceptibilities and requirements of the two systems. Morphologically, both myelins are grossly similar in their fundamental features and they appear to perform the same function. Important differences in the protein composition (Table 2) should be emphasized more so than differences in the lipid. PNS myelin lacks PLP and has instead a high concentration of P_0, a glycoprotein (Fig. 1) which spans the membrane and extends into the aqueous space on either side. MBP appears to be less abundant in PNS than in CNS myelin and studies in mutant mice indicate that MBP is not important for maintaining compact PNS myelin. MBP, called P_1 in the PNS, is not encephalitogenic when PNS myelin is used as antigenic material. Therefore, this suggests that the organization and function of MBP differs in PNS and CNS myelin (for a review, see Brostoff, 1984).

Myelin assembly

It can be assumed that myelin is synthesized, as reported for other membranes, through precursor vesicles, directly transported to and fused into plasma membranes. Since the composition of myelin differs somewhat from that of oligodendroglial plasma membrane, it can be postulated that myelin assembly is a process more complicated than the mere fusion of membrane precursor vesicles with the growing oligodendroglial plasma membrane (Morell and Toews, 1984). Myelin assembly and maintenance must result from a sequential process in which the interaction between the axon, the oligodendrocyte, the astrocyte and the environment modulates the expression of a basic genetic program. In humans, several genes are essential for normal myelin formation. Therefore, current research on demyelinating diseases addresses molecular genetics in order to understand how myelin formation and maintenance are regulated.

Demyelination

The distal portion of a sectioned nerve degenerates (wallerian degeneration) and myelin is degraded. In the PNS, myelin is degraded quickly and as a unit. In contrast, in the CNS, demyelination is a slow and sequential process (Table 3). In MS, the mechanisms leading to myelin breakdown differ greatly from wallerian degeneration but the same chemical changes can be observed. The enzymes involved in myelin degradation are usually produced by glia, macrophages or infiltrating immune cells. However, proteolytic enzymes are also present in myelin. They could be involved in demyelinating

TABLE 3. DEMYELINATION FOLLOWING WALLERIAN DEGENERATION

SEQUENCE OF EVENTS

1. MAG CONTENT DECREASES AT DAY 2.
2. CHOLESTEROL ESTERS ARE DETECTABLE AT DAY 8.
3. EXTRA-MYELINIC CNP DECREASES AFTER DAY 16.
4. MBP IS DEGRADED AFTER DAY 32.
5. THE YIELD OF MYELIN DECREASES SIGNIFICANTLY ONLY
   AFTER DAY 90.

REF. REIGNER ET AL., 1981.

diseases. The activity of a neutral protease found in myelin, which degrades MBP and cleaves MAG is greater in MS myelin than in that from normal brains (Sato et al., 1982). As a consequence of myelin breakdown, intact or degraded myelin constituents can be recovered in the cerebrospinal fluid (CSF) of patients with demyelinating disorders (e.g. CNP and MBP).

References

Alexander, S., and Elder, J.H., 1984. Carbohydrate dramatically influences immune reactivity of antisera to viral glycoprotein antigens. Science 226:1328-1330.

Braun, P.E., 1984. Molecular organization of myelin. In: P. Morell (Editor), Myelin, 2.ed., Plenum Press, New York, pp. 97-116.

Brostoff, S.W., 1984. Immunological responses to myelin and myelin components. In: P. Morell (Editor), Myelin, 2.ed., Plenum Press, New York, pp. 405-439.

Itoyama, Y., Sternberger, N.H., Webster, H.deF., Quarles, R.H., Cohen, S.R., and Richardson, E.P.Jr., 1980. Immunocytochemical observations on the distribution of myelin-associated glycoprotein and myelin basic protein in multiple sclerosis lesions. Ann.Neurol. 7:167-177.

Laursen, R.L., Samiullah, M., and Lees, M., 1984. The structure of bovine brain myelin proteolipid and its organization in myelin. Proc.Natl. Acad.Sci. U.S.A. 81:2912-2916.

Lees, M.B., and Brostoff, S.W., 1984. Proteins of myelin. In: P. Morell (Editor), Myelin, 2.ed., Plenum Press, New York, pp. 197-224.

Matthieu, J.-M., and Omlin, F.X., 1984. Murine leukodystrophies as tools to study myelinogenesis in normal and pathological conditions. Neuropediatrics suppl. 15:37-52.

Morell, P., and Toews, A.D., 1984. In vivo metabolism of oligodendroglial lipids. In: W.T. Norton (Editor), Oligodendroglia, Advances in Neurochemistry, vol. 5, Plenum Press, New York, pp. 47-86.

Murray, N., and Steck, A.J., 1984. Indication of a possible role in a demyelinating neuropathy for an antigen shared between myelin and NK cells. The Lancet 1 (8379):711-713.

Quarles, R.H., 1985. Myelin-associated glycoprotein in development and disease. Develop.Neurosci. in press.

Reigner, J., Matthieu, J.-M., Kraus-Ruppert, R., Lassmann, H., and Poduslo, J.F., 1981. Myelin proteins, glycoproteins, and myelin-related enzymes in experimental demyelination of the rabbit optic nerve: sequence of events. J.Neurochem. 36:1986-1995.

Sato, S., Quarles, R.H., and Brady, R.O., 1982. Susceptibility of the myelin-associated glycoprotein and basic protein to a neutral protease in highly purified myelin from human and rat brain. J.Neurochem. 39: 97-105.

30

The Cerebrospinal Fluid Immunoglobulins in Multiple Sclerosis

P. DELMOTTE

Early in the history of Multiple Sclerosis (MS) research, simple floc-
culation tests have drawn attention to some protein fractions imbalance in
the cerebrospinal fluid (CSF) of MS patients (Bauer, 1961). However, it was
the application of the successive electrophoretic techniques to the proteins of the CSF that played the major role in the evolution of what, until
now, approaches the nearest a laboratory test for MS. In the late fourties,
the crude techique of paper electrophoresis not only permitted to observe a
sporadious elevation of the gamma globulins in the CSF, but also an occasional hint of an abnormal distribution of the proteins in that region.
Since then, electrophoretic techniques have ondergone a tremendous evolution (Lowenthal, 1964; Delmotte, 1977; Delmotte, 1979). Now, 40 years later, using isoelectric focusing in thin layers of polyacrylamide gels, we
can put into evidence up to 30 or more sharply delineated oligoclonal fractions in the gamma globulin region of most of the CSF samples from MS patients.

Parallel with the study of the CSF proteins by electrophoretic techniques, a lot of research has been done on the quantitation of well defined
protein entities by chemical and immunochemical techniques. Refinements in
these methods, especially in the field of immunochemistry, has lead to easy,
specific and accurate methods for measuring proteins in biological fluids
(Mancini et al, 1965; Laurell, 1965; Schliep et al, 1978; Masson et al,
1981).

The influx of large numbers of data obtained with these methods stimulated several authors to evaluate the relationship of the most important

217

protein fractions, first among themselves in the CSF and later with respect to the corresponding fractions in the blood plasma. As it became evident that in some neurological diseases, especially MS, those more or less predictable values could be disturbed, even without alteration of the blood/brain barrier, several authors elaborated mathematical formulas permitting the estimation of the abnormal intrathecal synthesis of some protein fractions, especially the immunoglobulin G fraction (Rieder et al, 1980; Link et al, 1977; Tourtellotte et al, 1980; Reiber, 1979).

Regarding MS, the following conclusions are generally agreed upon:
- in the vast majority of MS patients, the CSF total protein content and/or the relative and absolute immunoglobulin concentrations are above normal with, in most cases, a normal blood/brain barrier.
- depending on the electrophoretic technique used, an abnormal oligoclonal distribution of the immunoglobulins in the CSF of between 80 and 95 percent of MS patients can be demonstrated.
- in all other neurological diseases together, a more or less identical observation can be made in between 6 and 8 percent of the cases.
- in contrast to normal individuals and the vast majority of patients with other neurological diseases, a continuous intrathecal biosynthesis of immunoglobulin G can be demonstrated in the vast majority of MS patients. Quantitative studies by capillary isotachophoresis (Delmotte, 1979) have confirmed these results and values up to several tens of milligrams per day are not uncommon.
- this elaboration of immunoglobulins, once established in a patient, seems to undergo little change, neither qualitatively nor quantitatively.

Parallel to the refinement of detection techniques for the abnormal distribution of the proteins in the gamma region of MS/CSF specimens, enormous efforts have been spent for the identification of these fractions. Classical immunoelectrophoresis (Kolar et al, 1980), crossed immunoelectrophoresis in combination with zone electrophoresis or isoelectric focusing (Siden, 1977), two dimensional electrohoresis with pore size gradient in the second dimension (Moulin et al, 1980), immunofixation, directly or after blotting (Mehta et al, 1981), radioimmunofixation (Chazot et al, 1980) and all their variants have been and are still being used for this purpose.

From these studies the following conclusions can be drawn:

- the abnormal proteins which present themselves as oligoclonal bands
  in the CSF of most of the MS patients, are complete immunoglobulins
  with heavy chains of the type G.

- concerning the light chain moiety of these immunoglobulins, it is
  generally admitted that the kappa/lambda ratio is elevated above
  normal, especially when compared to the same ratio in the blood
  plasma. Lymphocytes isolated from MS/CSF and from plaque material,
  also produce a relatively greater amount of kappa light chains
  (Esiri, 1977).

- it was found that in the total of IgG subgroups, the proportion of
  the type IgG-1 was significantly higher in an MS group while IgG-2
  was lowered with no difference for the groups IgG-3 and IgG-4
  (Eickhoff et all, 1979).

- Bollengier et al (1978) not only observed a higher than normal frequency of free light chains in the CSF of MS patients, but also concluded that this occurence somewhat correlated with the severity of
  immunological processes going on in the central nervous system.

Correlations between the CSF immunological findings and a battery of
clinical parameters have been sought after for many years. Helas, with not
too much succes. Some authors (Stendhal-Brodin et al, 1980; Moulin et al,
1983) could find evidence suggesting that patients with a low humoral response in the CSF tend to present a more benign course of the disease.
Others (Christensen et al, 1978; Verjans et al, 1983) could find only in-
consistant or no correlations between CSF findings and most of the common
clinical parameters. Trojaborg et al (1981) could find no relation between
presumed number of lesions and the rate of intrathecal IgG syntheses.
Jozefczyk et al (1984) conclude that MS patients with HLA-A3 and B7 antigens had a higher than predicted incidence of elevated kappa/lambda ratios,
suggesting an immunogenetic control mechanism influencing the CSF parameters. However, the HLA parameters did not correlate with the clinical data.
It has been reported that for patients suffering from optic neuritis, the
CSF data can give valuable prognostic information about wether or not they
run a high risk of getting MS later in live (Nikoskelainen et al, 1981).
However, normal CSF findings do not rule out the possibility of optic
neuritis progressing to MS.

Because of the persistent presence in the MS/CSF of large quantities of immunoglobulins with a peculiar electrophoretic distribution, a real chase for the corresponding antigen(s) has been going on for years. Due to certain analogies between subacute sclerosing panencephalitis and MS, measles virus has had for a long time the honour of being the number one suspect for causing MS. With radioimmunoassays it has been possible to show that, in MS, it is not only measles antibodies that show a slight elevation, but that the same is true for the antibodies against most of the common viruses. Therefore, MS must be seen more as a slight but continuous hyperactivation of the immune system, than as a special reaction against the presence of antigens from one or more viruses (Vandvik et al, 1976). In general, a good overall correspondance was usually found in the fluctuations of the different antiviral antibodies synthetized intrathecally. However, these fluctuations did not correlate with the clinical course of the disease and it can be concluded that the antiviral antibodies studied are not relevant to the ethiology of MS.

From studies set up to identify some or all of the oligoclonal IgG fractions in MS/CSF as antiviral antibodies it can be concluded (Roström, 1981) that there is a local antiviral antibody synthesis but also that this local biosynthesis is heterogeneous. In most cases, one or more of the IgG bands remained completely unidentified as antiviral immunoglobulin and on a quantitative basis, only an insignificant amount of the immunoglobulins could be considered as antiviral antibodies.

Experiments to lay a link between autoantigens (brain specific proteins) and the oligoclonal immunoglobulins have not met with much more succes. Recent studies by Gorny et al (1983) showed that antibodies against myelin or against oligodendrocytes can be identified in the CSF from patients with neurological diseases, but that these antibodies are a common feature of diseases of the central nervous system in which demyelinisation is a common component. The antibody-dependent cytotoxicity test against myelin basic protein must be seen in the same light (Frick et al, 1980). On the ground of its specificity and high frequency of positive findings, this test may be of diagnostic significance but it has no validity as a primary aetiological factor in MS.

In the field of physiology, attempts have been made to implicate the MS/CSF immunoglobulins directly in some mechanisms like slowing of nerve impulses (Trojaborg et al, 1981), myelinotoxicity (Stendhal Brodin et al,

1979) and tissue culture demyelinisation (Bornstein et al, 1965). No useful diagnostic test has come forth from these studies.

Allthough the interest in CSF immunoglobulins in MS centers mainly on those of type G, sporadious studies on those of other types have been made.

For the high molecular weight IgM, the following conclusions were reached for MS (Sindic et al, 1982):

- in nearly fifty percent of the patients an elevation of CSF/IgM concentrations was observed.
- the lack of correlation between the blood/CSF ratios for albumin and IgM lets suppose that a fraction of the CSF/IgM is produced intrathecally.
- the presence of oligoclonal IgM in the CSF of about 3 percent of the MS patients has been reported (Link et al, 1977).
- the lack of correlation between the CSF/IgM values and the clinical data undermine the interest of this determination.

Measurement of the immunoglobulin A concentrations in MS/CSF with the same technique led to the conclusion that in about 20 percent of the patients the local IgA biosynthesis reached values above the upper normal limit (Sindic et al, in print).

Serious data on the CSF/immunoglobulin E levels became available only recently (Sindic et al, 1984) and it was observed that most neurological patients with an elevation of the CSF/IgE values suffered from various infections of the central nervous system. Most of the MS patients studied had CSF/IgE values only slightly above the upper normal limit and no local biosynthesis could be detected.

Related to the immunoglobulins is the problem of the eventual presence of immune complexes. Allthough conflicting results have been published for MS patients, in a recent study, using the particle counting immunoassay (Sindic et al, 1984), no significant concentrations of immune complexes could be detected in MS/CSF.

REFERENCES

(note: no special parameters have been applied to select these few papers related to the subject of this review)

Bauer, H., 1961. Die cerebrospinal Flussigkeit - Neuere Methoden und Forschungsergebnisse als Grundlage der Deutung von Liquorbefunden. Internist (Berlin), 2, 85-94.

Bollengier, F., Rabinovitch N., Lowenthal A., 1978. Oligoclonal immunoglo-
    bulins, light chain ratios and free light chains in the cerebrospinal
    fluid and serum from patients affected with various neurological di-
    seases. J. Clin. Chem. Clin. Biochem., 16, 165-173.
Bornstein, M.B., Appel, H., 1965. Tissue culture studies of demyelinisa-
    tion. Ann. N.Y. Acad. Sc., 122, 280-286.
Chazot, G., Lasne, Y., Benzerara, O., Confafreux, C., Schott, B., 1980.
    Radio-immunofixation: une nouvelle technique de caractérisation des
    immunoglobulines dans le liquide céphalo-rachidien non concentré.
    Rev. Neurol. (Paris), 136, 783-786.
Christensen, O., Clausen, J., Fog, T., 1978. Relationships between abnor-
    mal IgG index, oligoclonal bands, acute phase reactants and some
    clinical data in Multiple Sclerosis. J. Neurol., 218, 237-244.
Delmotte, P., Gonsette, R., 1977. Biochemical findings in Multiple Sclero-
    sis IV. Isoelectric focusing of the CSF gammaglobulins in M.S. and
    other neurological diseases. J. Neurology, 215, 27-37.
Delmotte, P., 1979. The evaluation of the blood/CSF barrier permeability
    and the intrathecal IgG synthesis by capillary isotachophoresis.
    in 'Humoral immunity in neurological diseases', Nato advanced Study
    Institute, Antwerpen.
Eickhoff, K., Kaschka W., Skuaril, F., Thelkaes, L., Heipertz, R., 1979.
    Determination of IgG subgroups in cerebrospinal fluid of Multiple
    Sclerosis patients and others. Acta Neurol. Scand., 60, 277-282.
Esiri, M.D., 1977. Immunoglobulin containing cells in Multiple Sclerosis
    plaques. Lancet ii (n° 8036), 478-480.
Frick, E., Stickl, H., 1980. Antibody-dependent lymphocyte cytotoxicity
    against basic proteins of myelin in Multiple Sclerosis. J. Neurol.
    Sci., 46, 187-197.
Gorny M.A., Wroblewska, Z., Pleasure, D., Miller, S.L., Wajgt, A., Kopprow-
    ski, H., 1983. CSF antibodies to myelin basic protein and oligodendro-
    cytes in MS and other neurological diseases. Acta Neurol. Scand., 67,
    338-347.
Jozefczyk, P., Kelly, R.H., Rabin, B.S., 1984. Clinical significance of
    immunological and immunogenetic evaluation in MS. Immunol. Comm.,
    13 (4), 371-379.
Kolar, O.J., Rice, P.H., Jones, F.H., Defalque, R.J., Kincaid, J., 1980.
    Cerebrospinal fluid immunoelectrophoresis in Multiple Sclerosis.
    J. Neurol. Sciences, 47, 221-230.
Laurell, C.B., 1965. Antigen antibody crossed electrophoresis. Annal.
    Biochem., 10, 358-361.
Link, H., Tibblung, G., 1977. Principles of albumin and IgG analyses in
    neurological disorders. II. Relation of the concentration of proteins
    in serum and cerebrospinal fluid. III. Evaluation of IgG synthesis
    within the central nervous system in Multiple Sclerosis. Scand. J.
    Lab. Invest., 37, 391-401.
Lowenthal, A., 1964. Agar gel electrophoresis in neurology. Elsevier
    Publ. C°., Amsterdam.
Mancini, G., Carbonara, A.O., Heremans, J.F., 1965. Immunochemical quanti-
    tation of antigens by single radial immunodiffusion. Immunochemistry,
    2, 235-254.
Masson, P.L., Cambiaso, C.L., Collet-cassart, D., Magnusson, C.G.M.,
    Richards, G.B., Sindic, C.J.M., 1981. Particle counting immunoassay
    (PACIA). Methods in Immunology, 74, 106-139.

Mehta, P.D., Patrick, B.A., Wisniewski, H.M., 1981. Isoelectric focusing
    and immunofixation of cerebrospinal fluid and serum in Multiple
    Sclerosis. J. Clin. Lab. Immunol., 6, 17-22.
Moulin, D., Paty, D.W., Ebers, G.C., 1983. The predictive value of CSF
    electrophoresis in possible Multiple Sclerosis. Brain, 106, 809-816.
Nikoskelainen, E., Frey, H., Salmi, A., 1981. Prognosis of optic neuritis
    with special reference to cerebrospinal fluid immunoglobulins and
    measles virus antibodies. Ann. Neurol., 9, 545-550.
Rieder, H.P., Fritschi, J., 1980. Quotienten der Liquorproteinfraktionen
    und ihre labordiagnostische Bedeutung. Der Nervenarzt, 51, 704-707.
Reiber, H., 1979. Quantitative Bestimmung der lokal im Zentralnervensystem
    synthetisierten Immunoglobulin G Fraktion des Liquors. J. Clin. Chem.
    Clin. Biochem., 17, 587-591.
Roström, B., 1981. Specificity of antibodies in oligoclonal bounds in
    patients with Multiple Sclerosis and cerebrovascular diseases.
    Acta Neurol. Scand., Suppl. 86, Vol. 63.
Schliep, G., Felgenhauer, K., 1978. Rapid determination of proteins in
    serum and cerebrospinal fluid by Laser Nephelometry. J. Clin. Chem.
    Clin. Biochem., 16, 631-635.

Siden, A., 1977. Crossed immunoelectrofocusing of cerebrospinal fluid im-
    munoglobulins. J. Neurol., 217, 103-109.
Sindic, C.J.M., Cambiaso, C.L., Depre, A., Laterre, E.C., Masson, P.L.,
    1982. The concentration of IgM in the cerebrospinal fluid of neurolo-
    gical patients. J. Neurol. Sc., 55, 339-350, 1982.
Sindic, C.J.M., Magnussson, C.G.M., Laterre, E.C., Masson, P.L., 1984a.
    IgE in the cerebrospinal fluid. J. Neuroimmunology, 6, 319-324.
Sindic, C.J.M., Cambiaso, C.L., Depre, A., Laterre, E.C., Masson, P.L.,
    1984b. Immune complexes in the cerebrospinal fluid and serum of neuro-
    logical patients. J. Neuroimmunology, 6, 9-18.
Sindic, C.J.M., Delacroix, D.D., Vaerman, J.P., Laterre, E.C., Masson, P.L.
    Study of IgA in the cerebrospinal fluid of neurological patients
    with special reference to size, subclass and local production.
    In print.
Stendahl-Brodin, L., Link, H., Aristensson, K., 1979. Myelinotoxic activi-
    ty on tadpole optic nerve of cerebrospinal fluid from patients with
    optic neuritis. Neurology, 29, 882-886.
Stendahl-Brodin, L., Link, H., 1980. Relation between benign course of MS
    and low grade humoral immune response in CSF. J. Neurol. Neurosurg.
    Psych., 43, 102-105.
Tourtellotte, W.W., Potuina, R., Fleming, J.O., Murthy, K.N., Levy, J.,
    Syndulko, K., Potvin, J.H., 1980. Multiple Sclerosis: measurement and
    validation of central nervous system IgG synthesis rate. Neurology,
    30, 240-244.
Trojaborg, W., Böttcher, J., Saxtrup, O., 1981. Evoked potentials and
    immunoglobulin abnormalities in MS. Neurology, 31, 866-871.
Vandvik, R., Norrby, E., Nordal, H.J., Degre, M., 1976. Oligoclonal meas-
    les virus specific IgG antibodies isolated from cerebrospinal fluid,
    brain extracts and sera from patients with SSPE and MS. Scand. J.
    Immunol., 3, 979-992.
Verjans, E. , Theys, P., Delmotte, P., Carton, H., 1983. Clinical parame-
    ters and intrathecal IgG synthesis as prognostic features in MS.
    Part I. J. Neurol., 229, 155-165.

31

Multiple Sclerosis: A Two Stage Process?

D. INZITARI, G. VOLPI, A. CASTAGNOLI and L. AMADUCCI

INTRODUCTION

In order to confirm and to better define previously reported data
(Bartolini et al., 1982) (Inzitari et al., 1984) indicating an abnormal
IC pattern in a high number of Multiple Sclerosis(MS) patients, we
revaluated the result of IC study in 86 cases(49 male and 37 female)
affected by a definite form of MS and studied during the last 10 years
(1975-1985). Correlations were searched between IC abnormalities,
clinical and laboratory findings. Particular attention was drawn to the
possible relationship between changes of the CSF flow and symptoms in MS.

MATERIAL AND METHODS

99Tc-DTPA solution, 20 to 30 uCi per Kilogram of body weight (total
volume, 1 to 1.5 ml), was introduced into the spinal subarachnoid space.
Radiography was performed 1, 2, 6, and 24 hours after the injection. The
Cisternographic pictures were classified according to recent literature
(Wolinski et al., 1973):

Normal pattern: uninterrupted flow from the lumbar subarachnoid
space into the basal cisternes, around the brainstem, through the
tentorial notch into the Sylvian cisterns, and over the convexities
of the emispheres to the parasagittal regions. No ventricular
activity is observed.

Slow flow pattern (Dov Front, 1982): low ascent of the tracer over
the emispheric convexities, with persistent visualizations of the
basal cisterns at 24 hours, no ventricular activity is observed.
Mixed pattern:filling of the ventricular system 4 to 6 hours after
lumbar injection. At 24 hours ventricular activity may still be
seen, but normal flow over the hemispheric convexities is also
observed.

Ventricular pattern: Ventricular influx both early and late as long as radioactivity can be detected. Although there is no flow of isotope above the tentorial notch, one or both sylvian cisterns may occasionally be visualized; flow over the hemispheres to the parasagittal regions is not observed.

Diagnostic criteria of MS were those indicated by Poser (Poser et al., 1984). The different clinical courses were classified according to McAlpine's criteria (McAlpine et al.,1972) . The disability degree at the time of IC examination was assessed by means of the Kurtzke's expanded disability status scale (E.D.S.S.) (Kurtzke, 1983) . Mental impairment was evaluated using the item 14 of the Incapacity Status Scale (I.S.S.) of Kurtzke (Kurtzke, 1981) The IgG index was calculated according to Tibbling and Link (Link et al., 1977). The Agar-gel electrophoresis IgG pattern was carried out according to Lowenthal (Lowenthal et al., 1960).

RESULTS

In 28 (32%) of the 85 MS patients examined, the IC study showed an abnormal picture (Table 1). In 13 cases the IC was of "Slow flow" type, in 11 cases the pattern was defined as mixed and in 4 cases as ventricular. The abnormal IC was significantly more frequent among patients with a longer duration of the disease (Table 2), those with a chronic progressive course and those with a higher disability score (Table 3). Moreover an abnormal IC was significantly more frequent in the group of patients with mental impairment (Table 4). On the contrary no correlation was found with IgG index values and the occurrence of an cligoclonal pattern (Table 5).

Table 1: The Cisternographic pictures were classified as follows:

		N°of cases	N°of cases
NORMAL			57
ABNORMAL	Slow flow pattern	13	
	Mixed pattern	11	28
	Ventricular pattern	4	
	Total		86

Table 2: Correlations between cases with normal and abnormal IC pattern and sex, age and duration of disease.

Parameters		IC normal	IC abnormal	p
SEX	(M/F)	34/22	15/15	n.s.
AGE	(years)	36.9±9	43.5±9	n.s.
DURATION OF DISEASE	(years)	7.3±6	12.48±7	0.001

Table 3: Comparison between cases with normal and abnormal IC pattern in relation to clinical course, disability score and evolution.

	IC normal	IC abnormal	p
CLINICAL COURSE			
Remitting	27/57	4/27	
			0.001
Chronic-progressive	32/57	23/27	
DISABILITY SCORE (Expanded Disability Status Scale)			
E.D.S.S. ⟨ 4	23/57	2/27	
			0.001
E.D.S.S. ⟩ 4	34/57	25/27	

Table 4: Comparison between normal and abnormal IC groups by mental impairment as defined according to the Incapacity Status Scale (I.S.S.) (Kurtzke, 1981)

	IC normal	IC abnormal	p
Mental impairment	3/57	11/28	0.001

Table 5: Comparison among patients with normal and abnormal pattern
according to CSF findings

	IC normal	IC abnormal	p
Oligoclonal IgG pattern	18/27	9/27	
			n.s.
Normal IgG pattern	37/54	17/54	
IgG Index (Link)	0.9±0.5	1.05±0.9	n.s.

DISCUSSION

The hereby reported data of IC study in MS confirm on a larger series of cases the previously published findings of a significant correlation among IC abnormalities, severity of disability and progressive clinical course.

However the observation obtained in smaller series of cases indicating a correlation between the IC alterations and the IgG index values was not confirmed. It is possible that the larger number of milder cases included in the present report may contribute to this finding. On the other hand while in the previously reported cases the picture of the so-called ventricular pattern (corresponding to the normal pressure hydrocephalus pattern) had been never observed, we recently were able to detect this pattern in four cases of the present series.

Moreover it was of interest to find that the abnormal IC pattern was more frequent among patients with mental disturbances. These observations may further suggest that CSF flow disturbances may have a role in the clinical picture of MS, aggravating the functional disability and contributing to a progressive course.

Retrospective and Prospective studies are needed in order to confirm the prognostic predictive value of IC in MS; other methodologies such as Nuclear Magnetic Resonance (N.M.R.), enhanced C.T. and Cisternography with not ionic contrast media together with CSF pressure monitoring may add further elements on this ground, and are in progress.

Acknowledgements: This work was supported by a Grant from the Italian National Research Council (C.N.R.), Rome; Italy-Grant N°82027104

REFERENCES

1.Bartolini S., Inzitari D., Castagnoli A. and Amaducci L.. Correlation
  of Isotopic cisternographic patterns in multiple sclerosis with CSF IgG
  values. Ann.Neurol.,12,486, 1982.

2.Inzitari D., Capparelli R., Sità D., Barontini F., Marini P. and
  Amaducci L.. Isotopic Cisternogrphy in MS : possible correlation with
  diseases course. In "Multiple Sclerosis, Immunological and clinical
  aspect", Gonsette and Delmotte Eds, 1984.

3.Wolinsky J., Barnes B.B., Margolis M.T.: Diagnostic test in normal
  pressure hydrocephalus. Neurology(Minneap.)23:706-713, 1973.

4.Dov Front: Radionuclide Brain Image. Appleton Century Crofts/Norwalk,
  Connecticut: 104-134, 1982.

5.Poser C.M., Paty D.W., Scheinberg L., McDonald W.I., Davis F.A., Ebers
  G.C., Johnson K., Sibley W., Silberberg D.H. and Tourtellotte W.W.: New
  diagnostic criteria for Multiple Sclerosis: Guidelines for research
  protocols. Ann.Neurol. 13:227-231,1983.

6.McAlpine D., Lumsen C.E., Acheson E.D.: Multiple Sclerosis. A
  reapraisal. 2nd Edn.(Edinburgh, London: Churchill Livinstone), 1982.

7.Kurtzke J.F.: Rating neurologic impairemnt in Multiple Sclerosis: an
  Expanded disability status scale (EDSS). Neurology (Cleveland),
  33:1444-52, 1983.

8.Tibbling G., Link H.and Ohman S.: Principles of albumin and IgG
  analyses in neurological disorders. I. Establishment of reference
  values. Scand.J.Clin.Lab.Invest., 37: 385, 1977.

9.Lowenthal A., Van Sande M., Karcher D.,: The differential diagnosis of
  neurological diseases by fractionating electrophoretically the CSF
  proteins. J. Neurochem., 6: 51, 1960.

10.Kurtzke J.F.: A proposal for uniform minimal record of disability in
  multiple sclerosis. Acta Neurol.Scand.(Supll 87), 64:110-129.1981.

32

CSF Immunoglobulins and Clinical Course

H. LINK

INTRODUCTION

Establishment of a relation between any clinical variable of MS such
as disease activity or duration, and aberrations of CSF immunoglobulins
is hampered by several difficulties. Clinical variables are often difficult to define. Thus, an exacerbation may be simulated by changes of body
temperature, or plaques may develop in areas of white matter without
presenting any clinical signs and symptoms. One or two strategically located plaques may induce profound disability while, in other patients,
extensive dissemination of plaques may be accompanied by no or only
slight disability. Furthermore, various "treatment" protocols nowadays
used in many centres include drugs which modulate the immune response and
have long-lasting effects on e.g. Ig levels in CSF. These may be some of
the reasons why, in the vast literature on MS, few studies deal with relation between clinical variables and Ig aberrations in CSF even though
these aberrations after all might have importance for the pathogenesis of
the disease. Thus, modern laboratory tests such as nuclear magnetic resonance studies or determinations of myelin basic protein levels in CSF in

MS patients in order to establish disease activity more appropriately, have hitherto not been related to Ig concentrations in CSF.

IgG LEVELS AND NUMBERS OF IgG PRODUCING CELLS IN CSF

In a classical study from 1954 Yahr, Goldensohn and Kabat related the CSF IgG/total protein ratio (an indicator for IgG synthesis within the CNS) to a number of clinical variables among 244 patients. The IgG ratio was increased in 67%. Elevated ratios did not correlate to type of onset, acute or chronic, duration of disease (1-20 years) or occurrence of new symptoms. However, increased ratios were found in 80-100% of patients who had multiple attacks, multiple lesions and marked functional disability, while the lowest incidence, 47% was found in patients who had only one attack - so called benign MS. Others have confirmed this observation. In one study patients with no or slight disability after a duration of diseases >10 years showed a low frequency of abnormally high CSF IgG/ total protein ratios (Olsson et al., 1976). Adopting the IgG index equal to (CSF IgG/serum IgG):(CSF albumin/serum albumin) on 105 consecutive patients with MS, only 2 of 17 cases (12%) with malignant course (moderate to severe disability within 5 years after onset) displayed normal values compared to 9 of 19 patients (47%) with the most benign course (slight or no disability after 20 years) (Stendhal-Brodin and Link, 1980).

In a study comprising 64 patients with MS we were also unable to identify a correlation between clinical variables in the form of age at the time of lumbar puncture, duration of disease, exacerbation of symptoms and disability degree on one hand, and occurrence of elevated CSF IgG/ total protein ratio on the other (Link and Müller, 1971). However, in a subsequent study based on investigation of CSF and serum specimens obtained from 22 patients during exacerbations as well as remissions, thus enabling a more careful statistic evaluation and eliminating the difference between individual patients, we calculated a ratio between the concentrations of CSF IgG in the same MS patient (Olsson and Link, 1973). In this way, a significant increase of CSF IgG levels could be documented during exacerbations (Table 1). Significantly higher absolute values of kappa and lambda chains were also registered during exacerbations, which is in accordance with the elevated IgG levels.

Adopting a formula for calculation of IgG synthesis within the CNS per 24 h, Tourtellotte and Ma (1978) have reported higher IgG production in patients with a greater number of relapses, in those with active clinical definite MS, and to some extent in older patients and in those with a longer course of disease. On the other hand, no consistent effect on CSF IgG production was noted in regard to degree of disability or clinical status (exacerbating, stationary or remitting), except that production was reduced by administration of ACTH and/or steroid therapy.

TABLE 1   Concentrations of IgG, IgA, albumin and kappa and lambda light chain antigenic determinants and kappa/lambda ratios in CSF during exacerbation and remission of MS. Values are mean ± SEM. All CSF values are percentages of CSF total protein. Modified from Olsson and Link (1973).

CSF protein	Exacerbation	Remission	Exacerbation: Remission ratio
IgG	14.4 ± 0.84	13.6 ± 0.89	1.10 ± 0.04*
IgA	1.2 ± 0.11	1.0 ± 0.13	1.37 ± 0.12**
Albumin	57.3 ± 2.66	55.2 ± 2.58	1.04 ± 0.02
Kappa light chains	6.6 ± 0.67	6.3 ± 0.72	1.12 ± 0.05*
Lambda light chains	5.0 ± 0.56	4.6 ± 0.54	1.19 ± 0.02**
Kappa/lambda ratio	1.5 ± 0.19	1.7 ± 0.26	1.04 ± 0.03

*Significance level of $p < 0.05$. **Significance level of $p < 0.01$.

Enumeration of mature B cells, i.e. plasma cells secreting Ig, in CSF and peripheral blood has increased our knowledge about the humoral immune response in MS (Henriksson et al., 1981). Enumeration of Ig-secreting cells may be carried out by an indirect hemolytic plaque-forming cell assay which is based on the capacity of one single plasma cell to produce and secrete Ig molecules of a certain class. Adopting this assay on 37 patients with MS, 89% had cells in CSF producing IgG. Subgrouping the patients into active and stable MS did not reveal any differences (Table 2). As expected, the number of IgG producing cells was significantly higher in CSF than in peripheral blood (Henriksson et al., 1985).

In conclusion, evidence has been presented for elevated CSF IgG levels occurring more frequently in malignant compared to benign MS, and during exacerbations compared to remissions. Numbers of IgG producing cells per 20×10^3 lymphocytes are higher in CSF compared to peripheral blood.

IgA LEVELS AND NUMBERS OF IgA SECRETING CELLS IN CSF

Only a minority of MS patients present evidence for intrathecal IgA production when the IgA level is presented as CSF IgA/total protein ratio (Link and Müller, 1971; Mingeoli et al., 1978) or as IgA index (Stendahl-Brodin and Link, 1980). The study by Olsson and Link (1973) revealed, however, higher IgA levels in CSF during exacerbations compared to remissions (Table 1).

Further evidence for a local IgA response in MS has recently been obtained by enumeration of IgA producing cells. No less than 70% among 37 patients with MS displayed IgA secreting cells in CSF (Henriksson et al., 1985). No difference was found when the patients were subgrouped into active and stable MS (Table 2).

TABLE 2   Absolute numbers of plaque forming cells per 20 x 10^3 lymphocytes in peripheral blood and CSF from 37 patients with MS and after subgrouping in active and stable MS, in 20 patients with acute meningo-encephalitis (AM) examined within 10 days after onset, and in peripheral blood only from 27 healthy controls. From Henriksson et al., 1985.

Diagnosis and numbers of subjects		IgG		IgA		IgM	
		Blood	CSF	Blood	CSF	Blood	CSF
MS (n=37)	Range	2-26	0-858	0-135	0-94	0-27	0-307
	Median value	10	89	25	10	4	4
Active MS (n=13)	Range	2-19	0-858	8-95	0-60	0-27	0-77
	Median value	8	89	17	5	4	4
Stable MS (n=24)	Range	2-26	0-520	0-135	0-94	0-23	0-307
	Median value	10	91	25	10	4	3.5
AM (n=20)	Range	0-319	0-716	7-295	0-596	4-99	0-326
	Median value	31	16	83	29	17	9
Healthy controls (n=27)	Range	2-20	n.d.	4-42	n.d.	1-7	n.d.
	Median value	7		12		2	

n.d. = not done

IgM LEVELS AND NUMBERS OF IgM PRODUCING CELLS IN CSF

Modern technology has enabled determination of IgM in CSF under normal and pathological conditions. Williams et al. (1978) measured IgM levels in CSF by radioimmunoassay (RIA) and found raised CSF IgM/CSF albumin ratios in 46% of 56 patients with MS. Interestingly, 8 patients had elevated IgM ratio in presence of normal corresponding IgG ratio. No relationship was found between the CSF IgM level and clinical severity in MS, relapses or steroid therapy. Employing particle counting immunoassay (PACIA), Sindic et al. (1982) reported elevated IgM index in 32% of 80 patients with MS. Four of the patients had a high IgM index without either increase of IgG index or presence of oligoclonal bands. None of 10 patients with MS history >15 years had elevated IgM index. Otherwise, no significant influence of age of onset, interval between onset and sampling and clinical state was observed. Forsberg et al. (1984) used enzyme-linked immunosorbent assay (ELISA) and found elevated IgM index in 63% of 35 patients with MS. Two of the patients had elevated IgM index in the presence of normal IgG and IgA indices. Elevated values were registered in 11 of 15 patients with a duration of MS <5 years, in 8 of 10 patients after 5-10 years, in 3 of 6 after 10-15 years, and in none of 4 after 15 years. Similar frequencies of elevated levels were encountered in active and stable disease.

Further evidence for IgM synthesis within the CNS in MS has recently been obtained by determination of numbers of IgM producing cells. 57% of 37 patients had cells in CSF producing IgM and in 6 of them, IgM producing cells predominated in CSF (Henriksson et al., 1985). No difference was found between patients with active compared to stable MS (Table 2).

These studies indicate that IgM synthesis within the CNS is common in MS but may vanish in burnt-out cases. Systematic studies are warranted in order to establish the CSF IgM profile in relation to clinical variables in greater detail. Determination of IgM index might have a place in the routine characterization of the humoral immune profile of CSF in suspected as well as clinically definite MS. We have found evidence for presence of monomeric IgM in addition to pentameric IgM in MS CSF. The possible influence of the proportion between monomeric and pentameric IgM on IgM determination should be evaluated, and the significance of presence of monomeric IgM assessed.

OLIGOCLONAL RESPONSE WITHIN THE CNS

No clear evidence has been presented that the oligoclonal band pattern
changes in relation to clinical MS variables, irrespective of method used
for demonstration of bands. Our data (Olsson and Link, 1973) and those of
others (for review see Walsh et al., 1983) indicate that the oligoclonal
IgG band pattern in the individual patient does not change over the course
of MS, but may be influenced by immunomodulatory "treatments". We have
recently performed agarose isoelectric focusing on unconcentrated CSF adjusted to defined IgG levels, followed by transfer to cellulose nitrate
membrane and double-antibody avidin-biotin peroxidase staining (Olsson et
al., 1984). As many as 30 sharp oligoclonal IgG bands can be seen when MS
CSF is examined in this way. Simultaneous examination of consecutive specimens obtained from individual patients with MS covering exacerbations
and remissions revealed as principle feature a marked similarity of banding patterns in the individual patient. One or more weak band may wax
and wain, but whether this phenomenon is a result of technical pitfalls
or represents a biological phenomenon is not clear.

Lack of oligoclonal bands in CSF in patients with clinically definite
MS is accompanied by an improved prognosis. Fourteen out of 17 patients
(82%) with MS but lacking oligoclonal bands in CSF had no or slight disability after a mean duration of disease of 17 years, compared to 47 of
88 patients (53%) with oligoclonal bands after a mean duration of 13 years
(Stendahl-Brodin and Link, 1980). Absence of oligoclonal bands was only
rarely accompanied by elevated IgG index or abnormal CSF kappa/lambda
ratio.

TABLE 3   Frequencies of mononuclear pleocytosis, elevated levels of IgG, IgA and IgM and elevated numbers of IgG, IgA and IgM plaque-forming cells (PFC) per 20 x 10^3 lymphocytes in CSF in 31 patients with monosymptomatic paraesthesiae or hypasthesiae, subgrouped according to presence (group I) or absence (group II) of oligoclonal bands in CSF. From V. Kostulas, A. Henriksson and H. Link, manuscript in preparation.

CSF abnormality	Group I (n=20)		Group II (n=11)	
	sample 1	sample 2	sample 1	sample 2
Mononuclear cells $>$ 5	14	11	1	0
CSF IgG index $>$ 0.7	10	11	0	0
CSF IgA index $>$ 0.6	0	1	0	0
CSF IgM index $>$ 0.06	4/18	5/18	1	0
CSF IgG PFC $>$ 2	n.d.	12/16	n.d.	0/8
CSF IgA PFC $>$ 2	n.d.	5/16	n.d.	0/6
CSF IgM PFC $>$ 2	n.d.	5/15	n.d.	0.6
Normal CSF	2	2	10	11

n.d. = not done

In acute unilateral optic neuritis (Stendahl-Brodin and Link, 1983) and monosymptomatic sensory disturbances (V. Kostulas, A. Henriksson and H. Link, manuscript in preparation), demonstration of oligoclonal bands in CSF has also prognostic implications. This is exemplified in Table 3 for 31 patients with paraesthesiae or hypaesthesiae who were subjected to lumbar puncture at two occasions and subgrouped with regard to presence (group I) or absence (group II) of oligoclonal bands in CSF. The mean intervals between lumbar puncture No. 1 and 2 were 13 and 15 months, respectively. Among the 20 patients in group I, 19 displayed oligoclonal bands in both specimens while one had bands in No. 2 only. The 11 patients in group II were negative for bands at both occasions. Subsequent follow-up revealed that 8 of the patients of group I and none of those of group II had developed MS.

CONCLUDING REMARKS

Comparison of results obtained from determination of Ig levels and numbers of Ig producing cells in CSF have revealed discrepancies which are

most conspicious for IgA since elevated IgA levels were only rarely encountered in MS CSF while a majority of MS patients have IgA secreting
cells in CSF. It must therefore be anticipated that intrathecal IgA production is common in MS although not detectable by conventional CSF IgA
determinations. One explanation might be that free Ig's in CSF are bound
to the target and therefore difficult to detect at increased levels. This
might be one reason why reports regarding relations between levels of
free Ig's in CSF and clinical variables have been few and sometimes contradictory. It can be anticipated that enumeration of Ig producing cells
reflects the humoral immune response within the CNS-CSF compartment in a
more appropriate way. Similarly, determinations of levels of specific
antibodies in CSF might be inferior to enumeration of cells secreting
such antibodies. Systematic studies of numbers of Ig and specific antibody producing cells belonging to various classes and IgG subclasses over
the course of disease in individual patients with MS are highly warranted
to throw further light on the possible role of the humoral immune response within the CNS for the pathogenesis of MS. In order to circumvent
uncertainties inherent to more clinical evaluations, such studies should
include laboratory grading for disease activity such as determinations of
levels of myelin basic protein in CSF as well as nuclear magnetic resonance.

REFERENCES

Forsberg, P., Henriksson, A., Link, H. and Ohman, S., 1984. Reference
    for CSF-IgM, CSF-IgM/S-IgM ratio and IgM index, and its application to
    patients with multiple sclerosis and aseptic meningoencephalitis.
    Scand. J. Clin. Lab. Invest., 44: 7-12.
Henriksson, A., Kam-Hansen, S. and Andersson, R., 1981. Immunoglobulin-
    producing cells in CSF and blood from patients with multiple sclerosis
    and other neurological diseases enumerated by Protein-A plaque assay.
    J. Neuroimmunol., 1: 299-309.
Henriksson, A., Kam-Hansen, S. and Link, H., 1985. IgM, IgA and IgG pro-
    duction cells in cerebrospinal fluid and peripheral blood in multiple
    sclerosis. Ann. Neurol., submitted.
Link, H. and Müller, R., 1971. Immunoglobulins in multiple sclerosis and
    infections of the nervous system. Arch. Neurol. (Chic.), 25: 326-344.
Mingioli, E.S., Strober, W., Tourtellotte, W.W., Whitaker, J.N. and
    McFarlin, D.E., 1978. Quantitation of IgG, IgA and IgM in the CSF by
    radioimmunoassay. Neurology, 28: 991-995.
Olsson, J.E. and Link, H., 1973. Immunoglobulin abnormalities in multiple
    sclerosis - Relation to clinical parameters - Exacerbations and re-
    missions. Arch. Neurol. (Chic.), 28: 392-399.
Olsson, J.E., Link, H. and Müller, R., 1976. Immunoglobulin abnormalities
    in multiple sclerosis. Relation to clinical parameters: Disability,

duration and age of onset. J. Neurol. Sci., 27: 233-245.

Olsson, T., Kostulas, V. and Link, H., 1984. Improved detection of oligoclonal IgG in cerebrospinal fluid by isoelectric focusing in agarose,
  double-antibody peroxidase labeling, and avidin-biotin amplification.
  Clin. Chem., 30: 1246-1249.

Sindic, C.J., Cambiaso, C.L., Depré, A., Laterre, E.C. and Masson, P.L.,
  1982. The concentration of IgM in the cerebrospinal fluid of neurological patients. J. Neurol. Sci., 55: 339-350.

Stendahl-Brodin, L. and Link, H., 1980. Relation between benign course
  of multiple sclerosis and low-grade humoral immune response in cerebrospinal fluid. J. Neurol. Neurosurg. Psychiat., 43: 102-105.

Stendahl-Brodin, L. and Link, H., 1983. Optic neuritis: Oligoclonal bands
  increase the risk of multiple sclerosis. Acta Neurol. Scand., 67: 301-
  304.

Tourtellotte, W.W. and Ma, B.I., 1978. Multiple sclerosis: The blood-
  brain barrier and the measurements of de novo central nervous system
  IgG synthesis. Neurology (part 2), 28: 76-83.

Walsh, M.J. and Tourtellotte, W.W., 1983. The cerebrospinal fluid in
  multiple sclerosis. In: J.F. Hallpike, C.W.M. Adams, W.W. Tourtellotte
  eds., Multiple sclerosis. Williams and Wilkins, Baltimore, pp 275-358.

Williams, A.C., Mingioli, E.S., McFarland, H.F., Tourtellotte, W.W. and
  McFarlin, D.E., 1978. Increased CSF IgM in multiple sclerosis.
  Neurology, 28: 996-998.

Yahr, M.D., Goldensohn, S.S. and Kabat, E.A., 1954. Further studies on
  the gamma globulin content of cerebrospinal fluid in multiple sclerosis and other neurological diseases. Ann. N.Y. Acad. Sci., 58: 613-
  624.

33

Immunoglobulin Abnormalities for IgG, IgA and IgM in Cerebrospinal Fluid of Multiple Sclerosis Patients

K. J. B. LAMERS, W. VAN GEEL, J. C. N. KOK, O. R. HOMMES and B. FEENSTRA

INTRODUCTION

Increased IgG levels in CSF and oligoclonal pattern of the gamma-globulin fraction is characteristically found in MS patients (Laterre et al., 1970; Kjellin et al., 1974; Delmotte et al., 1977).
Already in 1958 Frick et al. demonstrated that a part of the IgG in CSF is produced within the central nervous system (CNS). Link et al. (1977) introduced the IgG index as a measure of IgG synthesis within the CNS. This index takes into account both an abnormal transsudation flow in case of a disturbed permeability of the blood brain barrier (BBB) and the actual serum IgG level. More than CSF IgG, the IgG index is a discriminating parameter for abnormal IgG production in the CNS.
Abnormal concentrations of IgA and IgM in CSF have also been described in MS patients. But IgA and IgM abnormalities in MS occur less frequently than IgG abnormalities. The results differ considerably in various MS studies (Glasner, 1975; Williams et al., 1978; Schuller et al., 1978; Sindic et al., 1982). It is assumed that the CSF IgG, IgA and IgM from non vascular origin is derived from production in the CNS (Frick et al., 1958; Tourtellotte, 1978).
Intrathecal production of IgM has also been reported in occasional patients with various inflammatory nervous system disorders such as neurosyphilis (Strandberg et al., 1982), meningoencephalitis (Link et al. 1971), Guillain Barré syndrome (Link, 1973). These data imply that intrathecal IgM production may be of importance for the pathogenesis in

inflammatory nervous system disorders. In order to establish the occurrence of the immunoglobulin abnormalities in CSF of MS patients we have
collected data on IgG, IgA and IgM in CSF and serum and the oligoclonal
aspect of CSF gammaglobulins in definite MS patients.
A patient group with other neurological diseases (OND) was also included
in the study.

MATERIALS AND METHODS

Subjects

In the MS group results of 98 definite MS patients, diagnoses according to the criteria, described in the study of Schumacher et al. (1965)
were used.
Most of the MS patients had the chronic progressive form of MS. All
patients were hospitalized between 1983 and the end of 1984 in the
Radboud University Hospital, Department of Neurology, University of Nijmegen. In order to compare the data of MS patients with OND patients,
217 OND patients were analyzed. Patients where the CSF was contaminated
with blood elements (red blood cells $> 1000/3 \ mm^3$) were excluded from the
study. Some of the MS patients have received an intensive immunosuppressive treatment years before. However, comparison of the immunoglobulin
levels between both patient groups (treated and untreated) did not give
obvious differences for IgM and IgA. The OND patients could be subdivided
into 16 different neurological groups. Five of these are included here:
infections in CNS (n=17), polyradiculitis/polyneuropathy (n=20), degenerative diseases (n=15), primary tumors and metastases (n=15), vascular
diseases (n=35). The reference group is a patient group (n=48) with cranial
nerve and spinal root disturbances, including HNP.

Biochemical methods

IgG, IgA and Albumin in unconcentrated CSF were measured by means of
an automated kinetic turbidimetric method on a centrifuged analyser. The
reaction time was approximately 2 min. Sheep antihuman IgG and IgA
(Boehringer, Mannheim) and rabbit antihuman Albumin (Behringwerke,
Marburg) were used. Serum was always diluted (1:400) with saline and
both specimens (CSF and serum) were run in the same batch.

IgM was measured on a Hyland laser nephelometer with goat antihuman IgM, (Hyland Diagnostics, USA). The reaction time was 2 hours. A sample blanc was always measured. Serum was diluted (1:100) for the IgM determination. Serum and CSF were determined in the same batch. The detection limit for IgM was 0,1 μg/ml. CSF protein electrophoresis was performed on cellulose acetate (cellogel). We used a tris, EDTA, borate buffer Ph 9,0 (high separation capacity for detecting oligoclonal bands). CSF proteins were always concentrated by ultrafiltration for electrophoresis. For the determination of abnormal immunoglobulin production in the CNS we have used the Ig indices:

$$\text{Ratio Q Alb} = \frac{\text{CSF Alb}}{\text{serum Alb}} \; ; \quad \text{Ratio Q Ig} = \frac{\text{CSF Ig (G, A or M)}}{\text{serum Ig (G, A or M)}} \; ;$$

$$\text{Immunoglobulin index is the quotient} = \frac{\text{Q Ig (G, A or M)}}{\text{Q Alb}}$$

Statistical methods

The upper and lower 2,5 percentiles are generally accepted as limits for reference range (Reed et al., 1971). Only the upper reference limit is of interest for detecting intrathecal immunoglobulin synthesis. To determine the upper 2,5 percentile we tested the Gaussian distribution with the chi-square goodness of fit method.

RESULTS

Reference values of Ig indices

For the neurological control group (n=48) the individual values of Q Alb are plotted versus Q IgG, Q IgA and Q IgM in fig. 1, 2 and 3 respectively. There is a good correlation between Q Alb on the one hand and Q IgG and Q IgA on the other hand (fig. 1 and 2). The absence of a clear

correlation between Q IgM and Q Alb (fig. 3) and the slight correlation between CSF IgM and IgM index (fig. 4) might suggest that CSF IgM is regulated in a manner different from that of IgG and IgA.
The upper normal limits for the three immunoglobulin indices of the reference group are:

for IgG index : 0.58

for IgA index : 0.39

for IgM index : 0.20

Indices above the upper normal limits are indicative for intrathecal immunoglobulin production in CNS.
In literature there is a conflicting discussion about the most suitable parameter for discriminating intrathecal IgM synthesis: the IgM index or the CSF IgM level. We have observed also indications for a difference in regulation for IgM in comparison with CSF IgA and IgG. Therefore, for IgM, both the IgM index (> 0.20) and a CSF IgM level (> 1.0 mg/l) are used in our study for determining abnormal IgM production in CNS.

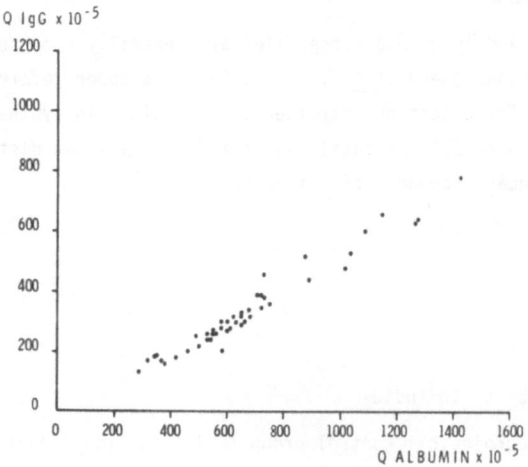

Fig. 1   Relationship between Q. albumin and Q IgG in 45 patients of the reference group

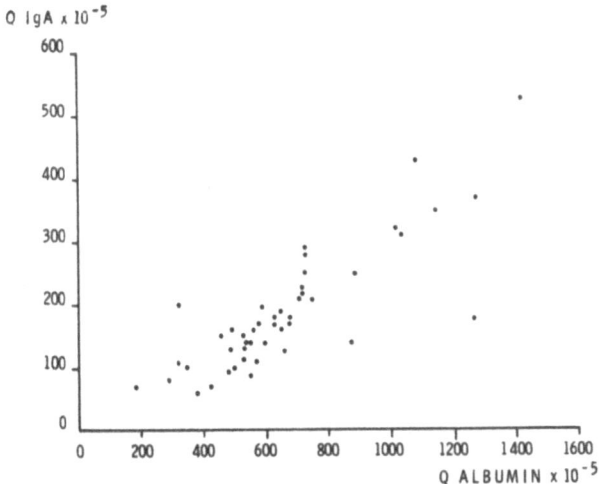

<u>Fig. 2</u>   Relationship between Q albumin and Q IgA in 46
patients of the reference group

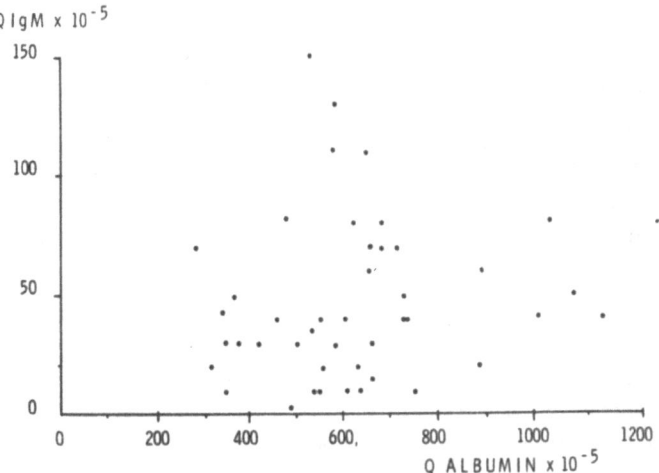

<u>Fig. 3</u>   Relationship between Q albumin and Q IgM in 45
patients of the reference group

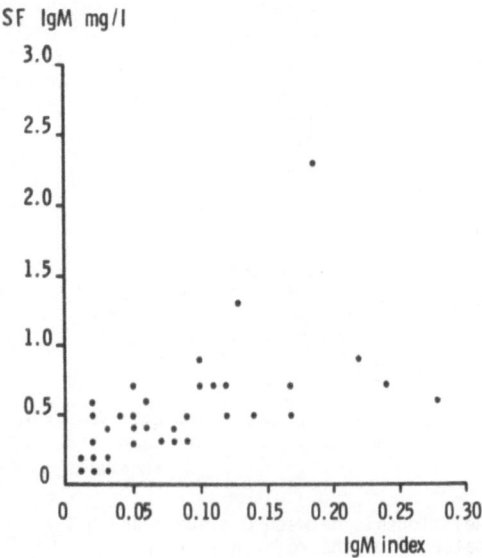

Fig. 4   Relationship between IgM index and CSF in 35
          patients of the reference group

Comparison of abnormalities for immunoglobulin indices and oligoclonal pattern in MS- and OND patients

The median values of both the indices for IgG, IgA and IgM and the
CSF IgM concentration are presented in Table 1. Furthermore, the percentages abnormalities for these parameters and the oligoclonal pattern are
given in this Table. In fig. 5 the abnormalities are graphically represen-
ted for the different neurological patients groups.
From these results it is evident that intrathecal IgG production and CSF
oligoclonal gammabands in definite MS patients are nearly always present
in CSF in contrast to abnormal IgA and IgM production. Moreover, all CSF
specimens in MS with an abnormal IgG index show an oligoclonal pattern.
This phenomenon demonstrates that the abnormal IgG in CSF of MS patients
has an oligoclonal gamma pattern. The CSF specimens with an abnormal IgM
show always an abnormal IgG.

TABLE 1

Immunoglobulin abnormalities in neurological patients

Patient groups	Number	IgG index		IgA index		IgM index		CSF IgM in mg/l		Oligoclonal aspect
		Median	Abnormal in %	Median	Abnormal in %	Median	Abnormal in %	Median	Abnormal in %	Abnormal in %
Definite MS	98	0.82	87	0.28	11	0.08	15	0.50	12	93
Possible MS	15	0.61	66	0.27	20	0.07	6	0.60	6	85
Infections in CNS	17	0.54	47	0.34	37	0.16	35	1.10	53	40
Polyradiculitis/ polyneuropathy	20	0.52	15	0.32	26	0.11	20	0.80	40	20
Degenerative diseases	15	0.49	20	0.28	7	0.10	20	0.50	20	23
Primary tumores and metastases	15	0.49	20	0.30	0	0.07	6	0.60	13	31
Vascular diseases	35	0.47	2	0.26	0	0.08	11	0.50	8	10
Controls: Cranial nerve and spinal root disturbances	48	0.49	9	0.28	2	0.06	8	0.40	6	5

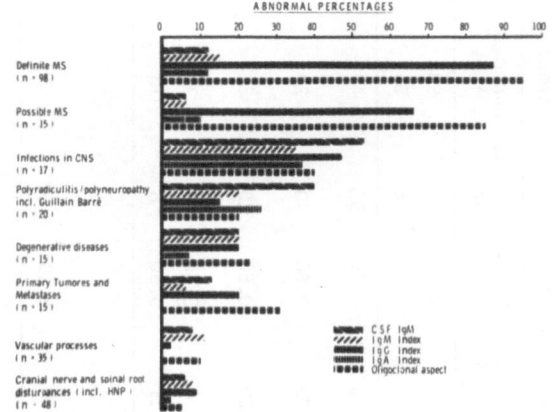

Fig. 5   Abnormal percentages of Ig indices and oligo-
         clonal pattern in 8 distinct neurological
         patient groups

Furthermore, with respect to infections in the CNS, it is obvious that the
percentages abnormalities in CSF immunoglobulins and the oligoclonal
pattern are all about 40%. 50% of the CSF specimens with an abnormal IgM
also show an abnormal CSF IgG. In the groups polyradiculitis/polyneuro-
pathy and degenerative diseases the percentages abnormalities are about
20%. Also in these groups about 50% of the CSF with abnormal IgM has also
abnormal IgG.

DISCUSSION

     The findings in this study of abnormal CSF IgG in MS patients are in
agreement with other observations (Laterre et al., 1970; Kjellin et al.,
1974; Delmotte et al., 1977). Furthermore, the CSF specimens with an abnormal IgG in MS demonstrates an oligoclonal pattern. CSF IgM abnormalities are rarely observed (15%). In different MS studies increased CSF
IgM values were found frequently ranging from 19% to 66% (Williams et al.,
1978; Schuller et al., 1978; Sindic et al., 1982; Glasner, 1975). The
variability in abnormal CSF IgM findings in MS patients can possibly be
explained by a combination of factors as differences in the measurement
of low level CSF IgM, the detection limits for CSF IgM determinations and

differences in the various MS populations (chronic progressive forms and exacerbating forms). Most of the MS patients in our study suffered from the chronic progressive form, without distinct exacerbations. While IgM production mostly appears at the beginning of an (acute) immunological reaction, the low incidence of CSF IgM abnormalities in our study can partly be explained by the choice of our MS population.

On the contrary, in the group of (acute) infections in the CNS we observed a shift in the humoral respons in CSF in comparison with the MS group by a lower IgG respons (47%) and a higher IgM respons (35% CSF index, 53% CSF IgM). IgA and IgM show a comparable pattern with respect to CSF abnormalities. Longitudinal studies of CSF IgM, IgA and IgG, especially in MS patients with the exacerbating form, might be important for the understanding of the immunological process in MS.

REFERENCES

Delmotte, P. and Gonsette, R.J., 1977. Biochemical findings in multiple sclerosis. IV. Isoelectric focusing of the CSF gammaglobulins in multiple sclerosis (262 cases) and other neurological diseases (272 cases). J. Neurol., 215: 27-37.

Frick, E. and Scheid-Seydel, L., 1958. Untersuchungen mit I^{131} markierten Albumin über Austauschvorgange zwischen Plasma und Liquor cerebrospinalis (Klin. Wochenschr., 36: 857-863.

Glasner, H., 1975. Barrier impairment and immune reaction in cerebrospinal fluid. Eur. Neurol., 13: 304-314.

Kjellin, K.G. and Vesterberg, O., 1974. Isoelectric focusing on CSF proteins in neurological diseases. J. Neurol. Sci., 23: 199-213.

Laterre, E.C., Callewaert, A., Heremans, J.F. and Sfaello, Z., 1970. Electrophoretic morphology of gammaglobulin in cerebrospinal fluid of multiple sclerosis and other diseases of the nervous system. Neurology, 20: 982-990.

Link, H. and Müller, R., 1971. Immunoglobulines in multiple sclerosis and infections of the nervous system. Arch. Neurol., 25: 326.

Link, H., 1973. Immunoglobulin abnormalities in the Guillain Barré syndrome. J. Neurol. Sci., 18: 11.

Link, H. and Tribbling, G., 1977. Principles of albumin and IgG analysis in neurological disorders: Relation of the concentration of the proteins in serum and cerebrospinal fluid. Scand. J. Lab. Invest., 37: 391-401.

Reed, A.H., Henry, R.J. and Mason, W.B., 1971. Influence of statistical method used on the resulting estimate of normal range. Clin. Chem., 17: 275.

Schuller, E., Delasucrie, N., Hilary, M. and Lefèvre, M., 1978. Serum and cerebrospinal fluid IgM in 203 neurological patients. Eur. Neurol., 17: 77-82.

Schumacher, G.A., 1965. Problems of experimantal trials of therapy in multiple sclerosis. Ann. NY. Acad. Sci., 122: 552.

Sindic, C.J.M., Cambiasso, C.L., Depré, A., Laterre, E.C. and Masson, P.L. 1982. The concentration of IgM in cerebrospinal fluid of neurological patients. J. Neurol. Sci., 55: 339-350.
Strandberg Pedersen, N., Kam-Hansen, S., Link, H. and Mavra, M., 1982. Specificity of immunoglobulines synthesized within the central nervous system in neurosyphilis.
Tourtellotte, W.W., 1978. Multiple sclerosis: The blood brain barrier and the measurement of the novo central nervous system IgG synthesis. Neurology, 28 (9) part 2: 76-83.

34

Immunoglobulin IgG Abnormalities and the Oligoclonal Pattern of IgG in Multiple Sclerosis Brains

K. J. B. LAMERS, W. VAN GEEL,
R. A. WEVERS and O. R. HOMMES

INTRODUCTION

Elevated IgG distributed in oligoclonal bands is often observed in the CSF of MS patients. There is evidence that the abnormal IgG in CSF of MS patients is derived from intrathecal IgG production. Already in 1967 Tourtellotte et al. reported elevated IgG concentrations in both plaques and apparently normal white and grey matter of MS brains. Other studies in MS brains have confirmed the existence of elevated unbound IgG in plaque and non-plaque material (Link, 1972; Gilden et al., 1977; Mehta et al., 1981). Furthermore cell surface-bound IgG can also be eluted from MS brains with help of acid or alkaline extraction of brain material (Gilden et al., 1979; Mehta et al., 1981). Isoelectrofocussing (IEF) in combination with IgG immunofixation (IF) of MS brain extracts has frequently revealed an oligoclonal pattern of IgG (Link, 1972; Mattson et al., 1980; Mehta et al., 1981).
Comparative studies of IgG levels and the oligoclonal aspect inside and outside plaques and in different brain areas in MS patients are very scarce. Therefore we have studied in 3 autopsy MS brains the presence of bound and unbound IgG in different plaques and in brain sections outside plaques. Moreover we have analysed the oligoclonal pattern of IgG in these brain extracts in order to determine the possible origin and nature of the (abnormal) IgG and to compare the gammabanding in both IgG fractions (bound and unbound) and in different plaques.

MATERIALS AND METHODS

For the study of brain, autopsy brain material of 3 MS patients and one non neurological control person was examined.
The specimens consisted of brain sections including cortex, pons and spinal cord. Pieces (0.5-1.5 gr) of plaque and non plaque material of grey or white matter were used. Signs of cellular activity were rarely observed upon microscopic examination in any of the plaques.
Astrocytosis was present, while oligodendrocytes and myeline were generally absent in the plaque. The tissue was stored at -70°C until use.

Extraction of brain homogenates was performed according to the method described by Mehta et al., (1981). The (0,01 M PBS, pH 7,2) brain homogenate was centrifuged for 1 h at 100.000 x g. The clear supernatant (unbound IgG fraction) was collected. The residue was washed at least 8 times in 2,5 ml 0,01 M PBS each by centrifugation at 100.000 x g for 1 h and the washing procedure was ended if the last washing showed an undetectable IgG level (< 2,5 µgr/ml). The supernatants of the 2th to 8th washing step were collected and examined. After the last washing step a second extraction at pH 10,8 yielded the bound alkaline IgG fraction. For isoelectrofocussing (0,3-0,7 µgr) IgG was applied to the gel. For immunofixation 50 µl of rabbit antihuman IgG (DAKO, Denmark) was used. After 2 h incubation at 37°C, the gel was washed and stained with help of the B10 Rad Silver staining technique. IgG in (un) concentrated eluates was determined by means of an automated kinetic turbidometric method. Sheep antihuman IgG (Boehringer, Mannheim) was used. Protein determination of brain extracts was performed according to the method of Lowry et al. (1951).

RESULTS

Variation of IgG levels in MS plaques of one MS patient

The distribution of IgG within one extensive plaque (spinal cord) was studied by cutting out 9 small pieces of tissue. Furthermore, also the IgG level in 3 different plaques in one MS brain was examined (cortex, pons, spinal cord). The results are presented in Table 1. Form these results it is clear that the variation of IgG inside one plaque is minor in contrast to the variation between plaques for both fractions (bound and unbound).

TABLE 1   IgG levels in MS plaques

	No of specimens	Wet weight in gr (range)	IgG fraction	μgr IgG/gr wet weight		
				mean	sd	v.c.%
Inside one plaque	9	0.49 - 1.18	unbound bound	52.2 47.9	16.7 11.7	32 24
				mean	range	
Between plaques in one MS brain	3	0.20 - 0.70	unbound bound	170 174	52 - 338 48 - 370	

Variation of IgG levels in MS brain sections of various patients

The concentration of IgG inside different plaques and outside plaques of 3 MS patients and the distribution of IgG over both fractions (bound and unbound) were examined. The results are given in Table 2 and 3.

TABLE 2   Median IgG levels in MS brain

	Unbound IgG μgr/gr wet weight		Bound IgG μgr/gr wet weight	
	Inside plaque (7 plaques/2 brains)	Outside plaque (n = 10 in 3 brains)	Inside plaque (7 plaques/2 brains)	Outside plaque (n = 10 in 3 brains)
Median	120	94	47	30
Range	(0 - 668)	(27 - 158)	(0 - 370)	(0 - 1000)

TABLE 3   IgG levels in brain sections of MS patients

Brain localization	Position	No of plaques	No of patients	Mean μgr IgG/gr wet weight	
				unbound	bound
Cortex	inside plaque	5	2	94	113
Pons	inside plaque	1	1	668	103
Spinal cord	inside plaque	1	1	52	43
Cortex	outside plaque	9	3	91	38
Pons	outside plaque	1	1	101	1000
Cortex	control brain		1	37	9

The individual values of Table 2 are plotted in Fig. 1.
No obvious difference was found between the median unbound IgG level inside and outside plaques. A similar result was obtained for the bound IgG
fraction (Table 2). This is in contrast with the results of Mehta et al.
(1981).

Fig. 1   MEDIAN IgG LEVELS IN MS BRAINS

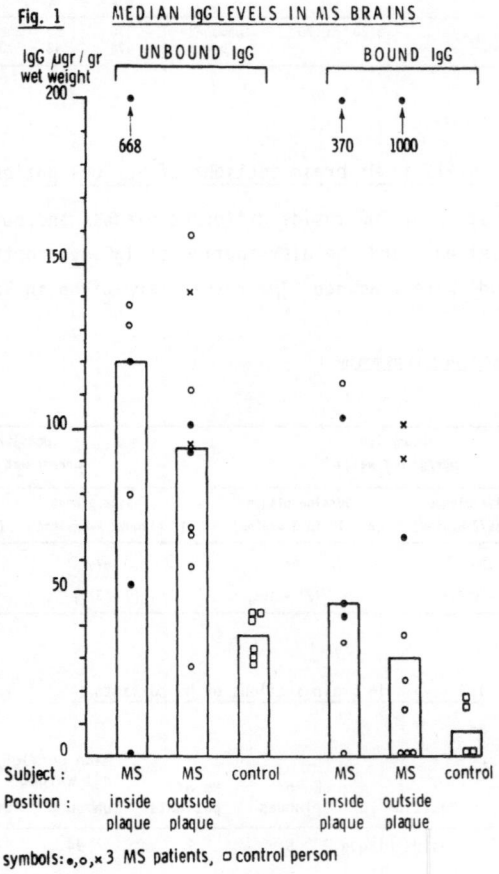

symbols: •, o, × 3 MS patients, □ control person

The median IgG concentration of the bound IgG fraction is lower than in
the unbound fraction (Table 2).
The highest value for both unbound and bound IgG is found in the pons
(Table 3).

The IgG levels (bound and unbound) in 3 MS brains are generally higher than in the control brain (Table 3).

Very low levels ($<$ 2,5 µgr/gr) as well as very high levels of bound IgG are sometimes found both inside and outside plaques in MS brain. Similar variations have been found for unbound IgG.

The oligoclonal aspect of IgG in MS brain

With help of the IF method we have studied the oligoclonal pattern of 9 different MS brain extracts from 3 MS patients and 4 brain extracts from 1 control person. The results are presented in Table 4. All investigated MS brain extracts showed an oligoclonal aspect for IgG. The 4 brain extracts of the control person had a normal (serum like) IgG pattern.

We have also characterized the identity of the banding pattern in different brain sections of one patient. In one experiment the banding pattern of unbound IgG inside a plaque was identical with the unbound IgG fraction of a brain section at a 2 cm distance outside this plaque. Furthermore, 2 specimens (outside plaque sections) in one MS brain showed both common and unique bands. Non-identical bands were observed on comparing bound and unbound IgG inside one plaque.

TABLE 4   Oligoclonal aspect of IgG in different brain sections with help of immunofixation

No of patients	Localization	IgG fraction	No of specimens with IF investigations	No of specimens with an oligo-clonal aspect	No of specimens with a serum like aspect	percentage oligoclonal aspect (%)
2	inside plaque	unbound	3	3	0	100
3	outside plaque	unbound	5	5	0	100
1	outside plaque	bound	1	1	0	100
1	control brain	unbound	4	0	4	0

DISCUSSION

The findings in this study of abnormal IgG concentrations in bound and unbound brain fractions of MS patients are in agreement with other observations (Link, 1972; Gilden et al., 1979; Mehta et al., 1981). In contrast to the results of Mehta et al. (1981) we found comparable IgG levels inside and outside plaques. A possible explanation for this difference can be given by the fact that signs of cellular activity were rarely observed in any of the plaques in our material. This observations do raise the question about the origin and significance of abnormal IgG in inactive plaques, especially the bound IgG fraction.

With respect to the oligoclonal pattern, we can confirm the results of other studies about the oligoclonal nature of abnormal IgG in MS brain (Link, 1972; Mattson et al., 1980; Mehta et al., 1981). We have observed abnormal gamma banding in the bound IgG fraction of a tissue sample (outside plaque). The banding pattern was not identical with the pattern in the unbound IgG fraction. There are also indications that in different brain areas of one MS patient both common and unique bands are present in the unbound fractions. Similar results have been found by Mattson et al., (1980).

Several explanations for this observation can be given. Old inactive plaques might contain plasma cell clones differing from clones in more recent plaques. Another possibility is that a single agent can undergo antigenic shifts leading to different antibody responses in time. Finally, the presence of both specific and nonsense antibodies in individual plaque has been suggested (Mattson et al., 1980). The specificity of antibodies in MS has not yet been established. Antibodies to known and unknown brain substances, oligodendrocytes or viruses have been thought to play a role in the humoral respons in MS brain.

Investigation of the location and nature of IgG in MS brain extracts can be important for an understanding of the pathogenesis of MS.

REFERENCES

Gilden, D. and Tachovsky, T., 1979. Immunoglobulin elution from multiple sclerosis brain. J. Neurosci. Methods, 1: 133-142.
Link, H., 1972. Oligoclonal immunoglobulin G in multiple sclerosis brains. J. Neurol. Sci., 16: 103-114.
Lowry, O.H., Rosenbrough, N.J., Farr, A.L. and Randall, R.J., 1951. Protein measurements with the folin phenol reagent. J. Biol. Chem., 193: 265-275.
Mattson, D.H., Roos, R.P. and Arnason, B.G.W., 1980. Isoelectric focusing of IgG eluted from multiple sclerosis and subacute sclerosing panencephalitis brains. Nature, 287: 335-337.
Mehta, P.D., Frisch, S., Thormar, W.W., Tourtellote, W.W. and Wisniewski, H.M., 1981. Bound antibody in multiple sclerosis brains. J. Neurol. Sci., 49: 91-98.
Tourtellotte, W.W. and Parker, J.A., 1967. Multiple sclerosis. Correlation between immunoglobulin G in cerebrospinal fluid and brain. Nature (London), 214: 683-686.

35

IgG Synthesis in Multiple Sclerosis

D. CAPUTO, P. FERRANTE, S. PROCACCIA,
M. ZAFFARONI and C. L. CAZZULLO

INTRODUCTION

Although the pathogenesis of multiple sclerosis (MS) is still today unknown, many lines of evidence suggest that an aberrant immune
response is involved (Weiner et al., 1982). The most important data supporting this point of view are the finding of an intrathecal IgG production of restricted heterogeneity, the presence of a mononuclear and
plasmacell perivascular infiltration in areas of acute demyelination,
the finding of autoantibodies directed at myelin basic protein or other
brain antigens, the prevalence of certain HLA haplotypes closely to the
genetic locus of immune response control and finally the pathogenetic
mechanism of the demyelinating disease of experimental models in animals.
The humoral immune system abnormalities were the first to be noted but
still awaits elucidations. We studied in several directions immunoglobulins, immunocomplexes and viral antibodies in MS patients.

MATERIALS AND METHODS

All MS patients had a clinically definite diagnosis according to the
criteria of Mc Donald and Halliday (1977). Other neurological diseases
included: spondylotic myelopathies, brain tumors, spinal cord tumors,
ALS, cerebellar atrophies, spino-cerebellar ataxias, essential tremor
etc. i.e. non-inflammatory, non immune-related neurological diseases.

Cerebrospinal fluid (CSF) IgG synthesis: (a) the IgG index was calculated according to Link; (b) the CNS de novo synthesis was calculated according to the empiric formula proposed by Tourtellotte. Normal values
were less then 3.3 mg/24 hrs; (c) CSF and serum isoelectrofocusing (IEF)
were performed on thin layer 5% polyacrylamide gels containing ampholines
with pH range 3.5 - 9.5 by a LKB-Multiphor equipement, according to the
manufacturer's instructions; (d) CSF and serum protein quantitation was
performed by single radial immunodiffusion according to Mancini (1965);
(e) analytic capillary isotachophoresis (ITP) was performed by Delmotte's
method on a LKB 2127 Tachophor apparatus; slow IgG percentages and intrathecal synthesis rate by ITP (mg/24 hrs) were previously described by
Zaffaroni et al. (1983); immune complexes assay was performed by Procaccia et al. (1983) using three different methods: C_{1q} binding test
(C_{1q} BA); polyethylenglycol precipitation test (PEG-prec.); monoclonal
rheumatoid factor inhibition test (MRF-1); virological studies: the
antibodies to measles rebella, mumps, parainfluenza 1, herpes simplex
type 1 and 2 were titred as described in Caputo et al. (1981), Ferrante
et al. (1982).

RESULTS

Intrathecal IgG synthesis. The evaluation of intrathecal IgG synthesis by different methods (Table 1) demonstrated that IEF of CSF is
the most reliable index, once other causes of oligoclonal IgG synthesis

Tab. 1: IgG syntheis in MS and OND patients: percentages of pathological
findings

		IgG INDEX	IgG DE NOVO SYNTH.	IEF
MS DEFINITE	n. 32	80.8%	84.6%	93.7%
OND	n. 17	35.7%	21.4%	11.7%
		n.v. 0.8	n.v. 3.3 mg/24hrs.	
STUDENT'S T-TEST		$P < 0.01$	$P < 0.01$	

are excluded (SSPE viral encephalitides, neurosyphilis, paraproteinemia).
ITP analysis demonstrated that CSF from MS patients are significantly
characterized by high percentages of slowly migrating IgG fractions
(Fig. 1, 2). The high concordance of this parameter with Tourtellotte's

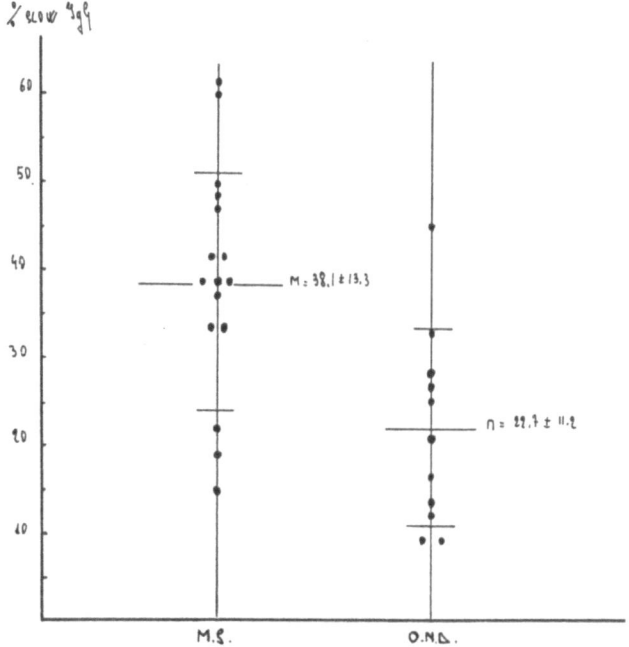

Fig. 1. = "Slow IgG" percentages in the CSF of patients with M.S. and O.N.D. lines represent mean value ± S.D.

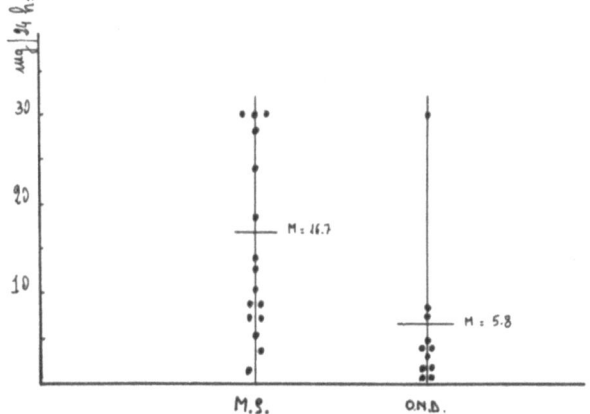

Fig. 2: = Slow IgG synthesis rate in patients with M.S. and O.N.D.

empiric formula (Fig. 3) suggests that these "slow IgG's" are intrathecally synthesized.

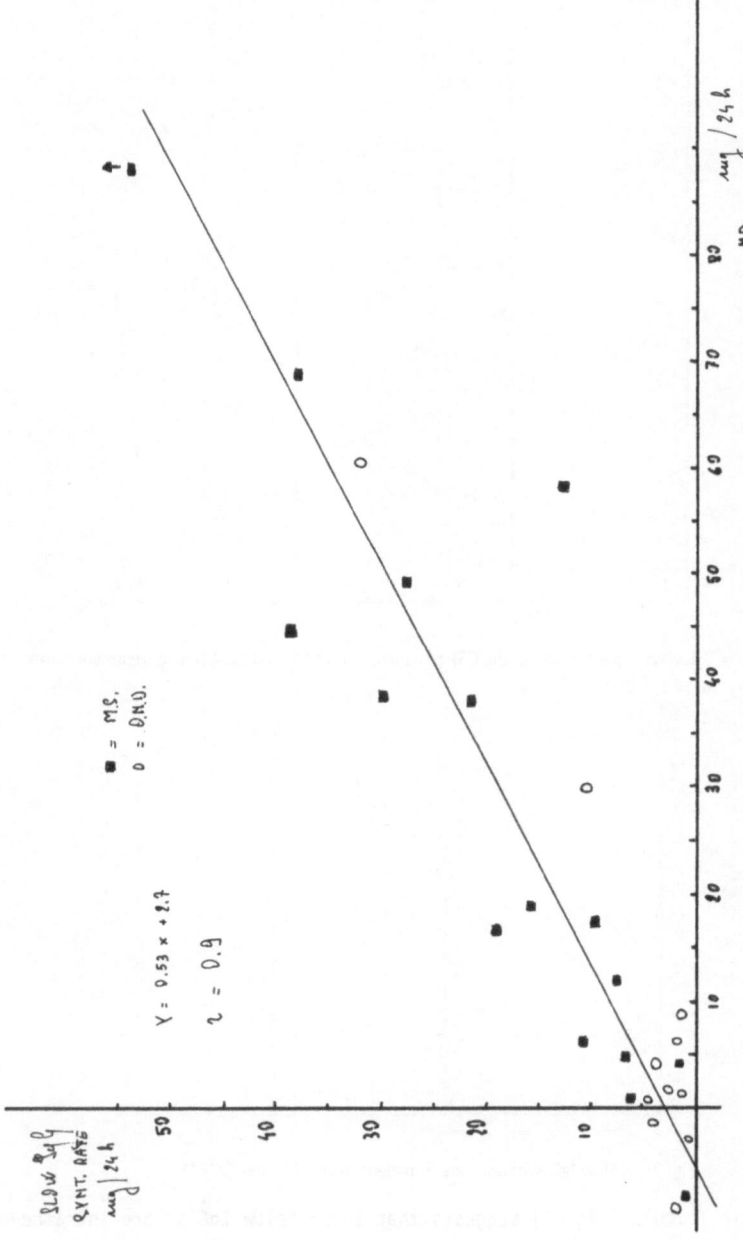

Fig. 3. = Concordance between Tourtellotte's empiric formula (E.F.) Slow IgG synthesis rate.

Immunocomplexes. IC levels, determined by the three methods for
each sample are illustrated in Fig. 4. If we consider our MS population,
we can outline that 17/30 patients had increased levels of IC when

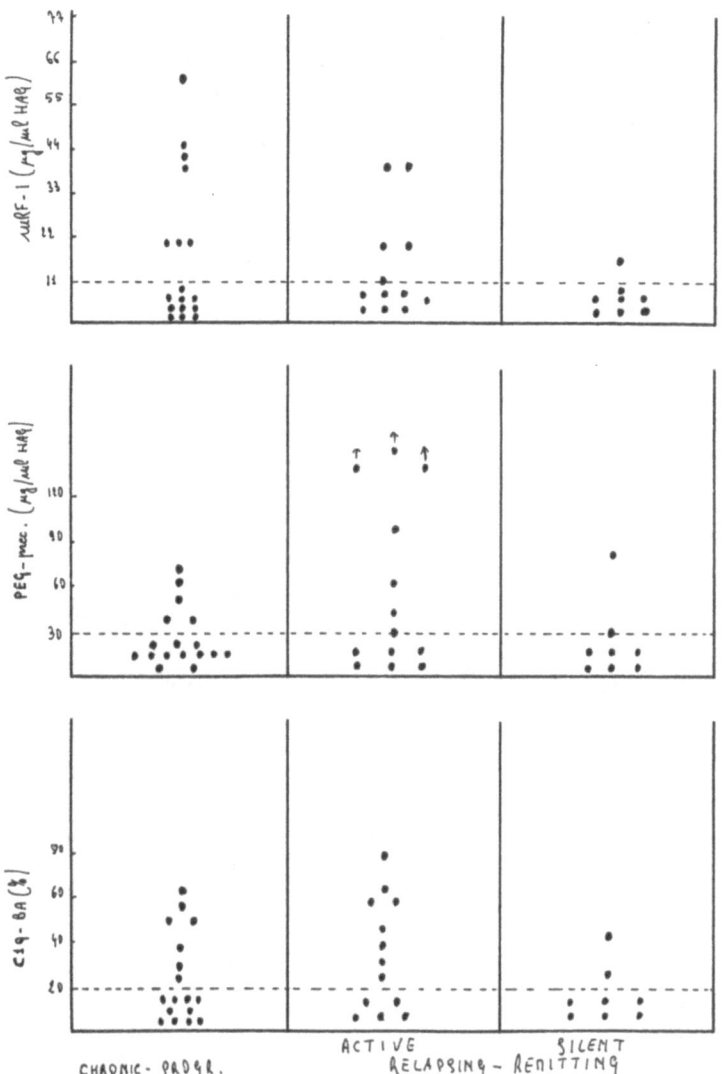

Fig. 4. = Circulating immune-complexes in M.S. patients.

measured by C_{1q} BA. This frequency is lower for the PEG-prec. test and for the MRF-1 assay (Fig. 4). We can, first of all, outline that our MS patients reveal the well known high frequency increased titres of measles antibodies which are constantly higher in patients with increased levels of IC. Particularly the correlation is statistically significant ($P < 0.01$) for the PEG-prec. test. We stress the finding that patients with the highest IC levels (PEG-prec. test defined) show simultaneously the highest anti-measles virus antibody titres (Table 2).

Tab. 2: Correlation between circulating immune complexes (IC) and viral antibodies (geometric means).

	Measles	Rubella
PEG $\geqslant$ 30	1:23.1 *	1:38.2 o
PEG $<$ 30	1:10.8	1.38.9
C_{1q}-BA $\geqslant$ 20	1:14.6 o	1:32.9 o
C_{1q}-BA $<$ 20	1:12.9	1:45.4
C_{1q}-BA + PEG	1:15.7 o	1:39.0 o
pos./neg.	1:12.6	1:41.7

* p $<$ 0.01 (Wilcoxon test)

o = N.S.

Anti-viral antibodies. In previous studies we found that MS patients differ from controls as it concerns antibody titres against two paramixoviruses first of all measles, secondly mumps (Table 3, 4). We are

Tab. 3: Antibodies antimeasles levels in M.S. patients and controls. (M.S. patients have been divided in treated and untreated with immunosuppressive drugs).

Antibodies	Subjects	No. examined	No. positivity (%)	P (1)
HIT	treated patients	151	136 (90.0)	
	untreated patients	32	30 (93.7)	$<$ 0.05
	controls	153	139 (90.8)	
CFT	treated patients	151	145 (96.0)	
	untreated patients	32	31 (96.8)	$<$ 0.001 (2)
	controls	153	116 (75.8)	

(1) At x^2 test, according to Yates remark, comparing frequencies of patients under treatment, untreated and controls (2 g.l.).

(2) Comparison patients examined versus controls P $<$ 0.001 (1 g.l.). Comparison patients not examined versus controls 0.05 $>$ P $>$ 0.01 (1 g.l.).

Tab. 4: Viral antibodies in sera from MS patients and controls.

Test (1)		MS patients Treated (N=146)		MS patients Untreated (N=30)		Controls (N=150)		x^2 (2)
		% Positive	Geometric (3) mean titers	% Positive	Geometric (3) mean titers	% Positive	Geometric (3) mean titers	
Mumps	HI	61.0	1:7.5	63.3	1:8.6	30.7	1:7.6	P<0.001(4)
	CF	72.6	1:5.5	60	1:4.8	75.8	1:5	n.s.
Parainfluenza 1 (Sendai)	HI	26.0	1:7.2	16.7	1:6.6	34.6	1:7	n.s.
(Sendai)	CF	63.0	1:5.6	43.3	1:5.4	52.9	1:5	n.s.
Rubella	HI	90.4	1:43.6	86.7	1:39.1	92.1	1:44	n.s.
Herpes Simplex type 1	CF	93.1	1:26.1	93.3	1:27.3	82.8	1:22.9	0.01>P≈0.001(5)

(1) HI_2: Haemoagglutination inhibition; CF: complement fixation.

(2) x^2 Test, with Yates correction, comparing frequencies of patients under treatment, untreated and controls (2 d.f.)

(3) for each test GMT of the three groups were compared with t student test

(4) treated patients versus controls P < 0.001; untreated patients versus controls P < 0.01 (1 d.f.)

(5) treated patients versus controls 0.01 > P > 0.001; untreated patients versus controls P < 0.05 (1 d.f.)

carrying out a case control study in which the antibodies against several viruses are checked in the sera of MS cases, of one patients' sibling
and of one patients' childhood friend. Table 4 reports the preliminary
results of 45 triplets. A significant difference has been observed for
HSV-2 antibodies between the patients and the other two groups. This
finding is very interesting especially if we consider that both the two
control groups are probably overmatched with the MS cases (Table 5).
This fact confirms the previously suggested role of HSV-2 virus in the
aetiology of MS (Martin, 1981).

Tab. 5: Are reported the reciprocal of the antibody titers or
optical density (OD) observed in the three groups.

		GMT AND MEANS OF ANTIBODIES IN		
		MS CASES	SIBLINGS	PLAYMATES
MEASLES	CFA	12	12	12
MEASLES	HIA	15.5	11.7	10
MEASLES	EIA	15.18	13.91	14.01
MUMPS	CFA	3.8	3.8	4.5
RUBELLA	HIA	27	27	18
HSV-1	EIA (OD)	1.23	1.18	1.20
HSV-2	EIA (OD)	0.69*	0.63	0.61

GMT: Geometric Mean Titers

* P < 0.05 Between the patients and other two groups.

CONCLUSIONS

The finding of intrathecally synthesized oligoclonal IgG is the
most evident abnormality of humoral immunity in MS; so important that it
is often used for diagnostic purpose, even if not pathognomonic for MS.
Beside this, we do not know yet the antigenic specificity of this abnormal IgG synthesis. It has been also reported the presence of abnormally
high titres of circulating antibodies against some viruses, particularly
against measles virus. Unfortunately this finding is reported also in
other diseases such as chronic active hepatitis. Perhaps, rather than

matching different populations it will be more useful to further investigate populations at risk: for example the period of life since birth up
to fourteen years (which has been stressed by epidemiologists) and the
period of disease onset. Recently, this kind of study has brought to
formulate hypothesis that HSV_1 may be a protective factor toward HSV_2
infection, considered as the putative aetiological agent of MS (Martin,
1981). Again, we must continue to study circulating immunocomplexes not
only in the terms of "presence or absence", but in order to characterize
both the anticorpal and the antigenic component. Immunocyte abnormalities
certainly play an important role in MS immune system imbalances. In
chronic-progressive form of MS, as during the clinical exacerbations of
the relapsing-remitting form, our and several other laboratories have
found a reduction of number of T-cells mediating a suppressive/cytotoxic
immune activity (Zaffaroni et al., 1985). If we admit that the enhanced
IgG synthesis is caused by such a reduced suppressive activity, two main
questions raise: (1) is this an aspecific event or is this anticorpal
synthesis directed.toward a restricted number of antigens? (2) Is there
a specific environmental factor or could any factor in certain periods
of life trigger this over-production of IgG, which is somehow related
to the pathogenesis of MS? It has been recently reported that certain
viral agents can infect and selectively alter T-lymphocyte activity (see
AIDS). Thus we must consider the possibility that unknown viruses or unknown viral effects may cause immunological imbalances, (even transitory), which constitute the background for other factors able to trigger
the pathogenetic mechanisms of MS. In this regard we must remember the
well-known hypoergic phase following measles infection. An interesting
line of research is the attempt to find specific antibodies produced by
cloned lymphocytes from MS patients. We must moreover stress here the
recent finding that T-lymphocytes from some MS patients are highly cytotoxic for measles infected HLA-specific human cells (Jacobson et al.,
1984). This finding is the in vitro demonstration of a not new but still
actual hypothesis of MS pathogenesis: a genetically determined aberration
of immune response which reacts abnormally versus measles infection.

REFERENCES

Caputo, D., Ferrante, P., Fasan, M. and Procaccia, S., 1981. Measles
    antibodies in MS patients. Boll. Ist. Sieroter. Milan., 60: 57-60.

Caputo, D., Zaffaroni, M. and Procaccia, S., 1982. CSF immunoglobulins in
    MS. Boll. Ist. Sieroter. Milan., 61: 393-403.
Ferrante, P., Caputo, D. and Fasan, M., 1982. Viral antibodies in MS.
    Ital. J. Neurol. Sci., 2: 115-118.
Jacobson, S., Richert, J.R., Biddison, W.E., Sabinsky, A., Hatzman, R.J.
    and McFarland, H.F., 1984. Measles virus-specific T4+human cytotoxic
    T-cell clones are restricted by class II HLA antigens. J. Immunol.,
    133: 754-757.
Mancini, G., Carbonara, A.O. and Heremans, J.F., 1965. Immunochemical
    quantitation of antigens by single radial immuno-diffusion. Immuno-
    chemistry, 2: 235-254.
Martin, J.R., 1981. HSV type 1 and 2 and multiple sclerosis. Lancet II:
    777-781.
Mc Donald, W.I. and Halliday, A.M., 1977. Diagnosis and classification
    of multiple sclerosis. Br. Med. Bull., 33: 4-8.
Procaccia, S., Caputo, D., Ferrante, P., et al., 1983. Circulating
    immune-complexes and viral antibodies in MS. In: C.L. Cazzullo, D.
    Caputo, A. Ghezzi (editors), New trends in MS research. Masson Italia
    pp 63-73.
Zaffaroni, M., Caputo, D., and Cazzullo, C.L., 1983. Isotachophoresis
    evaluation of synthesis of intrathecal IgG subfractions in MS.
    J. Neurol., 229: 55-60.
Zaffaroni, M., Caputo, D., Ghezzi, A. and Cazzullo, C.L., 1985. T-cell
    subsets in MS: relationship between peripheral blood and cerebro-
    spinal fluid. Acta Neurol. Scand., (in press).
Weiner, H.L. and Hauser, S.L., 1982. Neuroimmunology. Immunoregulation
    in neurological diseases. Ann. Neurol., 11: 437-449.

ACKNOWLEDGEMENTS

    Supported by the CNR grant no. 84-01839.52".

36

Antigenicity of Galactosylceramide

B. ZALC, M. MONGE, C. LUBETZKI and N. A. BAUMANN

INTRODUCTION

Galactosylceramide (GalC) is the major glycolipid of the central nervous system (CNS) and in adult human myelin it accounts for 23% of the total lipids. The immunological properties of GalC were first detected during the search for a solution to the problem of the immunological specificity of brain lipids. Brandt et al. in 1926 reported that an antiserum against bovine brain reacted highly with the total brain lipid extract from other mammalian, but not with lipid extracts from other organs. It took 35 years before Joffe et al. (1963) demonstrated that the so called " lipid hapten of CNS " is in fact GalC. Another line of evidence for the immunological properties of GalC came from the work by Niedieck et al. (1963) showing that the serum of rabbits developing allergic encephalomyelitis reacted with GalC. Since, antisera against GalC have been produced by immunization with the purified lipid. In this report we will present data on the production of antiGalC antibodies, the serological tests allowing their detection, and the use of these antibodies both in basic and clinical research.

METHODS

Preparation of antiGalC antibodies

As stated above, antibodies against GalC are present in sera from animals immunized with whole brain or spinal cord or myelin. If total brain lipid extracts or pure GalC are injected, one need to add a carrier for the mixture to become immunogenic. Indeed, GalC, as other lipids, is a hapten. But contrary to usual haptenic molecules, the coupling of GalC to the carrier does not have to be covalent; simple mixing of GalC with the carrier is sufficient. Most probably, binding of GalC to the protein carrier occurs by binding of the two aliphatic chains of GalC via hydrophobic bonds. This lets the antigenic determinant of GalC, i.e. its hydrophilic moiety, accessible to the immunocompetent cells. Most frequently, antiGalC antisera have been raised by immunizing rabbits (or mice) with a mixture of GalC, carrier (usually serum albumin) and complete Freund adjuvant (CFA). In our laboratory, we prefer to use the immunization procedure described by Dupouey et al. (1976). This involves repeated intravenous injection of a mixture of GalC-cholesterol-human (or bovine) serum albumin in the respective weight ratio 0.2 : 1 : 4. The antisera thus obtained displayed a high affinity and specificity,(Zalc et al. 1981).

More recently, monoclonal antibodies (mAb) to GalC have been produced in different laboratories. Ranscht et al. (1982) immunizing mice with synaptic membranes produced a mAb which target antigen was shown to be GalC. Similarly, among a battery of mAb produced by injection of bovine corpus callosum, Schachner (1982) reported two of them to be directed against GalC. More recently, Rostami et al. (1984) have generated an antiGalC mAb following immunization of mice with a mixture of purified GalC and bovine serum albumin in CFA.

Affinity purification of antiGalC antibodies

For the purification of anti-glycolipid antibodies, several immunoadsorbents have been used. One involves incorporation of glycolipids into a polyacrylamide gel (Marcus 1976), others involve covalent attachment of glycolipid to different supports such as aminoalkyl-agarose or glass beads, or aminopropyl silicagel (Laine et al. 1974, Kundu and Roy 1979, Uchida and Nagai 1980). Alving and Richards (1977) have purified antiGalC antibodies by adsorbtion of the antiserum to GalC containing liposomes followed by either elution with 1M NaI or extraction with a saline-chloroform mixture. All these methods still have their own drawbacks in reproducible preparation of adsorbents or in their yield of purification. In our hands the most satisfactory procedure to purify antiGalC antibodies has been the one developed by Coulon-Morelec (1972). The immunoadsorbent is prepared by adsorbtion of GalC to cholesterol particles dispersed in 0.15M NaCl. The immunoadsorbent is centrifuged and the pellet resuspended in the antiGalC antiserum with stirring for 30 min at room temperature. The immunoadsorbent is washed twice in saline before beeing treated with 0.01M H_3BO_3 for 45 min. The specific antibodies are eluted by stirring 15 min in a $NaCl-BaCl_2$ solution (2.5 and 0.01M respectively)

The immunoadsorbent is then separated from the purified antibodies by dissolving the former in ether containing 0.5% lecithin.

Immunological detection of antiGalC antibodies

With regards to GalC (as well as to others glycolipid haptens) the assay of specific antibodies is more difficult than with usual water soluble antigens. Most, if not all, of the classical serological techniques have to be adapted in order to circumvent the problems due to the hydrophobicity of GalC. Before solid phase immunoassays had been developed, the most commonly used techniques were precipitation in agar, passive agglutination and complement fixation (CF). For all these assays, GalC had to be mixed with *auxiliary lipids*, i.e. lecithin and cholesterol. The role of auxiliary lipids has been discussed in details in the remarkable review by Rapport & Graf (1969). One explanation, though probably incomplete, is that the mixing of lipidic hapten in a water phase with cholesterol (hydrophobic) and lecithin (amphiphilic) forms mixed micelles where the carbohydrate of the hapten protudes and is more accessible to the antibodies. Among these assays, we found CF the most sensitive, specific and reproducible.

Complement-mediated lysis of liposomes (CLL) containing GalC also needs auxiliary lipids (Alving et al. 1974). Although sensitivity of CLL can be greatly influenced by the choice of entrapped marker, it remains usually in the same range as CF, and in our hands CLL has not been much more performant as CF. Comparing these two assays, one peculiar fact is noteworthy: antiGalC and antimonogalactosyldiglyceride antisera cross react completely with their respective haptens in the CF test. This cross reactivity is not observed when the antisera are reacted with biological membranes containing one or the other hapten (Dupouey et al. 1976). Similarly, each antiserum, in the CLL test, reacts only with liposomes containing the specific hapten but not the other (Alving et al. 1974). This suggests that in the CLL, the presentation of the hapten to the antibodies matches very closely the one occuring in vivo in natural membranes.

More recently, solid phase immunoassays have been introduced. For RIA or ELISA, microtitration plates are coated by evaporation of GalC solutions either in ethanol (polystyrene) or in methanol: chloroform 1:1 (polyvinyl). In our hands these types of assays have been found to be more sensitive than CF by a factor of 2 to 5. They are usually less adapted to detect cross reactivities and unspecific sticking of some sera or antibodies (especially IgM) to the plastic is a frequent, difficult to overcome, encountered problem.

An interesting opening has been the introduction by Magnani et al (1980) of immunodetection on thin-layer chromatogram (TLC). This technique, first developed for detection of GM_1 by ^{125}I-labeled cholera toxin is in many respects the equivalent for lipids of "western blot" for proteins. It is thus the ideal technique to study the cross reactivity of any antiglycolipid antibody. As a total lipid extract can be screened in one experiment. A major drawback of the technique is that its sensitivity varies considerably from one lipid to another. For instance, comparing one $antiGM_1$ and one antiGalC antisera having the same titer in the CF test, the $antiGM_1$ could detect ng amounts of GM_1 spoted on the TLC, while the antiGalC could not detect less than 100ng of GalC (unpublished data).

Immunolocalization of GalC

Contrary to what we have described for serological assays, immunolocalization of GalC on dissociated cells or cultures, is not more difficult as for a protein antigen.

In the case of localization on tissue sections, few methodological points are worth to be stressed. As GalC is a lipid, any microtomy technique involving dehydratation of the tissue by organic solvent which solubilizes GalC is out of question. This excludes for instance paraffin embbeding.

Fixation, although not compulsory, is advisable as it insures a better preservation of the sections. Our best results have been obtained with paraformaldehyde (4% in buffer). One should avoid commercially available formaldehyde as this chemical is stabilized with 10% methanol.

Accessibility of antiGalC antibodies to the myelin sheaths has been a delicate problem to solve (Zalc et al. 1981). We now preincubate the sections for 1 min in ice cold ethanol (Zalc et al. 1983 and 1984). This brief and mild ethanol treatment was found more satisfactory than the Triton X-100 treatment we had first developed (Zalc et al. 1981). It solubilizes part of myelin phospholipids and cholesterol, but not GalC, allowing thus a better penetration of antiGalC antibodies to their target hapten.

RESULTS

AntiGalC antibodies as a probe for basic research

Use of GalC as an oligodendrocyte marker in culture has first been pointed out by Raff et al. (1978). It has since been widely used in many laboratories. In isolated myelinated axons preparations, we have shown that GalC was present at the surface of the myelin sheath (Dupouey et al. 1979). On brain tissue sections, we have reported that GalC was present only in myelin and oligodendrocytes (Zalc et al. 1981). GalC was found in the whole thickness of the myelin sheath. In the myelinated tracts isolated oligodendrocytes and intrafascicular oligodendroglial cells were GalC positive. Outside myelinated tracts, satellite oligodendrocytes were also GalC positive. Interestingly enough, we found that subependymal cells, in the close vicinity to corpus callosum,were also positive for GalC. This suggested that, in adult animals, immature oligodendrocytes start synthetizing GalC before their migration in the corpus callosum. In culture, GalC seems to be the first known myelinic marker synthetized by oligodendrocytes (Abney et al. 1981). During development, in dissociated cell preparations, comparing different myelin constituents, we found that oligodendrocytes first express GalC, then Wolfgramm protein W1, then myelin basic protein (MBP) and proteolipid protein (PLP). This sequence was always respected, whatever brain area was explored. The absolute timing of appearance of GalC differed from one area to another, respecting the caudo-rostral timing of myelination (Monge et al. in preparation).

AntiGalC antibodies in clinical research

Studies on in vitro and in vivo antibody-mediated immunopathologic reactions of the CNS and PNS, with antiGalC antibodies have recently been reviewed by Lisak 1984. Sera from animals with experimental allergic encephalomyelitis (EAE) induced .with CNS tissue or myelin, usually contain antiGalC antibodies, and most of the in vitro effects of these sera can be i) reproduced with antiGalC antibodies alone, and ii) be inhibited by adsorbtion with GalC. On the contrary, there have not been convincing data showing a significant increase of antiGalC antibodies in sera from patients with multiple sclerosis (MS), in comparison to sera from controls.

AntiGalC antibodies can cause demyelination in vitro, in CNS or PNS cultures, and in vivo after intra neural injection in the optic nerve or the sciatic nerve. These demyelinating effects are complement dependent. As GalC is a surface hapten of oligodendrocyte and myelin sheath, demyelinating power of antiGalC antibodies was predictable. This observation taken together with the absence of antiGalC antibodies in MS patients make the pathogenic implication of antiGalC antibodies, in MS, doubtfull.

It remains, nevertheless, that antiGalC antibodies can be a powerfull tool to study human demyelinating diseases, for instance as a marker for oligodendrocytes. The presence of autoantibodies to oligodendrocytes in sera or CSF from MS patients has been controversial for the past few years. Using a double label approach with antiGalC antibodies and CSF from MS patients, on rat and human oligodendrocytes in culture, we have been able to demonstrate that binding of MS-CSF immunoglobulins occurs, in our cultures, on some cells (probably microglial cells) but not on oligodendrocytes defined as GalC positive cells (Lubetzki et al. submitted).

REFERENCES

BRANDT R., GUTH H. and MÜLLER R. Zur Frage der organspezifität von lipoid antikörpen. Klin. Wschr.(1926)5:655.

JOFFE S., RAPPORT MM. and GRAF L. Identification of an organ specific lipid hapten in brain. Nature (1963)197:60.

NIEDIECK B. and PETTE E. Immunochemische untersuchungen zur identifierung eines äthanollöslichen myelinhaptens. Klin. Wschr. (1963)41:773.

DUPOUEY P., BILLECOCQ A. and LEFROIT M. Comparative study of the immunochemical properties of galactosyldiglyceride and galactosylceramide included within natural membranes. Immunochemistry (1976)13:289-294.

ZALC B., MONGE M., DUPOUEY P., HAUW JJ. and BAUMANN NA. Immunohistochemical localization of galactosyl and sulfogalactosyl ceramide in the brain of the 30-day-old mouse. Brain Res. (1981)211:341-354.

RANSCHT B., CLAPSHAW PA., PRICE J., NOBLE M. and SEIFERT W. The development of oligodendrocytes and Schwann cells studied with a monoclonal antibody against galactocerebroside. PNAS (1982)79:2709-2713.

SCHACHNER M. Cell type-specific surface antigens in the mammalian nervous system. J. Neurochem. (1982)39:1-8.

ROSTAMI A., ECCELSTON PA., SILBERBERG DH., HIRAYAMA M., LISAK RP., PLEASURE DE. and PHILLIPS SM. Generation and biological properties of a monoclonal antibody to galactocerebroside. Brain Res. (1984)298:203-208.

MARCUS DM. Applications of immunological techniques to the study of glycosphingolipids. In: Glycolipids methodology. LA. Witting,Ed., Am.Oil Chem. Soc., Champaign III.(1976) 233-245.

LAINE RA., YOGEESWARAN G. and HAKOMORI SI. Glycosphingolipids covalently linked to agarose gel or glass beads. J. Biol. Chem. (1974)249:4460-4466.

KUNDU SK. and ROY SK. Aminopropyl silicagel as a solid support for preparation of glycolipid immunoadsorbent and purification of antibodies. J. Lip. Res. (1979)20:825-833.

UCHIDA T. and NAGAI Y. Affinity chromatographic purification of anti-glycolipid antibodies and their application to the membrane studies. J. Biochem. (1980)87:1829-1841.

ALVING CR. and RICHARDS RL. Immune reactivities of antibodies against glycolipids -I. Immunochemistry (1977)14:373-381.

COULON-MORELEC MJ. Purification des anticorps anti-haptène lipidique. Ann. Inst. Pasteur(Paris)(1972) 123:620-640.

RAPPORT MM. and GRAF L. Immunochemical reactions of lipids, Prog. Allergy (1969)13:273-331.

ALVING CR., FOWBLE JW. and JOSEPH KC. Comparative properties of four galactosyl lipids as antigens in liposomes. Immunochemistry (1974)11:475-481.

MAGNANI JL., SMITH DF. and GINSBURG V Detection of gangliosides that bind cholera toxin: direct binding of ^{125}I-labeled toxin to thin-layer chromatograms. Anal. Biochem. (1980) 109:399-402.

ZALC B., MONGE M., LACHAPELLE F. and BAUMANN NA. Galactosylceramide and sulfogalactosylceramide as central nervous system markers. In: XXXth colloquium on protides of the biological fluids (1983):123-126.

ZALC B., COLLET A., MONGE M., OLLIER-HARTMANN MP., JACQUE C., HARTMANN L. and BAUMANN NA. Tamm-Horsfall protein, a kidney marker is expressed on brain sulfogalactosylceramide positive astroglial structures. Brain Res. (1984) 291:182-187.

RAFF MC., MIRSKY R., FIELDS K., LISAK RP., DORFMAN S., SILBERBERG DH., GREGSON NA., LEIBOWITZ S. and KENNEDY MC. Galactocerebroside is a specific cell surface antigenic marker for oligodendrocytes in culture. Nature (1978) 274:813-816.

DUPOUEY P., ZALC B., LEFROIT-JOLY M. and GOMES D. Localization of galactosylceramide and sulfatide at the surface of myelin sheath. Cell. Mol. Biol. (1979) 11:269-272.

ABNEY ER., BARTLETT PP. and RAFF MC. Astrocytes, ependymal cells and oligodendrocytes develop on schedule in dissociated cell cultures of embryonic rat brain. Develop. Biol. (1981) 83:301-310.

LISAK RP. Antibodies to galactocerebroside: probes for the study of antibody-determined neurologic damage. In: Neuroimmunology, Behan P. and Spreafico F. eds. Raven press, New York (1984) 167-177.

37

Immune Complexes and Complement in Multiple Sclerosis

H. JANS

INTRODUCTION

Immune complexes (IC) have been demonstrated in both serum
(Tachovsky et al. , 1977) and cerebrospinal fluid (CSF) (Glickmann et al. ,
1980) from patients with multiple sclerosis (MS). Weak but promising
relations between clinical progression, the occurrence of circulating
immune complexes (CIC) (Patzold et al. , 1980) and fluctuations in the
levels of complement factors C4, C3A and C3 (Jans et al. , 1982) have
been observed. Furthermore, hypocomplementaemia with low levels of
C2, C3 and C3B (Trouillas & Betuel, 1977, Jans et. al. 1979), low levels of
C4 and C9 in CSF (Jans et al. , 1984; Morgan et al. , 1984) and alterations in
phenotypes of C4, C3 and C3B (Jans & Særensen, 1980, Fauchet et al. ,
1984) have been reported.

This variety of features in MS indicates a great heterogeneity in the
group of patients. Therefore, the aim of this presentation is an attempt
to interpret possible relations between the different observations and
the clinical appearance of MS.

MATERIAL AND METHODS

In 4 different series, 144 patients with clinically definite MS according
to Schumacker et al. ,(1965) and with signs of progression were investigated as follows:

1. 53 patients were investigated for IC, total hemolytic activity of complement (THC), complement factors Clq, C4, C3, C5, C9 and activation products (AP) of C4 and C3 in serum, (Jans et al., 1979).

2. 60 patients were investigated for IC, C3 and C3-phenotypes (C3FF, C3FS, C3SS) in serum, (Jans & Sørensen, 1980).

3. 21 patients were investigated monthly in a longitudinal study of serum samples collected during one year for IC, THC, CI-inactivator (INA), C4, C3, C3A, C5, C9, C4 and C3AP and correlated to concomitant values of total neurological deficit (TND) (Fog & Raun, 1976), (Jans et al., 1982).

4. 31 patients were investigated for IC, C4, C3, C4 and C3AP in serum and CSF, (Jans et al., 1984).

All laboratory methods have been described in detail in the references mentioned above. As a supplementary clinical parameter, the patients were typed according to the main site of their neurological lesion (cerebral, cerebellar, brainstem, pyramidal, spinal, disseminated) (Fog, T., personal communication).

RESULTS

CIC occurred in 81 (56%) of the 144 patients with concomitant appearance of C4 and C3 AP in 71 ($p < 0,01$).

Low levels of C3 was found in 48 (33%) of the 144 patients, with a concomitant absence of CIC in 43 ($p < 0,001$).

CSF-IC were found in 9 (29%) of 31 patients and with a strong correlation to a low level of CSF C4 (p 0,01).

The distribution of CIC positive individuals in the various topographical groups of lesions is shown in Table 1.

The longitudinal study demonstrated as follows (Fig 1): A. Negative regression of TND on C4 (p = 0,03) and on C3A (p = 0,04) from one month previously. B. A concomitant negative regression of TND on C3 (p = 0,01). C. A positive regression of CIC one month subsequently on TND (p= 0,02).

D. A predominance of rapidly progressing cases among patients with high prevalences of CIC (p = 0, 05, one tailed).

C3-phenotyping disclosed gene frequencies of C3F = 0, 275 (controls = 0, 172), of C3S = 0, 725 (controls = 0, 825), p 0, 05. The relative risk incidence (RRI) of the disease (Woolf, 1955) was 1, 89 for the C3D positive individuals. In the group of MS patients with CIC, the RRI was 4, 1 for C3F positive individuals.

TABLE I.   The distribution of 144 patients with multiple sclerosis in groups according to the topography of their neurological lesions, and with respect to the occurrence of circulating immune complexes (CIC) and immune complexes in CSF (CSF-ik).

	No	CIC	CSF-ik
Cerebral	6	2	0/0
Cerebellar	30	25	5/11
Brain-Stem	9	7	0/1
Pyramidal	21	16	0/3
Spinal	51	18	2/10
Disseminated	27	13	2/6
Total	144	81 (56%)	9/31 (29%)

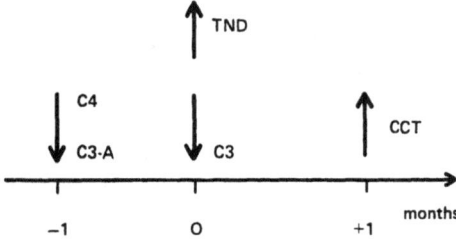

Fig 1. Covariation between the quantitative levels of the complement factors C4, C3-activator (C3-A), C3, the total neurological deficit (TND) and the level of immune complexes (CIC) detected by means of the complement consumption test (CCT).

CONCLUSIONS

CIC and complement alternations seems to be a persistent feature in MS and they might to a certain extent act as disease activity makers.

There seems to be a tendency of an increased prevalence of CIC in patients with lesions in the cerebellar, the brainstem and in the pyramidal area; and generally in cases with a high rate of progression. However,   the CIC seems to occur in the course of an increase in TND and thereby indicating the IC to be the product rather than the cause of the neurological lesions. Phenotyping of C3 disclosed increased frequencies of the C3F gene. The relative risk incidence of the disease in the group of MS patients with CIC was shown to be four times higher for C3F positive individuals when compared to a control group. Previously, the low levels of C3 have been suggested to be associated with HLA-specificities (Trouillas & Betuel, 1977). If so the corresponding absence of CIC could be due to compromised resolubilisations of TC because of a real C3-deficit. Therefore, it is most probable that several genetically determined immunological abnormalities coules predispose to MS.

REFERENCES

Fauchet, R., Madigand, M., Gueguen-Duchesne, M. Y., Papin, J., Sabouraud, O. and Genetet, B., 1984. Les marqueurs BF et C4 du complement dans la sclerose en plaques. Rev. Neurol (Paris), 140: 422-425.

Fog, T. and Raun, N. E., 1976. Computerized forms in multiple sclerosis for medical history and full neurological examination.. Kommune-hospitalet, DK 1399 Copenhagen

Glickmann, G., Svehag, S. -E., Hansen, E., Hansen, O., Husby, S., Nielsen, H and Farrel, C., 1980. Soluble immune complexes in cerebrospinal fluid of patients with multiple sclerosis and other neurological diseases. Acta Neurol. Scand., 61: 333-343.

Jans, H., Jersild, E., Taaning, E., Dybkjaer, E., Fog, T. and Heltberg, A., 1979. The occurrence of immune complexes in multiple sclerosis. In Protides of the biological fluids 26, ed. H. Peeters, Pergamon Press, Oxford and New York, pp 255-258.

Jans, H. and Sørensen, H., 1980. C3 polymorphism and circulating immune complexes in patients with multiple sclerosis. Acta Neurol. Scand. 62: 237-243.

Jans,H. , Heltberg,A. and Raun, N. E. , 1982. Circulating immune complexes and complement in the course of multiple sclerosis. Acta Neurol.
Scand. , 66:488-496.

Jans, H. , Heltberg,A. , Zeeberg, I. , Halkjaer Kristensen, J. , Fog, T. and
Raun, N. E. , 1984. Immune complexes and the complement factors C4
and C3 in cerebrospinal fluid and serum from patients with chronic
progressive multiple sclerosis. Acta Neurol. Scand. 69:34-38.

Morgan, B. P. , Campbell, A. K. and Compston, D. A. S. , 1984. Terminal
component of complement C9 in cerebrospinal fluid of patients with
multiple sclerosis. Lancet, i:251‑254.

Patzold, U. , Haller, P. , Baruth, B. , Liman, W and Deicher, H. , 1980.
Immune complexes in multiple sclerosis. J. Neurol. 222: 249-260.

Schumacher, G. A. , Beebe, G. , Kibler, R. F. , Kurland, L. T. , Kurtzke,
J. F. ,   McDowell, F. , Nagler, B. , Sibley, W. A. , Tourtellotte, W. W. ,
and Willmon, T. L. , 1965. Problems of experimental trials of therapy
in multiple sclerosis: report by the panel on the evaluation of experimental trials of therapy in multiple sclerosis. Ann. New York Acad.
Sci. , 122: 552-568.

Tachovsky, T. G. , Lisak, R. P. , Koprowski, H. , Theofilopoulos, A. N. ,
and Dixon, F. J . , 1976. Circulating immune complexes in multiple
sclerosis and other neurological diseases. Lancet, ii: 997-999.

Trouillas, P and Betuel, H. , 1977. Hypocomplementaemic and normo-
complementaemic multiple sclerosis. J. Neurol. Sci. , 32: 4?5-435.

Woolf, B. , 1955. On estimating the relation between blood group and
disease. Ann. Hum. Genet. 19:251-253.

38

Myelin Basic Protein Like Reactivity in Normal Serum

T. A. OUT, P. C. DRIEDIJK and J. BAAS

INTRODUCTION

The determination of myelin basic protein in cerebrospinal fluid
(CSF) can be used for the detection of demyelination. Thus acute
exacerbations of the disease Multiple Sclerosis, and damage of myelin
upon cerebrovascular accidents can be assessed (Cohen et al., 1980,
Whitaker, 1977) When the determination of MBP is applied to sera, only
extremely severe demyelination can be discriminated from the normal state
(Palfreyman et al., 1978). On the other hand Paterson et al., 1981, by
applying their dual dilution RIA, showed the occurence of MBP serum
factors. The nature and the concentrations of these MBP serum factors
were related to the activity of the diseases Multiple Sclerosis and
Acute Disseminated Encephalomyelitis. In our study on the determination
of MBP in CSF (Nagelkerken et al.,1983) we showed that the amount of MBP

277

in CSF as determined by a competitive radioimmunoassay corresponded to
that determined by a two-site immunoradiometric assay.In this study the
results of the determination of MBP in sera by our radioimmunoassays are
reported.

RESULTS

The preparation of MBP and of fragments of MBP.

The purification of myelin basic protein(MBP) was performed as
follows. A pH 3 extract from the white matter of human brain tissue was
prepared according to Deibler et al.,1972. The extract was freeze-dried
and MBP was purified by ion exchange chromatography at 4°C with the use
of CM52-cellulose (Deibler et al.,1973). Fractions were pooled as
indicated in Fig. 1.

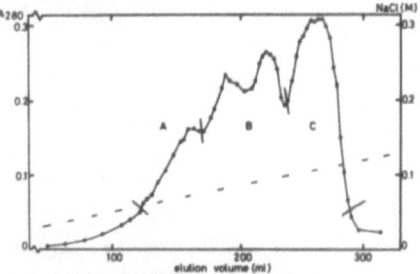

Fig. 1. CM-cellulose chromatography
of the pH3 extract.

The pools were desalted,
freeze-dried and redissolved
in 10 mM HCl. MBP was further
purified by gelpermeation
chromatography at 4°C with
the use of Sepharose G 150 or
ACA 44, and 10 mM HCl as
elution buffer. In the latter
case it was found that intact
MBP was retarded by the column
material resulting in the
elution of small fragments of MBP and other contaminants in front of
intact MBP. The SDS-PAGE analysis of the material before and after gel-

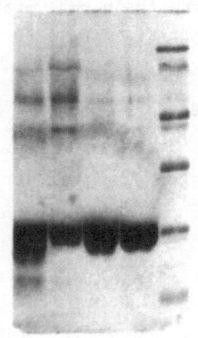

10 11 12 13 14

Fig. 2.

filtration is shown in Fig.2. The material before
gelfitration (pool C from Fig. 1) and the
fractions after gelfiltrationare shown in lane 11
and in lanes 12 and 13, respectively. MBP and
smaller proteins (lane 12) eluted at 115 to 130
ml. Material that shows a homogeneous band of
about 20kD (lane 13) eluted at 131 to 160 ml. It
should be noted that the bed volume of the column
was only 90 ml. From these results we conclude
that MBP can be purified from the white matter
of human brain to a state that shows a single
band in SDS-PAGE analysis.

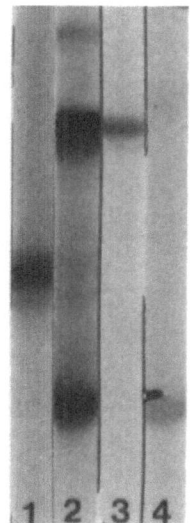

For the preparation of fragments, MBP was degraded by pepsin at pH 3.5 following the procedure of Whitaker, 1977. The degraded material was separated into different fragments (Whitaker, 1977). In Fig. 3 the electrophoretic analysis (Benuck et al., 1975) of the fragments is shown. The preparation in lane 3 contains the peptides with aminoacids 39 to 88, and probably 43 to 88, according to the results of the aminoacid analysis (not shown). The preparation shown in lane 4 possibly contains the peptide with aminoacids 1 to 36. No other peptides were obtained by this procedure.

The determination of MBP in cerebrospinal fluid and serum.

The procedure that we use for the determination of MBP in the cerebrospinal fluid (CSF) is described earlier (Nagelkerken et al., 1983). By that assay the amount of MBP that is demonstrated in CSF is in general below 0.11 ng/100 µl of CSF, when CSF's of patients not having neurologic diseases are studied.

Fig. 3.
Electrophoretic
analysis of MBP
fragments

Table 1 The determination of MBP in paired serum and CFS samples.

serum	CSF	MBP -	MBP +
MBP -		7	4
MBP +		4	18

Fisher exact test: p < 0.03

Sera from normal healthy persons caused 0% to 50% inhibition in the assay, corresponding to 0 to 0.4 ng MBP like material per 100 µl of serum. The nature of the immunoreactive material in sera is however not clear and we cannot exclude that non specific inhibitory effects by serum play a role. To analyse this reactivity in serum we determined MBP in paired serum and CSF samples, the results of which are shown in Table I. MBP in CSF was measured by the competitive RIA described earlier (Nagelkerken et al.,1983). For the determination of MBP in serum we applied a RIA in which immunoaffinity purified antibodies reactive with peptide(s) 37-88(43-88) were used

together with labelled intact MBP. Although there was a significant
association between the occurence of positive MBP scores for CSF with
those for serum it can be seen from Table I that several individual cases
did not correspond.Among these high CSF MBP values concurred with
negative MBP values in the paired serum sample and vice versa. These
results made us conclude that the determination of MBP in serum is
complicated by unknown interfering factors.

To investigate whether
particular serum proteins interfere with the determination of
MBP in serum we separated sera
from normal persons into fractions
by gelpermeation chromatography
and measured the effect of the
different fractions in the RIA of
MBP. In Fig. 4 the results of such
analysis is shown. It can be seen
that considerable to complete
inhibition of the binding of

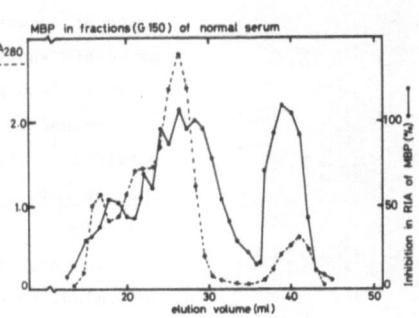

Fig. 4.

labelled MBP to the anti-MBP is caused by a large number of fractions.
Before gelfiltration of the serum under investigation only a minor
inhibitory effect of the serum in the RIA was observed.

Besides the effect shown in Fig. 4 for the RIA of intact MBP similar
inhibitory effects of the serum fractions were observed in RIA 's of
peptides of MBP. (RIA of peptide(s) 37-88(43-88) and RIA of the second
peptide in Fig.3).The MBP reactive material in the various fractions was
calculated from the response in the RIA of intact MBP, assumming that
intact MBP was measured, and amounted to about 5 μg/ml of serum.

The pattern of inhibition as it is distributed over the fractions
shown in Fig. 4 was found to depend on the following variables: invidual
serum, pretreatment of the serum at various temperatures, nature of the
column material, and type of RIA.

CONCLUSIONS

1)It is possible to obtain a preparation of MBP from human brain tissue that shows a single band in SDS-PAGE analysis.

2)The determination of MBP in sera is complicated by unknown factors.

3)MBP like reactivity, as measured by different types of RIA, is present in normal serum. This reactivity is masked, but unmasking can be obtained by gelpermeation chromatography.

REFERENCES

Benuck, M., Marks, N. and Hashim, A., 1975. Metabolic instability of myelin proteins. Eur. J. Biochem., 52: 615-621.

Cohen, S.R., Brooks, B.R., Jubelt, B. and McKhann, G.M., 1980. A diag nostic index of active demyelination: myelin basic protein in cerebrospinal fluid. Ann. Neurol., 8: 25-31.

Deibler, G.E., Martenson, R.E. and Kies, M.W., 1972. Large scale prepara tion of myelin basic protein from central nervous tissue of several mammalian species. Prep. Biochem., 2: 139-165.

Deibler, G.E. and Martenson, R.E., 1973. Chromatographic fractionation of myelin basic protein. J. Biol. Chem., 248: 2392-2396

Nagelkerken, A.M., Van Zoonen-van Exel, M., Aalberse, R.C., Van Walbeek, H.K. and Out, T.A., 1983. Comparison of a non-competitive two-site RIA and an inhibition RIA for the detection of myelin basic protein in cerebrospinal fluid. J. Neuroimmunol., 5: 157-170.

Palfreyman, J.W., Thomas, D.G.T. and Ratcliffe J.G., 1978. Radioimmunoassay of myelin basic protein in tissue extract, cerebrospinal fluid and serum and its clinical application to patients with head injury. Clin. Chim. Acta, 82: 259-270.

Paterson, P.Y., Day, E.D., Whitacre, C.C., Berenberg, R.A. and Harter, D.H., 1981. Endogeneous myelin basic protein-serum factors (MBP-SFs) and anti-MBP antibodies in humans. J.Neurol. Sci., 52: 37-51.

Whitaker, J.N., 1977. Myelin encephalitogenic protein fragments in cerebrospinal fluid of persons with multiple sclerosis. Neurology, 27: 911-920.

39

Blood-Brain Barrier in Experimental Allergic Encephalomyelitis and Multiple Sclerosis. A Minireview

J. J. HAUW and J. M. LEFAUCONNIER

Increasing evidence of damage to the Blood-Brain Barrier (BBB) in Multiple Sclerosis (MS) has been reported. However, little is known of the significance of this damage. Is it relevant to the pathogenesis of the disease ? Or is it, on the contrary, a secondary phenomenon ?

The Blood-Brain-Cerebrospinal Fluid System

There are several sites of exchange between blood and the various compartments of the central nervous system. At the interface between blood and the extracellular space (ECS), the vascular endothelium is characterized by : 1) "very tight" junctions ; 2) absence of pores ; 3) low vesicular transfer and pinocytosis ; 4) numerous endothelial mitochondria ; and 5) close contact with astrocytic foot processes. There is 1) nearly total exclusion of solutes of high molecular weight ; 2) necessity of a transcellular route for solutes of small molecular weight ; 3) a cellular polarity with asymmetry in the respective roles of the luminal and abluminal membranes, most active transport taking place in the brain to blood direction. Differences in the endothelial permeability of various parts of the vascular tree have been demonstrated. Arterioles and venules are more permeable than capillaries. For example, it has been shown that exogenous myelin basic protein injected into the CSF was found on the luminal surface of endothelial cells of the cerebral and meningeal veins (Vass et al., 1984). The main surface between blood and cerebrospinal fluid (CSF) is the choroid plexus, where CSF is secreted. In this structure, capillaries are permeable for

most tracers. In contrast, solute transport is restricted by tight intercellular junctions. These are, however, more permeable than those of endothelial cells of brain vessels. A second interface is situated at the arachnoid
villi. It allows only a CSF to blood flow. The interface between CSF and
ECS (pia mater, subpial astrocytes and ependymal cells) is devoid of a
patent barrier.

Water exchange between plasma and brain is similar to that which occurs
across lipid bilayers and most epithelia. The permeability to water of the
choroid plexus is higher than that of brain capillaries. CSF and ECS elec-
trolytes composition is strictly regulated, due to the low ionic permeability of brain vessels and to the Na^+-K^+ dependant ATPase of the abluminal
membrane of capillaries and of the apical membrane of the choroid plexus
epithelium. Blood-Brain transport of non-electrolytic substances of low molecular weight occurs either by diffusion through the membrane lipids (li-
pophilic molecules) or by means of a protein carrier system (some hydrophilic molecules like most metabolic substrates).

Pathology of the BBB

Non selective increase in the permeability of the BBB is most often
accompanied by the generation of cytoplasmic vesicles or of transendothe-
lial channels, less often by an obvious opening of intercellular junctions.
Whatever the significance of these lesions, there is an increase in CSF concentration of those solutes normally deficient relative to blood plasma,
and a decrease of those usually in excess. Brain tissue is the site of va-
sogenic edema. Large injury may lead to necrosis of endothelial cells, with
extravasation of erythrocytes. Once the opening of the barrier to protein
has occured, the latter may be taken up by astrocytes. Whether primary abnormalities of astrocytes may induce changes in the permeability of the
barrier remains hypothetical.

Increased permeability of the BBB has been described in various inflammatory disorders of the meninges and of the brain. Meningites - and particularly subacute or chronic ones-mediate severe barrier breakdown. In non-
cerebral tissues, the increased permeability associated with inflammation
is known to be related to histamine and other vaso-active compounds. Histamine administered in the carotid circulation increases the number of vesicles in endothelial cells and the permeability to sucrose and aminoisobu-
tyric acid (Dux and Joó, 1982, Gross et al., 1982). In addition, the injection of large doses of serotonin, noradrenalin or cyclic AMP through the

cerebral ventricules has induced enhanced vesicular transport across arterioles and venules.

Experimental Allergic Encephalomyelitis (EAE)

In acute forms, the electron dense horseradish peroxydase escaped from
capillaries into the ECS. Transfer vesicles were numerous. Free passage
though interendothelial junctions was not seen (Hirano et al., 1970). Clinical symptoms, increased amounts of ^{14}C-mannitol and lymphocytic infiltration occured at the same time (Oldendorf, 1979). However, increase in BBB
permeability to ions was seen in spinal cord one day before the onset of
clinical symptoms and 2 days before that of perivascular cuffs (Juhler et
al., 1984). In chronic relapsing EAE of the juvenile Hartley guinea-pig,
BBB damage was localized in demyelinated plaques and in blood vessels with
vasculitis. It was massive in active lesions, and minimal or absent in inactive ones. Elevated CSF albumin was a reliable indicator for BBB damage
if the changes were located near the inner or outer surface of the CNS. On
the contrary, focal and deep BBB damage may not be accompanied by detectable CSF protein changes (Kitz et al., 1984).

Multiple Sclerosis (MS)

Since the early descriptions, the presence of vascular changes has
been debated, as the plaque seems to follow one or two veins during their
course through the white matter. Most authors agree today that there are
few significant changes in vessels. However, some hyaline changes in old
plaques (Jellinger, 1969) or in normal appearing white matter (Allen, 1984)
have been described. Morphometric studies of acute or subacute plaques did
not show abnormalities of junctions but pinocytic vesicles were markedly
increased (Brown, 1978).

Several studies demonstrate increased permeability of the BBB in the
MS plaque. 1) Post-mortem perfusion with trypan blue stained the plaque
(Broman, 1947). 2) Immunohistochemical visualisation of albumin in plaques
has been reported (Lumsden, 1971). 3) The study of albumin concentration in
the CSF had initially shown only a small percentage (20 - 30 %) of patients
with moderate BBB damage (Tourtelotte et al., 1984), more marked in long
duration disease (Schuller et al., 1973). Recent studies have shown that
increased permeability of the BBB was constant when Haptoglobin polymers
were detected in CSF (Takeoka et al., 1983). 4) Reports on CT scan studies
in MS have shown an enhancement by contrast media of some low-density or

isodense lesions. Such enhancement presumably resulted from BBB disturbances in active demyelination : the contrast-enhancing vasoactive lesion was
a transient phenomenon that closely correlated with clinical exacerbation
(Sears et al., 1981). Ebers et al. (1984) have shown that, in 125 MS patients, one or more enhancing lesions were found in 53 % of cases with acute exacerbation, in 41 % of active cases and in 13 % of inactive cases.
High volume delayed scanning revealed enhancing lesions even more frequently (in 63, 50 and 13 % of cases, respectively). However, precise correlations between the type (demyelinating, acute..) and evolution of plaques
and the disturbances of the BBB are lacking. Magnetic Resonance Imaging
(MRI) studies will bring new data on BBB disturbances in MS (Johnson et
al., 1984, Tourtelotte et al., 1984).

Aknowledgments : We thank Dr H. Baron for reviewing the English manuscript and Mrs Bethermin for the dactylography. This work has been supported
by Association pour la Recherche sur la Sclérose en Plaques.

References
Allen, I,V,, 1984, Demyelinating disease. In : J, Hume Adams et al. (Eds),
    Greenfield's Neuropathology, Edward Arnold, London, pp. 338-384,
Bradbury, M., 1979. The concept of the Blood-Brain Barrier. John Wiley and
    Sons, Chicester.
Broman, T., 1947. Supravital analysis of disorders in the cerebral vascular
    permeability. II, Two cases of multiple sclerosis. Acta Psychiat.
    Neurol, Scand. supp. 46 : 58 - 71.
Brown, W,J., 1978. The capillaries in acute and subacute multiple sclerosis
    plaques : a morphometric analysis. Neurology, 28 : 84-92.
Dux, E., Joó, F., 1982. Effects of histamine on brain capillaries. Exp,
    Brain Res,, 47 : 252-258.
Ebers, G.C., Vinuela, F.V., Feasby, T., Bass, B., 1984. Multifocal CT en-
    hancement in MS. Neurology, 34 : 341-346,
Gross, P,M., Teasdale, G.M., Giraham, D.I., Angerson, W.J., Harper, A.M.,
    1982, Intra-arterial histamine increases blood-brain transport in rats.
    Am. J. Physiol., 243, H 307 - H 317,
Hirano, A., Dembitzer, H.M., Becker, N.H., Levine, S., Zimmerman, H.M.,
    1970, Fine structural alterations of the blood-brain barrier, J, Neuro-
    path. exp, Neurol., 33 : 616-631.
Johnson, M,A,, Li, D.K.B., Bryant, D.J., Payne, J,A., 1984. Magnetic Reso-
    nance Imaging : serial observation in Multiple Sclerosis. Amer. J.
    NeuroRadiol., 5 : 495-499.
Juhler, M., Barry, D.I., Offner, H., Konat, G., Klinken, L., Paulson, O,B,,
    1984. Blood-Brain and blood-spinal cord barrier permeability during the
    course of Experimental Allergic Encephalomyelitis in the rat. Brain Res.
    302 : 347 - 355.
Kitz, K., Lassmann, H,, Karcher, D., Lowenthal, A,, 1984. Blood-Brain bar-
    rier in Chronic Relapsing Experimental Allergic Encephalomyelitis,
    Acta Neuropathol. (Berl.) 63 : 41 - 50,
Lumsden, C.E., 1971. The immunogenesis of the multiple sclerosis plaque,
    Brain Res., 28 : 385-390,

Schuller, E., Delasnerie, N., Deloche, G,, Loridan, M., 1973. Multiple
sclerosis, A two phase disease. Acta Neurol, Scand., 49 : 453 - 460.

Sears, E.S., Mc Cammon, A., Bigelow, R,, Hayman, L.A., 1982. Maximizing
the harvest of contrast enhancing lesions in multiple sclerosis.
Neurology, 32 : 815 - 820 .

Takeoka, T., Shinohera, Y., Furumi, K., Mori, K., 1983. Impairment of
blood-cerebrospinal fluid barrier in Multiple Sclerosis. J. Neurochem,,
41 : 1102-1108.

Tourtelotte, W.W,, Shapshak, P., Baumhefner, R.W., Stangaitis, S,M.,
Syndulko, K., 1984. Laboratory aids in the diagnosis of Multiple Sclerosis (MS). In : Experimental Allergic Encephalomyelitis : a usefull
model for Multiple Sclerosis, Alan R. Liss, New York, pp. 313-321.

Vass, K,, Lassmann, H,, Wisniewski, H.M,, Iqbal, K., 1984. Ultracytochemi-
cal distribution of myelin basic protein after injection into the cerebrospinal fluid. J. Neurol. Sci., 63 : 423-433.

40

The Possible Role of Viral Infections in Multiple Sclerosis

V. TER MEULEN

The possibility that a virus infection may be the etiological basis for multiple sclerosis (MS) has mainly been derived from epidemiological studies as well as from the analysis of virus-specific immune responses in patients with the disease (ter Meulen and Stephenson, 1983). The epidemiological data are based on age-specific onset curves, geographic distribution of the disease, studies on migration and familiar clustering of MS cases. These data suggest that an infectious agent to which an MS patient is exposed to at or shortly after puperty could be responsible for this disease. The determination of viral antibodies in MS patients in comparison to those of a control population have proven that the majority of MS patients do reveal a statistically significant increase in viral antibody titers in serum and CSF material against a variety of viral agents such as measles, mumps, parainfluenza III, influenza C, herpes simplex, varizella zoster or rubella virus. These viral antibodies are often locally produced in CNS tissue by invading lymphocytes. Yet, all attempts to isolate or identify a particular virus as the causative agent have failed and the various virus isolates derived from MS material could not be unequivocally associated with the disease. Despite these failures to find a viral agent for multiple sclerosis, the available immunological and virological circumstantial evidence supports the hypothesis of an association between MS and a viral infection. Moreover, investigations of other human and animal CNS diseases have shown that viruses can induce demyelination, do persist over years in CNS tissue and may cause a chronic disease process different

289

from the well known viral induced acute infection (ter Meulen and Hall, 1978). Especially the slow virus diseases associated with conventional viruses have shown that a progressing CNS disease even with relapsis can develop after an incubation period of many years. It is therefore not surprising that these observations have been frequently cited in support of a possible viral etiology in MS.

In recent years, virological studies on a number of demyelinating diseases in animals associated with the virus infection have yielded interesting data which could be of importance for MS research (Dal Canto and Rabinovitz, 1982). Especially the murine coronavirus JHM infection in rats has demonstrated a new mechanism of virus induced demyelination (Wege et al., 1983). Inoculation of weanling rats with ts mutants of JHM virus causes a subacute demyelinating (SDE) disease after an incubation period of several weeks. The disease is clinically characterized by moderate hindleg weakness with ataxic gait which increases to a hindleg paralysis. In such a state no voluntary movement of the hind limbs is possible and approximately 60-70 % of the diseased animals die within a few days after onset of disease, whereas the surviving animals recover completely or have a stabilized disability. The most prominent histological finding consists of distinct demyelinating plaques located in the white matter primarily of the optic nerve, midbrain, pons, cerebellum and spinal cord (Koga et al., 1984). Within the demyelinating plaques, axons are well preserved. In addition, cell infiltrations and perivascular cuffings are observed, consisting of lymphocytes, plasma cells and macrophages. Infectious virus can be isolated by conventional methods and viral antigens are easily detectable in glial cells in the neighbourhood of demyelinating plaques. Of particular interest is the observation that the marked infiltrations of lymphocytes in affected brain areas resemble to some extent the changes seen in experimental allergic encephalopathy (EAE). This observation led to immunological studies which have proven that lymphocytes of SDE animals are sensitized against myelin basic protein (MBP) (Watanabe et al., 1983). In in vitro assays, a proliferation response was obtained with purified MBP and adoptive transfer experiments with restimulated lymphocytes led to clinical and histological CNS changes in the recipient rats. These animals showed clinical signs such as weight loss, abnormal sensitivity to touch or

slight ataxic gait. Histologically, perivascular mononuclear cell infiltrations were observed in the dorsal area of the spinal cord white matter,
in the pons and in the cerebellar white matter and thalamus. Since no JHM
virus could be detected in stimulated lymphocytes or in brain material of
recipient animals the possibility could be excluded that the transferred
lesions are the result of replicating JHM virus.

Another important aspect of this animal model is the observation that
some of the animals which survived and recovered from SDE, later came down
with a second attack of this disease 40 - 200 days after the first attack
(Wege et al., 1984). The clinical picture of the second attack was similar
to the first, except the course seemed to be more severe. Histopathological
studies showed fresh demyelinating lesions with infiltrations of mononuclear cells primarily located in spinal cord and brain stem. In the same
animals, old lesions could be seen in the pons, thalamus, cerebellum or
spinal cord. The old lesions in the white matter revealed extended remyelination of the CNS and/or PNS type. Viral antigens could only be located in
the neighbourhood of fresh lesions but attempts to reisolate infected JHM
virus were in the majority of cases unsuccessful indicating a defect of
viral replication.

These animal experiments demonstrate that in the course of a viral
infection an inflammatory demyelinating relapsing CNS disease can develop
in association with an immune response against myelin basic protein. This
observation poses the question how a viral infection can trigger an autoimmune response, either humoral or cellular, toward neuroantigens. There
is a number of possibilities which are currently discussed. First, the
virus infection could induce changes in the target cell membrane or lead to
a release of sequestered antigens which would appear as foreign to the
immune system. Second, the virus could directly activate a subpopulation
of lymphocytes resulting in the development of cell clones which recognize
host antigens and/or synthesize autoantibodies. Third, it is conceivable
that structural proteins of viruses possess antigenic similarities with a
host cell protein or lipid, referred to as "molecular mimicry". An immune
response to the virus infection would automatically trigger an autoimmune
response. Fourth, anti-idiotypic antibodies are formed which recognize a
common determinant or structural configuration shared by both a host cell
membrane antigen and the antiviral antibody.

So far, none of the suggested different mechanisms have been proven to lead to autoimmunity but evidence is mounting which would suggest that virus induced autoimmunity is not an epiphenomenon, but could play a pathogenetic role in certain diseases. The observation made with coronavirus infection in rats demonstrates for the first time that an infection of CNS cells triggers an autoimmune response to brain antigens. Whether similar events take place in multiple sclerosis is unknown but conceivable. Obviously, many virological and immunological aspects have to be studied before the complexity of a virus-host relationship in demyelinating diseases can be interpreted.

Acknowledgment

Supported by Deutsche Forschungsgemeinschaft. I thank Helga Kriesinger for typing the manuscript.

References

Dal Canto, M.C. and Rabinovitz, S.G., 1982. Experimental models of virus-induced demyelination of the central nervous system. Ann. Neurol. 11: 109-127.

Koga, M., Wege, H. and ter Meulen, V., 1984. Sequence of murine coronavirus JHM induced CNS changes in rats. J. Neuropathol. Appl. Neurobiol. 10: 173-184.

ter Meulen, V. and Hall, W.W., 1978. Slow virus infections of the nervous system: virological, immunological and pathogenetic considerations. J. Gen. Virol. 41: 1-25.

ter Meulen, V. and Stephenson, J.R., 1983. The possible role of viral infections in MS and other related demyelinating diseases. In: J.F. Hallpike, C.W.M. Adams, W.W. Tourtellotte (Eds) "Multiple Sclerosis" Chapman & Hall, London, pp. 241-274.

Watanabe, R., Wege, H. and ter Meulen, V., 1983. Adoptive transfer of EAE-like lesions by BMP stimulated lymphocytes from rats with coronavirus-induced demyelinating encephalomyelitis. Nature 305: 150-153.

Wege, H., Watanabe, R. and ter Meulen, V., 1983. Murine coronavirus infection of the central nervous system in rats. In: C.A. Mims, M.L. Cuzner and R.E. Kelly (Eds.) "Viruses and Demyelinating Diseases", pp. 67-79.

Wege, H., Watanabe, R. and ter Meulen, V., 1984. Relapsing subacute demyelinating encephalomyelitis in rats in the course of coronavirus JHM infection. J. Neuroimmunol. 6: 325-336.

Section IV
HLA, Epidemiology,
Genetics

41

Multiple Sclerosis Cooperative Etiological Study in Italy

C. FIESCHI

INTRODUCTION

A cooperative nation wide etiological study on multiple sclerosis (MS) was started in December 1983 in Italy, promoted by the Neuroepidemiology Section of the Italian Neurology Society. The specific aim for this study is to verify the existence of a different risk of disease among migrants with respect to non-migrants and to look to this eventually found different risk in terms of causality (ethnical origin, multiple moves). Italy has been considered a "medium" risk area and higher prevalence rate have been reported in Northern Italy than in Southern Italy. New studies (Dean et al., 1979; Granieri et al., 1982) have shown high rates in Southern Italy this putting in doubt the previous reported pattern of MS distribution in Italy. In our country there was a large migratory flow from Southern to Northern Italy in the fifties and sixties years. For this reason it is now possible for us to explore the effect that migration and the age at which migration occurred, has on MS risk. Under the hypothesis of a protective effect of migration from Southern to Northern Italy we will explore successively the influence of ethnic and environmental factors. Secondly the possible association of MS with some infectious viral diseases hypothesized, in the literature, to be cause(s) of MS (measles, herpes virus 1 and 2, mononucleosis) (Alter, 1976; Martin, 1981; Warner, 1981) is investigated. Thirdly the association with some other variables possibly related to the disease (alcohol consumption, occupational exposure to neurotoxic agents, tonsillectomy) is explored.

MATERIAL AND METHODS

A case-control design was chosen. Cases are diagnosed according to McDonald's criteria, revised by our clinical committee. All the hospitalized MS patients, newly diagnosed from 1 December 1983, living in 19 Italian provinces are interviewed. All the cases are included regardless the level of diagnosis certainty (definite, probable, possible and suspected MS). All the included cases are followed-up at least every six months. All the included cases perform lumbar puncture and cerebral CT-scan or myelography, according to their clinical signs and symptoms, in order to exclude neurological diseases other than MS.

Two sets of controls are recruited, neurological controls from the same hospital, neurological departments as the cases, non neurological controls from other specialistics and non specialistic departments of the same hospitals as the cases. Controls are randomly selected among patients suffering from diseases lasting no longer than 5 years. No matching is performed, controls are recruited with an estimated case/control ratio of ¼ and with an age and sex distribution based on the expected number and age and sex distribution of the cases. These estimates have been evaluated for every participating centre during a previous feasibility study.

Exposure variables are anamnestically investigated through questionnaire by skilled interviewers. The interview is performed, whenever possible, in the presence of the patient's mother. relative risks estimate and statistical significance is evaluated by the Mantel-Haenszel method for stratified data. Data are stratified for age (5 strata), sex and residence when appropriate (3 strata).

RESULTS

Present analysis is limited to migration, ethnic origin and multiple moves. The data refer to 400 consecutive patients, 86 cases, 183 neurological and 131 non-neurological controls, recruited during the first 6 months of the study.

At present 1069 patients are included in the interview study, 243 cases, 438 neurological and 388 non-neurological controls. None of the relative risk estimates that will be presented, is statistically significant.

In table 1 the age and sex distribution of the 400 cases and controls included in the analysis is shown. The case distribution in the 4 diagnostic categories shows that of the 86 cases interviewed only 31 (36%) are definite MS (table 2).

TABLE 1   Case and control, age and sex distributions among 400 (out of 743) consecutive patients recruited during the first 6 months of the study.

Age		⩽ 20	21-30	31-40	41-50	50+	Total
Cases	♂	5	13	7	8	2	86
	♀	3	20	13	7	8	
Neurol.	♂	14	12	14	31	31	183
Ctrls	♀	5	14	11	27	24	
Non neurol.	♂	21	19	8	20	10	131
Ctrls.	♀	10	6	12	12	13	

TABLE 2   Case classification

	Definite	Probable	Possible	Suspected	n.s.*
No	31	19	8	20	8
%	36.0	22.1	9.3	23.0	9.3

*not specified

Looking at migration (table 3) we can see that the Odds Ratio (O.R.s) for migrants from Southern Italy are less than 1 for both sets of controls and that they are further reduced when restricting the analysis to definite MS cases.

TABLE 3   Migration from Southern Italy.
Residents in Northern Italy with 4 grandparents born in
Southern Italy.

Neurological controls

	Non-migrants	Migrants
Observed cases (%)	5 (31.3)	11 (68.7)
Observed ctrls (%)	3 (7.5)	37 (92.5)
ODDS ratio	1	0.3

Non-neurological controls

	Non-migrants	Migrants
Observed cases (%)	5 (31.3)	11 (68.7)
Observed ctrls (%)	8 (29.6)	16 (71.4)
ODDS ratio	1	0.3

For ethnic origin, which was analysed as birth places of grandparents
we observe a pattern of the O.R.s similar to the one observed for migration (table 4). A reduced risk of disease among subjects with 4 grandparents born in Southern Italy was found when compared to subjects with

TABLE 4   Grandparents birthplace.
Residents in Northern Italy.

Neurological controls

	4 Grandparents born in Northern Italy	4 Grandparents born in Southern Italy	Any other combina-tion of birth-places
Observed cases (%)	37 (58.7)	16 (25.4)	10 (15.9)
Observed ctrls[+] (%)	77 (56.2)	39 (28.5)	21 (15.3)
ODDS ratio*	1	0.6	0.7
Observed def. cases (%)	15 (60)	6 (24)	4 (16)
ODDS ratio*	1	0.5	0.6

*age and sex adjusted

Non-neurological controls

	4 Grandparents born in Northern Italy	4 Grandparents born in Southern Italy	any other combina- tion of birth- places
Observed cases (%)	37 (58.7)	16 (25.4)	10 (15.9)
Observed ctrls[++](%)	46 (54.1)	26 (30.6)	13 (15.2)
ODDS ratio[*]	1	0.6	1.1
Observed def. cases (%)	15 (60)	6 (24)	4 (16)
ODDS ratio[*]	1	0.5	1

[*]age and sex adjusted

+for 11 and ++5 controls it was not possible to assess the birthplace of grandparents.

4 grandparents born in Northern Italy. But as migration from Southern Italy is associated itself with having 4 grandparents born in Southern Italy this last result could be due again to migration. Therefore we restricted the analysis of migration to subjects with 4 grandparents born in Southern Italy. This analysis correspond to a comparison of the risks of disease between the first and the second generation of migrants. Again migration is negatively associated with the disease (table 5).

TABLE 5   Migration.
         Residents in Northern Italy.

Neurological controls

	Non-migrants	Migrants from Central Italy	Migrants from Southern Italy
Observed cases (%)	45 (71.4)	5 (7.9)	13 (20.6)
Observed ctrls	96 (64.9)	12 (8.1)	40 (27.8)
ODDS ratio[*]	1	1.4	0.6
Observed def. cases (%)	18 (72)	2 (8)	5 (20)
ODDS ratio	1	-	0.5

[*]age and sex adjusted

Non-neurological controls

	Non-migrants	Migrants from Central Italy	Migrants from Southern Italy
Observed cases (%)	45 (71.4)	5 (7.9)	13 (20.6)
Observed ctrls (%)	64 (71.1)	2 (2.3)	24 (26.6)
ODDS ratio*	1	3.3	0.5^x
Observed def. cases (%)	18 (72)	2 (8)	5 (20)
ODDS ratio*	1	-	0.3^{xx}

*age and sex adjusted   xp = 0.13;   xxp = 0.18

For the age of migration (table 6) surprisingly we have not found any difference between the risk of subjects who migrated before and after the age of 15 in the comparison with both control groups. Wischer and Detels (1981) found among migrants affected by MS a higher prevalence of multiple moves than among controls. They concluded that multiple moves could both explain the high risk of their migrants and/or multiple moves could belong to a different causal chain than the one of migration. Following this last suggestion, although our migrants are at a lower risk than non migrants, we nevertheless analyzed multiple moves as an independent

TABLE 6   Age of migration from Southern Italy.
           Residents in Northern Italy.

Neurological controls

	No migration	Before 15 years	After 15 years
Observed cases (%)	45 (71.4)	7 (11.1)	6 (9.5)
Observed ctrls (%)	96 (64.9)	11 (7.4)	29 (19.7)
ODDS ratio	1	0.6	0.6

Non-neurological controls

	No migration	Before 15 years	After 15 years
Observed cases (%)	45 (71.4)	7 (11.1)	6 (9.5)
Observed ctrls (%)	64 (72.7)	10 (11.1)	14 (15.6)
ODDS ratio	1	0.6	0.6

variable from migration (table 7). These preliminary data do not seem to reproduce in a consistent way the association found by Wischer and Detels but this could represent the result of some confounding effect due to the fact that migration is positively associated with multiple moves.

TABLE 7   Multiple moves.

Neurological controls

	0-1 moves	2-4 moves	5 or more moves
Observed cases (%)	56 (65.1)	22 (25.6)	8 (9.3)
Observed ctrls (%)	108 (59.0)	57 (31.2)	18 (9.8)
ODDS ratio	1	1.2	1.1

Non-neurological controls

	0-1 moves	2-4 moves	5 or more moves
Observed cases (%)	56 (65.1)	22 (25.4)	8 (9.3)
Observed ctrls (%)	92 (70.2)	29 (22.1)	10 (7.6)
ODDS ratio	1	1.2	1.4

Move = residence change, lasting longer than 6 months, outside previous municipality.

CONCLUSIONS

Our results on migration have to be discussed in view of a possible healthy migrant effect. This bias seems unlikely at least for three reasons. (1) The controls and not only the cases are affected by a disease. (2) None but 2 of the controls migrated at an age in which the disease was present in the age and sex corresponding cases. (3) The negative association is stronger for definite MS as one would expect for any real association.

The results on migration is in agreement with the prevalence studies that have shown a decreasing with latitude risk of disease. As migration is negatively associated with MS also among subjects with the same ethnic origin our data suggest stronger environmental than genetic determinants of the disease. Finally more data are required to analyse multiple moves adjusting for migration.

ACKNOWLEDGEMENTS

This study is supported by the National Research Council Project "Preventive and Rehabilitative Medicine", subproject "Degenerative Diseases of the Nervous System".

REFERENCES

Alter, M., 1976. Is multiple sclerosis an age-dependent host response to measles? Lancet, 1: 456.
Dean, G., Grimaldi, G., Kelly, R., Karhausen, L., 1979. Multiple sclerosis in Southern Europe I: prevalence in Sicily in 1975. J. Epid. Comm. Health, 33: 107-110.
Granieri, E. Rosati, G., 1982. Italy: a medium or high risk area for multiple sclerosis? An epidemiological study in Barbagia, Sardinia, Southern Italy. Neurology, 32: 466-472.
Martin, J.R., 1981. Herpes simplex virus type 1 and 2 and multiple sclerosis. Lancet, 2: 777-781.
McDonald, W.I., Halliday, A.M., 1977. Diagnosis and classifications of multiple sclerosis. Br. Med. Bull., 33: 4-9.
Warner, H.B., Carp, R.I., 1981. Multiple sclerosis and Epstein Barr virus. Lancet, 2: 1290.
Wischer, B.R., Bunnell, D.H., Detels, R., 1981. Multiple sclerosis and multiple moves: an etiologic hypothesis. Am. J. Epidem., 113: 140-143.

Coordinating Center: G. Filippini, M.D. (Principal Investigator), M. Musicco, M.D., B. Bordo, M.D., S. Molinari and A. Tronci (Co-investigators) Neurological Institute C. Besta Milan.
Clinical Committee: Prof. V. Cosi, Prof. S. Marforio, Prof. D. Zerbi.
Statistical Committee: M. Musicco, M.D., L. Bisanti, M.D., G. Filippini, M.D., A. Citterio, M.D.
Principal Investigators and Interviewers (Neurological Centers) G. Rossi, M.D., O. Pernisi (Dept. of Neurology "S. Chiara" General Hospital, Trento); D. Benedetti, M.D., G. Coccia, M.D. (Dept. of Neurology "Borgo Roma" General Hospital, Verona); L. Bevilacque, M.D. (Dept. of Neurology "Niguarda" General Hospital, Milan); N. Massetto, M.D. (Dept. of Neurology "S. Paolo" General Hospital, Milan); C. Mariani, M.D. (II Dept. of Neurology University of Milan); G. Mora, M.D. (III Dept. of Neurology University of Milan); G. Comi, M.D. (IV Dept. of Neurology University of Milan); E. Beghi, M.D. (Dept. of Neurology "S. Gerardo" General Hospital, Monza); M. Pederzoli, M.D. (Dept. of Neurology General Hospital Vimercate); Prof. S. Marforio, M. Moscheni (MS Center General Hospital, Gallarate); A. Citterio, M.D. (Dept. of Neurology University of Pavia); M.G. Cavallo, M.D. (I Dept. of Neurology University of Turin); P. Mortara, M.D. (II Dept. of Neurology University of Turin); L. Appendino, M.D. (III Dept. of Neurology University of Turin); C. Ravetti, M.D. (Dept. of Neurology "Nuova Astanteria" General Hospital, Turin); M. Francinetti Bressy, M.D. (Dept. of Neurology "Mauriziano" General Hospital, Turin); D. Giobbe, M.D. (Dept. of Neurology "Maria Vittoria" General Hospital, Turin); C. Gandoldo, M.D., R. Vecchia, M.D. (Dept. of Neurology University of Genoa); N. Dagnino, M.D. (Dept. of Neurology General Hospital,

Sestri Ponente); S. Salvarani, M.D. (Dept. of Neurology General Hospital, Sampierdarene); Prof. L. Garello (Dept. of Neurology "San Martino", Genoa); S. Cammarata, M.D. (Dept. of Neurology "San Paolo" General Hospital, Savona); B. Peluffo, M.D. (Dept. of Neurology General Hospital, Imperia); D. Visentini, M.D., A. Solari, M.D. (Dept. of Neurology University of Parma); Prof. E. Granieri, A. Altobelli, M.D. (Dept. of Neurology University of Ferrara); L. Fratiglioni, M.D., C. Groppi, M.D. (Dept. of Neurology University of Florence); G.M. Malentacchi, M.D., A. Tiezzi, M.D. (Dept. of Neurology General Hospital, Arezzo); G. Meucci, M.D., A. Lippi, M.D. (Dept. of Neurology University of Pisa); M. D'Ettore, M.D. M. Mondelli, M.D. (Dept. of Neurology University of Siena); S. Bernardi, M.D., L. Pacifici, M.D. (Dept. of Neurology University of Rome); M. Troiano, M.D., G. Logroscino, M.D. (Dept. of Neurology University of Bari); G. Giuliani, M.D., F. Scataglini, M.D. (Dept. of Neurology General Hospital, Ancona); G. Savettieri, M.D., M.P. Castiglione (Dept. of Neurology University of Palermo).

National Research Council Contract No. 83.0264456.

42

A Multicenter Study of the Incidence of Multiple Sclerosis in Italy. Design of the Study

G. COMI

INTRODUCTION

Although the etiology of multiple sclerosis (MS) is still obscure, epidemiological studies have shown a geographical distribution correlated to latitude, with three zones of high, medium and low frequency (Kurtzke, 1980). Italy, extending from 37° to 46° North latitude, lies just below the borderline between the first two zones. The results of about 30 prevalence studies carried out in Italy between 1962-1980, using large population groups (Table 1) (Rossi 1980; Marforio et al., 1980; Mamoli et al., 1980; Caputo et al., 1979; Borri et al., 1976; Nardi, 1979; Tavolato et al., 1974; Rosati et al., 1981; Macchi et al., 1962; Paci et al., 1980; Megna et al., 1980; Palma et al., 1981; Rosati et al., 1977; Bramanti et al., 1978; Savettieri et al., 1978; Reggio et al., 1979) indicate ratios from 7.2 to 27.1/100.000 (Granieri and Rosati, 1982). These figures classify Italy as a medium risk area fro MS. However, more recent studies with smaller population groups (Table 2) (Rossi et al., 1980; Granieri et al., 1982: Savettieri et al., 1981; Dean et al., 1979) have reported prevalence figures from 30.2 to 65.3/100.000. These results shift Italy into an area with high frequency of MS. The difference between these prevalence figures may be partially explained by more com-

TABLE 1　MS prevalence investigation carried out in Italy using large population groups

Authors	Study area	Latitude	Population	Probable MS prevalence rates per 100.000	95% CI	Standardized prevalence rates per 100.000
Rossi (1980)	Trento	46°	442.873	27.1	22-32	-
Marforio (1980)	Varese	45°	790.046	24.2	21-28	-
Mamoli (1980)	Bergamo	45°	891.153	15.8	13-19	-
Caputo (1979)	Novara	45°	507.394	19.5	16-24	-
Borri (1976)	Torino	45°	2.287.016	17.1	15-19	-
Nardi (1979)	Venezia	45°	831.657	18.6	16-22	-
Tavolato (1974)	Padova	45°	760.649	16.0	13-19	17.8
Rosati (1981)	Ferrara	44°	386.896	26.9	22-33	24.8
Macchi (1962)	Parma	44°	389.276	11.6	8-15	-
Borri (1976)	Firenze	43°	1.146.367	10.6	9-13	-
Borri (1976)	Perugia	43°	552.136	17.0	14-21	-
Paci (1980)	Terni	43°	229.034	17.9	13-24	-
Megna (1980)	Bari	41°	1.351.288	15.5	13-18	-
Palma (1981)	Avellino	40°	433.864	7.6*	5-11	-
Palma (1981)	Napoli	40°	2.812.996	9.1*	8-10	-
Rosati (1977)	Sassari	40°	397.891	16.6	13-21	17.6
Rosati (1977)	Nuoro	40°	273.021	15.8	12-21	17.9
Rosati (1977)	Cagliari	39°	802.888	9.5	8-12	10.2
Bramanti (1978)	Messina	38°	673.791	12.6	10-15	-
Savettieri (1978)	Palermo	38°	666.175	12.3	10-15	13.1
Reggio (1979)	Catania	37°	938.273	7.2	6-9	-

*Includes possible MS

TABLE 2   MS prevalence investigations carried out in Italy using limited population groups

Authors	Study area	Latitude	Population	Prevalence rates per 100.000
Rossi et al., 1980	Bassa Valsugana	46°	24.570	44.8
Rosati et al., 1980	Copparo	44°	45.153	31.1
Rosati et al., 1980	Ozieri	40°	56.294	30.2
Granieri et al., 1982	Barbagia	40°	51.611	40.7
Savettieri et al., 1981	Monreale	38°	25.403	43.0
Dean et al., 1981	Agrigento	37°	49.979	32.0
Savettieri et al., 1981	Caltanisetta	37°	60.022	38.0
Dean et al., 1979	Enna	37°	28.189	52.9

plete case ascertainment in smaller populations (Kurland et al., 1965), but there are other possible causes. Particular methodological and local regional problems could influence the results. Accessibility and quality of the sources for case collection, medical records, collaboration of practitioners, level of socio-sanitary organization are very different from region to region. The surveys employ different criteria for inclusion, classification of MS cases and modalities of case collection. Thus the epidemiological data presently available do not enable us to compare the frequencies of MS in different areas of Italy.

In addition to latitude, other exogenous factors may play important roles in the etiopathogenesis of MS, as seen from the regional and temporal clustering of cases (Alperovitch and Bouvier, 1982; Wikström and Palo, 1975; Kurtzke et al., 1982, Kurtzke and Hyllested, 1979) and the migration between areas at different risk (Dean and Kurtzke, 1971; Alter et al., 1966). Finally, there are some factors whose influence on MS is controversial: socio-economic (Kurtzke et al., 1979, Beebe et al., 1967), urban-rural (Millar, 1971), exposure to toxic agents at work (Amaducci et al., 1982). The Section of Neuroepidemiology of the Italian Society of Neurology organized a Multicenter Study of the Incidence of Multiple Sclerosis in Italy in January 1982. The organization phase was finished in June 1983; in September of the same year the operation phase started, and this will be completed in June 1985.

The aims of the study are to evaluate incidence of MS in different areas of Northern, Central and Southern Italy and to investigate the effects on the risk of some of the variables mentioned above.

MATERIAL AND METHODS

Design of the study

The study is multicenter and retrospective. We preferred a multicenter study because the local research units know better the public health organization of the region and have easier access to the sources of material: this means more complete ascertainment of the cases. In addition, most local research units have had previous experiences with MS. However, multicenter studies have problems of homogeneity. To overcome these problems, a group of well-trained neurologists will review all the cases before definitive inclusion to guarantee homogeneity of all cases included. In April 1983, a course for all the physicians involved in the

study informing them about all methodological problems, was organized. A
register, in which all the possible sources for the identification of
potential cases are listed, was created. The physicians must sign for
each source the names of the potential cases of MS. A common questionnaire will be used for uniform collection of anagraphic and clinical
data. This questionnaire has already been applied to a series of at
least ten MS in patients at each center and the results examined by the
scientific committee with the neurologist incharged at each center, to
evaluate possible differences in the compilation.

We preferred a retrospective study, because of some of the characteristics of the natural history of MS. The disease is difficult to diag-
nose at onset, because its evolution is highly variable. The interval
between episodes in the remitting and relapsing type can be as long as
ten years, so a definite or probable diagnosis can be made only after
long observation. Therefore diagnosis is often made late after the onset
of the disease. An incidence prospective study should include a follow
up for at least five years after the end of data collection. The relatively low frequency of the disease also makes it necessary that the study
covers a good number of years to have enough patients.

The period selected was 1 January 1971 to 31 December 1980. The
choice was determined by the poor quality of clinical records before
that. Moreover, on the ground of studies of mortality among MS patients
(Hyllested, 1961; Kurtzke et al., 1971), fewer than 15% of cases occurring in that period should have died before 1985, which will permit clinical re-examination of most of the patients. In effect, since the period
examined is close to the time of the evaluation, some problems in the
classification of cases incident in the last few years considered could
arise, which means that in these years there may be an overestimation of
possible cases and an underestimation of definite and probable cases. We
should take this into account during the evaluation of the results and
will probably be necessary to re-examine these cases successively.

We preferred an incidence study because prevalence studies are likely
to be biased by several variables, such as natural evolution of the
disease, migratory flux, available medical services and accessibility to
the neurological unit, making the measure of the prevalence unsuitable
for comparing MS prevalence rates in different areas. Moreover, incidence
studies are a better approach to etiological problems (Mc Alpine et al.,
1972).

Diagnostic criteria

All patients who had the onset of symptoms of MS while living in the areas investigated will be included. Patients will be classified into groups of definite, probable and possible MS, according to the criteria of Rose et al. (1976). Time of onset of the disease is defined as the year of appearance of the first symptom later ascribed to the disease. Symptoms rarely occurring as initial symptoms in MS are accepted as initial symptoms only when they precede by less then one year the appearance of the commonly accepted symptoms (Mc Alpine et al., 1972). The diagnostic criteria for inclusion and classification of cases are based only on clinical symptoms and signs and are not influenced by selective use of modern supportive laboratory data, because these are not equally available in all the areas.

Areas of investigation

Fourteen different centers have participated in the study, each investigating one area. The latitudes of the area ranges between 37° and 46° North. Two areas lay between 37° and 40°, 7 between 41° and 43° and 5 between 44° and 46° (Table 3). The altitudes range from 0 to 2110 meters above sea level. The geographic, climatic, urban-rural and socio-economic characteristics are very variable from area to area. The total population in the areas investigated was on 21 October 1981 (12th General Census) 1.563.916. The area population varied from 43.651 (Anagni) to 356.211 (province of Ferrara). Seven areas had fewer than 100.000 inhabitans, 6 between 100.000 and 200.000. Medical organization is different from area to area, but all the areas have at least one neurological center.

Case collection and ascertainment

The poor homogeneity of the national public health system makes it difficult to specify possible sources for ascertainment of potential cases. To have a study as homogeneous as possible, we have individuated three kinds of sources: sources located within the area, sources in neighbouring areas and remote sources (national level center for treatment of MS patients).

The following sources has to be examinated: archives of the hospitals and university clinics, records of the National Health Insurance, archives of the National Pension Institute, records of local sections of the

TABLE 3   Latitude and population in the investigated areas.

Areas	Latitude	Population
Valle D'Aosta	46^0	112.654
Valle Brembana	46^0	51.027
Gallarate	45^0	174.212
Seriate	45^0	118.402
Ferrara	44^0	356.211
Ancona	43^0	123.603
Arezzo	43^0	87.330
Siena	43^0	60.058
L'Aquila	42^0	102.121
Terni	42^0	130.103
Anagni	41^0	43.651
Caserta	41^0	66.754
Sassari	40^0	77.586
Enna	37^0	60.204
	Total	1.563.916

Italian Association for MS (AISM). All the neurologists, ophthalmologists and general practitioners in the area are contacted by letter and by phone. Private citizens, particularly MS patients, will be interviewed. Analysis of the archives will include not only the diagnosis of MS but also other diagnosis such as myelopathy, encephalitis, myelitis, paraplegia, optic neuritis etc.

All available medical documents and data relative to potential cases will be examined. Cases with a possible diagnosis of MS will be given neurological examinations and detailed interviews, with compilation of the questionnaire. Cases who have died or moved away prior to examination or refused it, may or may not be included, on the basis of all medical documents concerning them and of information obtained from immediate family and other relatives.

CONCLUSIONS

At this time all centers have completed the examination of the sour-

ces in the areas themselves and neighbouring areas. There are still to
be examined the archives of hospitals and rehabilitation centers specialized in MS farther from the area. Examination of the cases has already
started. At this time questionnaires relative to 132 cases have come to
the the scientific committee. The study should be completed within the
planned time.

This report is a part of a collaborative study of various centers
and the participants are:
G. Giuliani (Ancona), M.R. Tola (Ferrara), M. Prencipe (L'Aquila), B.
Jandolo (Anagni-Roma), G. Malentacchi (Arezzo), P.F. Ottaviano (Terni),
A, Mamoli (Aosta), S. Marforio (Gallarate-Milano), G. Rosati (Sassari),
G. Grimaldi (Enna), C.R. De Fanti (Seriate-Bergamo), D'Ettorre (Siena),
G. D'Ambrosio (Caserta), L. Frattiglioni (Firenze), L. Fera (Bergamo),
V. Martinelli (Milano), G. Comi (Milano).

REFERENCES

Alperovich, A. and Bouvier, M.H., 1982. Geographical pattern of death
    rates from multiple sclerosis in France. An analysis of 4912 death.
    Acta Neurol. Scand., 66: 454-461.
Alter, M., Lebovitz, V. and Speer, J., 1966. Risk of multiple sclerosis
    related to age at immigration to Isreal. Arch. Neurol., 15: 234-237.
Amaducci, L., Arfaioli, C., Inzitari, D. and Marchi, M., 1982. Multiple
    sclerosis among shoe and leather workers: an epidemiological survey
    in Florence. Acta Neurol. Scand., 65: 94-103.
Beebe, G.W., Kurtzke, J.F., Kurland, L.T., Auth, L.T. and Nagler, B.,
    1967. Studies on the natural history of multiple sclerosis: 3.
    Epidemiologic analysis of the army experience in world war II.
    Neurology (Minneap.), 17: 1-17.
Borri, P.,Tavolato,B.F., Ballatori, F. and Cazzullo, C.L., 1976. Epide-
    miological survey on multiple sclerosis in Italy. Riv. Pat. Nerv.
    Ment. 97: 205-210.
Bramanti, P., Messina, C., Scuderi, D. and Vita, G., 1978. An epidemiolo-
    gical study on multiple sclerosis in the province of Messina, Italy.
    Acta Neurol., 34: 133-141.
Dean, G. and Kurtzke, J.F., 1971. On the risk of multiple sclerosis
    according to age at immigration to South-Africa. Br. Med. J., 3: 725-
    729.
Dean, G., Grimaldi, G., Kelly, R. and Karhausen, L., 1979. Multiple
    sclerosis in south Europe. I: prevalence in Sicily in 1975. J. Epide-
    miol. Commun. Health, 33: 107-110.
Dean, G., Savettieri, G., Taibi, G., Monreale, S. and Karhausen, L., 1981.
    The prevalence of multiple sclerosis in Sicily. II: Agrigento City.
    J. Epidemiol. Commun. Health, 35: 118-122.
Granieri, E. and Rosati, G., 1982. Italy: a medium or high-risk area for
    multiple sclerosis? An epidemiologic study in Barbagia, Sardinia,
    Southern Italy. Neurology, 32: 466-472.
Hyllested, K., 1961. Lethality, duration and mortality of disseminated
    sclerosis in Denmark. Acta Psych. Scand., 35: 553-564.
Kurland, L.T., Stazio, A. and Reed, D., 1965. An appraisal of population
    studies of multiple sclerosis. Ann. N.Y. Acad. Sci., 122: 520-544.

Kurtzke, J.F., Kurland, L.T. and Golberg, I.D., 1971. Mortality and migration in multiple sclerosis. Neurology, 21: 1186-1197.
Kurtzke, J.F., Beebe, G.W. and Norman, J.E., 1979a. Epidemiology of multiple sclerosis in U.S. veterans: I. Race, sex and geographic distribution. Neurology, 29: 1228-1235.
Kurtzke, J.F. and Hyllested, K., 1979b. Multiple sclerosis in the Faroe Island: I. Clinical and epidemiological features. Ann. Neurol., 5: 6-21.
Kurtzke, J.F., 1980. Epidemiologic contribution to multiple sclerosis: an overview. Neurology, 30: 61-79.
Kurtzke, J.F., Gudmundsson, K.R. and Bergmann, S., 1982. Multiple sclerosis in Iceland: 1. Evidence of a postwar epidemic. Neurology, 32: 143-150.
Macchi, G., Sanginaro, M. and Valla, S., 1962. La sclerose en plaques dans la province de Parma, Italy. World Neurol., 3: 731-739.
Mamoli, A., Fera, L., Camerlingo, M. and Alfieri, R., 1980. Sclerosi multipla: indagine epidemiologica nella provincia di Bergamo (dati preliminari). 2nd Italian Meeting of Neuroepidemiology, Milan (Italy), December 12-13.
Marforio, S., Caputo, D., Zibetti, A., Ghezzi, A., Di Costanzo, M. and Palestra, A., 1980. Sclerosi multipla: ricerca epidemiologica in provincia di Varese. Arch. Sci. Med. (Torino), 137: 1-8.
Mc Alpine, D., Lumsden, C.E. and Acheson, E.D., 1972. Multiple sclerosis: a reappraisal. Churchill Livingstone, Edinburg.
Megna, G., 1980. Rilievi epidemiologici sulla sclerosi multipla nella provincia di Bari. 2nd Italian Meeting of Neuroepidemiology, Milan (Italy), December 12-13.
Millar, J.H.D., 1971. Multiple sclerosis: a disease acquired in childhood. Springfield, Illinois.
Nardi, P.G., 1979. Studio epidemiologico sulla sclerosi multipla nella provincia di Venezia. Riv. Pat. Nerv. Ment., 100: 121-142.
Paci, A., Ottaviano, P. and Freddi, A., 1980. La sclerosi multipla nella regione umbra: dati epidemiologici relativi alla provincia di Terni. 2nd Italian Meeting of Neuroepidemiology, Milan (Italy), December 12-13.
Palma, V., Ciambellini, M. and Buscaino, G.A., 1981. Indagine epidemiologica sulla sclerosi multipla nelle province di Napoli e Avellino. Acta Neurol., 42: 280-290.
Reggio, A., Pero, G. and Campo, G., 1979. Indagine geo-demografica sulla sclerosi multipla nella provincia di Catania: risultati di un primo censimento. Boll. Soc. Med. Chir. Catania, 46: 151-155.
Rosati, G., Pinna, L. and Granieri, E., 1977. The distribution of multiple sclerosis in Sardinia. Riv. Pat. Nerv. Ment., 98: 46-64.
Rosati, G., Granieri, E., Carreras, M. and Tola, R., 1980a. Multiple sclerosis in southern Europe: a prevalence study in the socio-sanitary district of Copparo, Northern Italy. Acta Neurol. Scand., 62: 244-249.
Rosati, G., Granieri, E., Carreras, M., Pinna, L., Tola, R. and Paolino, E., 1980b. Epidemiologia della sclerosi multipla in piccole comunità dell'Italia settentrionale ed insulare. 2nd Italian Meeting of Neuroepidemiology, Milan (Italy), December 12-13.
Rosati, G., Granieri, E. and Carreras, M., 1981. Multiple sclerosis in Northern Italy: prevalence in the province of Ferrara in 1978. Ital. J. Neurol. Sci., 2: 17-23.
Rose, A.S., Ellison, G.W., Myers, L.W. and Tourtellotte, W.W., 1976. Criteria for the clinical diagnosis of multiple sclerosis. Neurology, 26 (6: part 2), 20-27.

Rossi, G., Ferrari, G. and Dalri, E., 1980. Sclerosi multipla nella
    provincia di Trento: ricerca epidemiologica. 2nd Italian Meeting of
    Neuroepidemiology, Milan (Italy), December 12-13.
Savettieri, G., Piccoli, F. and Chiaravalle, E., 1978. Epidemiological
    survey on multiple sclerosis in the city of Palermo, Italy. Acta
    Neurol., 33: 526-531.
Savettieri, G., Karhausen, L. and Dean, G., 1981. The prevalence of mul-
    tiple sclerosis in Sicily. I: Monreale city. J. Epidemiol. Commun.
    Health, 35: 114-117.
Savettieri, G., Grimaldi, G., Giordano, D., Ventura, A. and Karhausen, L.
    La sclerosis multipla in Sicilia: altri dati epidemiologici (personal
    communication).
Tavolato, B.F., 1971. Multiple sclerosis in Padova province, Italy. Acta
    Neurol. Scand., 50: 76-90.
Wikström, J. and Palo, J., 1975. Studies on the clustering of multiple
    sclerosis in Finland. I. Comparison between the domiciles and place
    of birth in selected subpopulations. Acta Neurol. Scand., 51: 85-98.

43

HLA Markers and Course of Disease in Multiple Sclerosis

M. MERIENNE, O. SABOURAUD, R. FAUCHET, M. MADIGAND, G. SEMANA, M. GUEGUEN, G. DEJOUR and G. MOREL

INTRODUCTION

The relationship between multiple sclerosis (M.S.) and some specific HLA system antigens is now a proven fact, showing in the caucasoïds population an increase in B7 and DR2 alleles in the M.S. populations.

Nevertheless the question of a relationship between HLA system and the clinical aspects of the disease is asked ?

In a former study (Madigand et Al, 1982) including 261 patients tested for A and B loci and 91 patients tested in locus DR, we suspected 2 forms of M S : a remittent form, relatively moderate linked to B7 and DR2 antigens, and a progressive form, more severe linked to the B8 and DR3 antigens. The aim of this study is to show again our results which were not confirmed by some others authors (Engell et Al, 1982 - Wentzel et Al, 1984).

MATERIAL AND METHODS

HLA-A and HLA-B antigens were typed by the standart microlymphocyto-toxicity test with 36 antisera defining 16 locus A alleles, and 66 antisera defining 30 locus B alleles. DR determinents were defined on B lymphocytes using 50 antisera defining DR1 throught DRW10. Antigens frequency were compared with a healthy population of 200 controls typed between 1980 and 1983.

122 unrelated britton patients followed in the department of neurology university of Rennes have been included in this study ; compared with the study of 1982, we included 65 new patients, some patients of the former study have not been included because loss of sight.

Otherwise 49 of them were genotyped by family studies compared with 114 controls belonging to 57 healthy families.

The 122 patients according to the new diagnostic criteria of M S (Poser et Al 1982) were classified as definite M S : 108 patients and as probable : 14 patients. There were 87 females and 35 males.

Clinical subgrouping of the patients was as follow (table 1).

according to the severity of the disease using the Kurtzke disability status scale (K.S.) (Kurtzke 1983), the patients have been classified in 4 groups.

- Benign M S (groupe 1) where K S $\leqslant$ 4 with a disease of more than 10 years : 23 patients had benign form.
- Intermidiate M S (groupe 2) where K S $\geqslant$ 4 after 10 years : 37 patients had intermediate form.
- Severe M S (groupe 3) where K S $\geqslant$ 4 before ten years : 32 patients had severe form.
- Non classified M S (groupe 4) with a disease of duration less than 10 years with a K S $\leqslant$ 4 : 30 patients had non classified form.
. according to tempo of evolution.
- Remitting M S, there were defined as patients who had had distinct attacks of the disease even if subsequently they showed a progressive evolution, 92 patients were classified as remitting or remitting progressive.
- Progressive M S : they were defined as patients with progressive evolution in the absence of antecedents attacks, 30 patients had progressive M S.

MS POPULATION : 122 PATIENTS

— ACCORDING TO THE SEVERITY OF THE DISEASE

— GROUP 1 : BENIGN	23 PATIENTS
— GROUP 2 : INTERMEDIATE	37 PATIENTS
— GROUP 3 : SEVERE	32 PATIENTS
— GROUP 4 : NON-CLASSIFIED	30 PATIENTS

— ACCORDING TO TEMPO OF EVOLUTION

— REMITTENT MS	68	T 92 PATIENTS
— REMITTENT PROGRESSIVE MS	24	

— PROGRESSIVE MS	30 PATIENTS

Table 1

RESULTS

M S group as a whole (table 2). Results were found significantly increased in M S population for B7 (0. 37 vs 0.25   p< 0.03)

DR2 (0. 49 vs 0. 29   p < 0.0003)

HLA ANTIGENS PHENOTYPIC FREQUENCIES (%) IN MS PATIENTS AND CONTROLS

P VALUES AND COMPARISON WITH CONTROLS ARE GIVEN WHEN SIGNIFICANT

LOCUS	SPECIFICITY	% MS = 122	% CONTROLS = 200	P
	A2	.44	.47	
A	A3	.30	.24	
	A9	.19	.20	
	B7	.37	.25	< 0.03
B	B8	.26	.21	
	DR2	.49	.29	< 0.0003
DR	DR3	.28	.24	
	DR5	.22	.18	

Table 2

Results in patients subgroups.

. According to the severity of the disease (table 3) comparing the frequency of the severe group and the benign group, the study of the alleles showed a decrease (not significant) of : DR5 (15 vs 34, x^2 = 2.72).

MULTIPLE SCLEROSIS

PATIENTS SUBMITTED IN FOUR GROUPS ACCORDING TO THE SEVERITY OF THE DISEASE

LOCUS	SPECIFICITY	1 BENIGN N = 23	2 INTERMEDIATE N = 37	3 SEVERE N = 32	4 NON CLASSIFIED N = 30
	A2	.54	.51	.25	.46
A	A3	.22	.24	.43	.30
	A9	.18	.27	.21	.13
	B7	.27	.45	.46	.30
B	B8	.22.7	.21	.31	.30
	DR2	.47	.45	.56	.50
DR	DR3	.17	.24	.40	.32
	DR5	.34	.21	.15	.21

Table 3

and an increased frequency (not significant)of : A3 (43 vs 22, x^2 = 2.53) ;
B7 (46 vs 27, x^2 = 3.38) ; DR3 (40 vs 17, x^2 = 3.38). We emphasize that
the frequency of the DR2 allele does not change according to the gravity
of the disease and that the non significant values are probably due to the
small number of patients tested.

According to tempo of evolution (table 4). The results showed
an increase of DR3 allele frequency in the progressive form.

PHENOTYPIC FREQUENCIES ACCORDING TO TEMPO OF EVOLUTION

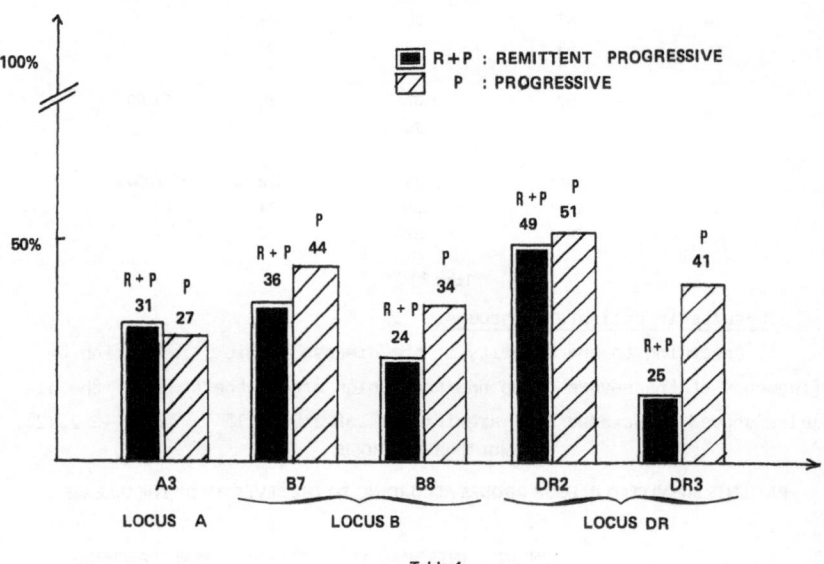

Table 4

- The study of the haplotypic associations were made with two kinds of
  results
. Phenotyped association (postulated from known linkage desequilibria among
the 122 patients (table 5) showed an increase of B7., DR2 (29, 5 vs 13
p < 0. 003 - S) A3, B7, DR2 (12.7 vs 6.5 p < 0.005-S) B8, DR3
(19.5 vs 9.5 p < 0.01 S) A1, B8, DR3 (14.5 vs 8.5 p < 0.08 N S).
among the subgroups we noted a difference of repartition between the benign

HAPLOTYPIC FREQUENCIES IN PHENOTYPED SUBJECTS

		PATIENTS PHENOTYPED N = 122	CONTROLS PHENOTYPED N = 200	P
B7	A3 B7	.15	.8	
	B7 DR2	.29	.13	$< 10^{-3}$
	A3 B7 DR2	⚡.12	.6	< 0.05
B8	A1 B8	.17	.12	
	B8 DR3	⚡.19	.9	< 0.01
	A1 B8 DR3	.14	.8	

Table 5

and the severe groups, the B8, DR3 association (table 6) is preferentially found in severe, intermediate and non classified group. We would like to point out the fact that the association DR2, DR3 is more frequent is our M S polutation that in controls patients (10 vs 1).
- genotyped association on 49 genotyped subjects compared to 114 genotyped
  controls calculated in haplotype frequency showed (table 7).
B7-DR2 (36.4 vs 18.4 $p < 0.05$-S) B3-B7-DR2 (12.2 vs 7.8   N S)
B8-DR3 (20.4 vs 15 N S)   A1-B8-DR3 (12.2 vs   12.2   N S).

LINKAGE DISEQUILIBRIUM

IN PATIENTS ACCORDING TO THE SEVERITY OF THE DISEASE

		1 BENIGN N = 23	2 INTERMIDIATE N = 37	3 SEVERE N = 32	4 NON CLASSIFIED N = 30
B7	A3 B7	.08	.13	.25	.14
	B7 DR2	.10	.35	.40	.25
	A3 B7 DR2	.09	.08	.20	.14
B8	A1 B8	.09	.16	.21	.25
	B8 DR3	.04	.18	.28	.28
	A1 B8 DR3	.00	.16	.18	.24

Table 6

HAPLOTYPIC FREQUENCIES IN GENOTYPED SUBJECTS

		PATIENTS GENOTYPED N = 49	CONTROLS GENOTYPED N = 114	P
B7	A3 B7	.12	11.4	
	B7 DR2	.36	.18	< 0.05
	A3 B7 DR2	.12	.07	
B8	A1 B8	.16	.17	
	B8 DR3	.20	.15	
	A1 B8 DR3	.12	.12	

Table 7

DISCUSSION

We confirmed in our brittany population, whatever the subgroups, the dominant increase of the DR2 antigen which confirms the postulate of a susceptibility gene on the sixth chromosome linked, either to DR loci, or to a linkage desequilibrium of the others class II loci (loci DQ, DP).That does not exclude the susceptibility gene location near the B f gene as it was postulated in a former study (Fauchet et Al 1984) for this reason we think of great interest the future studies not only on HLA products but chiefly on genes themselves.

The DR3 allele seems to be a gravity marker of the disease, it is found more frequently increased in the severe and progressive group, we note the progressive increase of its frequency in the benign, intermediate and severe forms. The average values of the non classified group is likely to signifie the unknow evolution of this group.

As a conclusion in the France area, we think that the DR2 antigen is a marker of the disease and the DR3 antigen a marker of gravity. The HLA markers in M S may be useful as prognostic estimate and a precious indicator to use or not the immunosuppressive treatment.

We are grateful to the ARSEP support.

REFERENCES

- Engell T., Raun N.E., Thomsen, M., Platz P. 1982
  HLA Heterogeneity of multiple sclerosis. Neurology 32, 1043-1046.
- Fauchet R., Madigand M., Gueguen-Duchesne MY., Papin J.,
  Sabouraud O., Genetet B., 1984.
  Les marqueurs Bf et C4 du complèment dans la sclérose en plaques
  140, 6-7 422-425.
- Kurtzke J.F.   1983.
  Rating neurologic impairment in M.S., an expanding disability scale.
  Neurology 33 p 1444-1452.
- Madigand M., Oger J., Fauchet R., Sabouraud O., 1982.
  HLA profiles in M.S. suggest two forms of disease and the existence
  of protective haplotypes.
  Journal of Neurological Sciences, 53, 519-529.
- Poser C., Paty D., Scheinberg L., Mc Donald WT et Al 1982.
  New diagnostic criteria of M S .
  Workshop Washington.
  Ann. Neurol. 13 : 227-231.
- Wentzel J., Roberts DF, Bates D. 1984.
  Multiple sclérosis, HLA and lymphocyte surface markers.
  Acta Neurol. Scand 69 : 65-73.

44

HLA-Antigens in Multiple Sclerosis Patients in the Benelux

H. CARTON, I. VAN DE PUTTE, J. M. MINDERHOUD,
J. M. BALEN, O. R. HOMMES, P. REEKERS, R. MEDAER,
M. DE BRUYÈRE, D. LATINNE and A. BOUCKAERT

INTRODUCTION

The association of multiple sclerosis (MS) with HLA-A3, B7 and DR2 is
well established in most northern European populations suggesting the
existence of an MS susceptibility locus closely linked to HLA. The demonstration of a negative association has been more problematic due to compensatory decreases in frequencies of antigens other than DR2 and antigens in
linkage disequilibrium. Attempts have also been made to correlate HLA
antigens and clinical characteristics including type of disease course and
rate of progression (Madigand et al. 1982, Meyer-Rienecker et al. 1982).

The objectives of this cooperative study were (1) to further examine
in a large and relatively homogeneous population the positive as well as
negative associations between HLA and MS, (2) to examine the possible
contribution of HLA antigens to well defined disease characteristics such
as age at clinical onset, progression rate and type of disease course, (3)
to examine a possible interaction between sex and HLA.

MATERIAL AND METHODS

Four hundred ninety eight MS patients from five different neurology
departments (Groningen, Nijmegen, Overpelt, Melsbroek and Leuven) have been
included in this study. All 498 patients were typed for HLA-A, B and C
but only 394 could be typed for HLA-DR. Available personal and clinical
data are date of birth, sex, age at first clinical symptom, disability
scored on Kurtzke's disability status scale, type of disease course
(relapsing-remitting, progressive following a relapsing-remitting onset,

323

or chronically progressive from onset), familial occurence of MS, and immunosuppressive therapy. The progression rate was calculated by dividing the disability score (0-10) by the duration of the disease in years.

HLA-A, B and C antigens were typed by the standard microlymphocytotoxicity test using 120 sera checked with the Eurotransplant serum set and defining 15 HLA-A, 28 HLA-B and 6 HLA-C antigens. Nine HLA-DR antigens were typed by the two colour fluorescence technique using 36 sera checked with the DR serum set. The normal control population consisted of 2728 blood donors typed for HLA-A, B and C and 780 blood donors typed for HLA-DR in Nijmegen, Leiden and Brussels. Statistical analysis was performed by the chi-square test and the student t test.

RESULTS

The mean age at onset of the disease was 30.5 years and not different for females and males. However the age at onset of female patients sharing HLA-DR1 was only 25.8 years versus 31.19 y for patients not sharing this antigen (p = 0.001). As shown in table 1, an increased frequency of HLA-A3,

TABLE 1

	INCREASED	FREQUENCY	
	DR2	B7	A3
% PATIENTS - % CONTROLS	54.8 % - 29.5 %	38.3 % - 24.5 %	36.5 % - 28.6 %
PC	$< 10^{-6}$	$< 10^{-7}$	0.005
RR	2.90	1.91	1.43
EF	0.36	0.18	0.13

	DECREASED	FREQUENCY	
	DR7	B12	A2
% PATIENTS - % CONTROLS	14.7 % - 24.5 %	16.6 % - 25.7 %	41.9 % - 49.9 %
PC	< 0.005	$< 10^{-5}$	< 0.05
RR	0.53	0.58	0.72
PF	0.12	0.14	0.02

	POSSIBLY	DECREASED	FREQUENCY
	DR5	DR6	
% PATIENTS - % CONTROLS	18.2 % - 26.2 %	17.0 % - 25.4 %	
PC	< 0.05	< 0.05	
RR	0.63	0.60	
PF	0.10	0.10	

TABLE 2   ASSOCIATION OF HLA-DR AND MULTIPLE SCLEROSIS

| | NUMBER | | FREQUENCY (%) | | P | P CORRECTED | |
	PATIENTS 394	CONTROLS 780	PATIENTS	CONTROLS		(1)	(2)
DR1+10	62	174	15.7	22.3	< 0.01	< 0.1	> 0.1
2	216	230	54.8	29.5	$< 10^{-7}$	$< 10^{-6}$	
3	91	189	23.1	24.2	NS		
4	88	184	22.3	23.6	NS		
5	72	204	18.2	26.2	< 0.005	< 0.05	$0.05 < P < 0.1$
6	67	198	17.0	25.4	< 0.005	< 0.05	$0.05 < P < 0.1$
7	58	191	14.7	24.5	< 0.0005	< 0.005	< 0.01
8	31	44	7.6	5.6	NS		
9	4	13	1.0	1.7	NS		
B1	102	133	26	17			

(1) P CORRECTED FOR THE NUMBER OF COMPARISONS MADE

(2) P CALCULATED TAKING INTO ACCOUNT THE COMPENSATORY DECREASE IN THE EXPECTED NUMBERS DUE TO THE INCREASED FREQUENCY OF DR2.

B7 and DR2 and a decreased frequency of HLA-A2, B12 and DR7 were found. HLA-DR5 and HLA-DR6 frequencies were also decreased in MS patients and these findings remained statistically significant after correcting for the number of comparisons made. However, when the P value was calculated taking into account the compensatory decrease in antigens other than DR2, only a tendency towards statistical significance was found (table 2). An increased frequency of B5 + BW53 (17.0 % versus 12.8 %) was also noted with a significance of p < 0.025 which became insignificant when corrected for the number of comparisons made. No difference in the distribution of HLA antigens was found in relation to sex. The relative risks and etiological or protective fraction carried by HLA-DR2 and DR7 were rather weak (Table 1).

The mean progression rate of the whole population was 0.50 (SD : 0.43). However the progression rate was approximately 20 % faster in females than in male patients (0.54 versus 0.45, p = 0.014). In the entire population, HLA-B7 carriers (but not DR2 carriers) had a more rapid disease course than patients not sharing HLA-B7 (0.56 versus 0.48, p = 0.046). On the other hand, HLA-B27 carriers had a less rapid evolution than B27 negative patients (0.32 versus 0.52, p = 0.036). In male patients, HLA-DR3 as well as B8 were associated with a 20 % more rapid progression (0.53 versus 0.43, p = 0.036 and 0.030 respectively). On the other hand, HLA-B8 was associated with a less rapid progression (0.39 versus 0.60, p = 0.009) in female patients.

The antigens HLA-DR2, B7, A3 and DR7, B12 or A2 did not affect the progression rate and neither did they influence the type of disease course. However increased frequencies of HLA-DR4 were found in patients having started the disease with exacerbations as opposed to patients having a slowly progressive disease course from onset (25.1 % versus 13.0 %, p < 0.01). The reverse was observed for HLA-DR5 carriers (15.2 % versus 28.2 %, p < 0.01).

DISCUSSION

An unequivocal increased frequency of HLA-DR2, B7 and A3 as found in this Benelux study has been well established in several other northern European populations. A decrease in the frequencies of B12 and DR7 has also been well documented. The strength of the association between HLA-DR2 and MS, as expressed by the relative risk or the etiological fraction, was rather low in the Benelux population : 2.90 and 0.36 respectively. Although the negative association between HLA-B12 and DR7 was statistically very significant, the clinical significance of this association is weak, as evident from the corresponding protective fractions (0.14 and 0.12 respectively). Nevertheless these latter associations appear to confirm Madigand's hypothesis that in addition to a susceptibility gene linked to HLA-DR2, a second gene linked to DR7 and/or B12 might protect against the occurence of MS (Madigand et al. 1982). On the other hand we were unable to confirm that DR1 and/or BW35 might be a protection marker as stated by Madigand et al. (1982) and by Ilonen et al. 1983) and neither could we confirm Bertrams et Kuwert's data (1976) of an increased frequency of DW3 and B8. Whether the tendency to association between MS and HLA-DR5 or HLA-DR6 as found in our study, is meaningful remains an open question. Doubts also persist as to whether correlations found between some HLA-haplotypes and clinical characteristics are real and meaningful findings since these correlations are often weak and the antigens involved often different in various studies. Increased frequencies of HLA-A1, A1-B8 and A1-B8-DR were found in the progressive form when compared with the relapsing form in Madigand's study, but not in our series where an increased frequency of DR5 and a decreased frequency of DR4 was noted in the chronic progressive form. Unlike Madigand's finding that the benign MS group was characterized by an increased B7, DR2 frequency, we found the disease progression of B7 carriers to be more rapid when compared to B7 negative patients. Furthermore, whereas severe disease was associated with DR3 and B8-DR3 in Madigand's study, we found HLA-DR3 and B8 to be associated with a more rapid disease course in males only. HLA-B8 in females was associated with a much slower or benign disease course. Since some antigens seem to influence age at onset or progression rate in one sex only, or in a different way in both sexes, it is tempting to speculate that an interaction of HLA and sex might be present in MS, as already suggested by Weitkamp (1983). However, several of these associations including some found in our study may be statistical artefacts due to the many possibilities of subdividing patient material.

REFERENCES

Bertrams, H.J., and Kuwert, E.K., 1976. Association of histocompatibility haplotype HLA-A3-B7 with multiple sclerosis. J. Immunol., 117 : 1906-1912.

Ilonen, J., Lagerstedt, A., Koskimies, S. and Reunanen, M., 1983. HLA-Dw1 and BfF as protective markers in multiple sclerosis. J. Neuroimmunol., 5 : 283-288.

Madigand, M., Oger, J.J.F., Fauchet, R., Sabouraud, O., and Genetet, B., 1982. HLA profiles in multiple sclerosis suggest two forms of disease and the existence of protective haplotypes. J. Neurol. Sci., 53 : 519-529.

Meyer-Rienecker, H.J., Wegener, S., Hitzschke, B. and Richter, K.V., 1982. Multiple sclerosis - relation between HLA haplotype A25,B18 and disease progression. Acta Neurol. Scand., 66 : 709-712.

Weitkamp, L.R., 1983. Multiple sclerosis susceptibility. Interaction between sex and HLA. Arch. Neurol., 40 : 399-401.

45

HLA Antigens and Multiple Sclerosis in Barbagia, Sardinia: Preliminary Results

P. L. MATTIUZ, C. CONIGHI, M. T. GRAPPA, R. TOLA and G. ROSATI

INTRODUCTION

In almost all populations so far studied, MS appears to be associated to the HLA antigen DR2/DW2: the increased frequency of B7 and A3 observed mainly in North Europe Caucasian patients is probably a secondary phenomenon due to the known linkage disequilibrium between DR2, B7 and A3 in the general population. As regards the Italian MS patients, the lack of association between MS and A3 and/or B7 (Cazzullo and Smeraldi, 1972) and the increased frequency of DW2/DR2 (Zibetti et al., 1977; Mattiuz et al., 1980) have been observed. These data have been confirmed by a more recent study (Conighi et al., 1985) performed in a geographical area in North Italy (the province of Ferrara) where, until a few years ago, malaria was endemic; the frequencies of A3 and B7 are respectively 19% and 17% in MS patients vs. 17% and 12% in controls, while the frequency of DR2 is 60% in affected vs. 28% in healthy individuals (P corrected < 0.001, RR = 3.87). Preliminary results of a study performed in a peculiar Italian population, living in Barbagia are here reported. Barbagia covers a hilly and montainuous area in the central part of Sardinia. To the Sardinians, Barbagia refers to "the barbarian communities" who lived and still live in this region. The original inhabitants may have come from Libya, settling in this interior and inacessible part

329

of the island after fleeing from the invasions that followed one after
the other throughout the ages. They were excluded from any contact with
the other ethnically distinct populations who occupied Sardinia, including the Chartaginians, Romans, Arabians, Ligurians, Tuscans,
Spaniards and Piedmontese. Some of the more frequent antigens in Cauca-
sians, such as HLA-A1 and B8, are almost absent in Barbagia's, whereas
the frequencies of HLA-A30 and B18 are unusually high. In the past,
malaria was endemic in Barbagia as it was in the province of Ferrara.
Based on 31 MS cases living in Barbagia on 24 October 1981 (49.022 inh.),
the prevalence per 100.000 was 65.3 (Granieri et al., 1983).

RESULTS AND DISCUSSION

So far, 25 patients have been examined (by the same clinicians who
examined the Ferrarese patients) and typed for the Caucasian HLA antigens
defined at the 9th Workshop; 19 of them have also been typed for DR1,2,3,
4,5 and 7; as control population, 220 healthy individuals (Contu et al.,
1984) have been considered. The frequencies of the "typical" Sardinian
antigens (A30/31 and B18) are similar in patients and in controls, thus
suggesting that both groups have the same ethnical origin. No statistically significant increase in A3, B7 and DR2 was observed among the
patients (4%, 8% and 37% respectively vs. 5%, 2% and 35% in controls);
the only statistically significant differencies between patients and
controls are the decrease in the frequencies of A2 and B17 in patients
(24% and 4% respectively vs. 53% and 24% in controls) but the P values
lose significativity after correction. The frequencies of DR1,2,3,4,5 and
7 in Barbagia and Ferrara's patients and in the respective controls are
shown in the table. The lack of association between HLA-A3, B7 and DR2
antigens and MS observed among Barbagi's patients is analogous to the
data concerning some non-Caucasian populations (Brautbar et al., 1977;
Tiwari et al., 1980) and the Hebridean inhabitants (Batchelor, 1985).
Several hypotheses have been put foreward (Brautbar et al., 1982) to
account for such "anomalous" behaviour:
1. The existence of disease susceptibility gene(s) not linked to HLA;
2. The possibility that in some populations environmental factors are
   sufficient to cause MS;
3. The MS susceptibility gene(s) is (are) linked to HLA, buth the strength
   of linkage disequilibrium with a particular HLA allele varies in

different populations.

Owing to the difficulties in testing the first two hypotheses, it has been suggested (Batchelor, 1985) that in future studies the patients and the controls should also be typed for the markers determined by alleles at the other D loci (in particular DQ), with which the linkage disequilibrium of the disease gene(s) could be stronger than it is with the DR alleles.

FREQUENCIES (x 100) OF HLA-DR ANTIGENS IN MS PATIENTS (P) AND IN CONTROLS (C) IN SARDINIAN AND FERRARESE POPULATIONS.

	Sardinia		Ferrara	
Antigen	P(N=19)	C(N=220)	P(N=73)	C(N=71)
DR1	15.8	18.1	13.7	21.1
DR2	36.8	35.0	60.3[a]	28.2
DR3	52.6	53.6	9.6	14.1
DR4	21.1	30.4	12.3[b]	2.8
DR5	26.3	23.1	35.6	33.8
DR7	0.0	7.2	17.8	21.1

a) x^2 = 15.025, P corrected $<$ 0.001, RR = 3.87
b) x^2 = 4.416, P corrected $>$ 0.05, RR = 4.85

ACKNOWLEDGEMENTS

    This work is supported partly by the funds of the Italian Ministry of Education and partly by a grant from the Bank of Sardinia.

REFERENCES

Batchelor, J.R., 1985. This conference.
Brautbar, C., Cohen, I., Kahana, E., Alter, M., Jørgensen, F. and Lamm, L. 1977. Histocompatibility determinants in Isreaeli Jewish patients with multiple sclerosis. Tissue Antigens, 10: 291-302.
Brautbar, C., Amar, A., Cohen, N., Oksenberg, J., Cohen, I., Kahana, E., Bloch, D., Alter, M. and Grosse-Wilde, H., 1982. HLA-D typing in multiple sclerosis: Israelis tested with European homozygous typing cells. Tissue Antigens, 19: 189-197.
Cazzullo, C.L. and Smeraldi, E., 1972. HLA-antigens and multiple sclerosis. Lancet II: 429-430.

Conighi, C., Granieri, E., Tola, R., Grappa, M.T., Sensi, A., Carreras, M. and Mattiuz, P.L., 1985. HLA antigens and multiple sclerosis in the province of Ferrara (North Italy). In preparation.

Contu, L., Cerimele, D., Pintus, A., Cottoni, F. and La Nasa, G., 1984. HLA and Kaposi's sarcoma in Sardinia. Tissue Antigens, 23: 240-245.

Granieri, E., Rosati, G., Tola, R., Pinna, L., Carreras, M., Manca, M. and Boldrini, P., 1983. The frequency of multiple sclerosis in Mediterranean Europe: an incidence and prevalence study in Barbagia, Sardinia, insular Italy. Acta Neurol. Scand., 68: 84-89.

Mattiuz, P.L., Baricordi, O., Conighi, C. et al., 1980. HLA antigens in Italian MS patients. Abstract, 8th Histocompatibility Workshop 1980, Los Angeles.

Tiwari, J.L., Morton, N.E., Lalouel, J-M., Terasaki, P.I., Zander, H., Hawkins, B.R. and Cho, Y.W., 1980. Multiple sclerosis. In: P.I. Terasaki (Editor), Histocompatibility Testing 1980, Los Angeles: UCLA Tissue Typing Laboratory, University of California, pp. 638-656.

Zibetti, A., Cazzullo, C.L., Smeraldi, E., Scorza-Smeraldi, R., 1977. HLA typing on Italian multiple sclerosis population. Boll. Ist. sierot. milan., 56: 539-543.

46

Clinical and Immunogenetic Data of 33 Double Case Families with Multiple Sclerosis: A Starting Point for Further Analyses on the DNA Level

H. ZANDER

INTRODUCTION

The sib-pair double case method of Penrose (1935) was used for association and linkage analyses between immunogenetic markers and multiple sclerosis (Zander et al. 1976).

MATERIALS AND METHODS

Families having two siblings affected with multiple sclerosis were recruited from all parts of West Germany. Patients of the Göttingen MS pool (H.J. Bauer) have been included. All of the patients were visited at home and neurologically re-examined and clinically documented by the author. All available hospital and consultant records were re-evaluated. The grading of the diagnoses into clinically definite, probable, and possible cases followed the Schumacher criteria (2nd. revision). Some patients' diagnoses could be upgraded from probable to definite MS after evoked potentials and NMR imaging of the brain had been arranged for. Families where patients were found to have Friedreich's disease, spinocerebellar inherited ataxia, spastic paraparesis, polio residues in combination with drug or alcohol addiction with polyneuropathia, etc., were excluded. Disability was scored according to Kurtzke. Thus, thirty-three sib-pair double case families were available for study, with 28 families having two siblings with clinically definite disease. In the other 5 families, one sib had definite MS and the other one probable or possible MS.

Heparinized blood from patients and relatives was taken by the author and sent to the laboratories by express mail or air cargo. Serum was centrifuged and frozen in liquid nitrogen within 90 min after bleeding.

333

Methods for the laboratory determinations of HLA-A,B,C,DR, GLO, complement factor polymorhisms of C2, C4, Bf, C3, C6, serum complement factor levels of C2, C4, C3, Bf, IgG heavy chain markers Gm, alpha 1-antitrypsin allotypes, natural killing (NK) activity and interferon (IFN) production are described in our publications (see references).

RESULTS AND DISCUSSION

Phenotypically, HLA-DR2 occurred in 24 out of 33 MS propositi (with the family's first patient in birth order being taken as a propositus) - i.e. in 72,7 % vs. 25,2 % in healthy Caucasian controls (chi-sqare = 14,9; p corr. = 0.0007). Genotypically, HLA-DR2 was present in 28 out of the 66 haplotypes of 33 MS propositi, i.e. its gene frequency in our MS family sample is 42,4 % vs. 13,3 % in Caucasian controls (chi-square = 13,9; p corr. = 0.002). Thus, HLA-DR2 seems to be even more frequent in familial than in nonfamilial cases (in a recent study of nonfamilial MS patients from the Würzburg and Hannover areas, 70/136 patients were positive for HLA-DR2; unpubl.data). This may point to genetic heterogeneity between familial and nonfamial MS. With regard to clinical features, however, the MS patients of this study did not differ from nonfamilial cases. When HLA haplotype sharing was analyzed, 5 affected sib-pairs shared 2 and 23 affected sib-pairs shared 1 haplotype. Thus, there was a considerable number of 5 exceptions from joint segregation of HLA and MS.

The first thirteen families of this sample - tested in 1979 - were incorporated into the HLA joint analysis of the 8th Intnl. Histocompatibility Workshop, Los Angeles, 1980 (Zander et al. 1980, Tiwari et al. 1980). Lateron, these 13 families were additionally analyzed for complement factor polymorphisms, complement factor levels in serum, IgG heavy chain markers Gm, and alpha 1-antitrypsin allotypes (Zander et al. 1981, Schröder et al. 1983; Zander, Weidinger, Jungwirth et al., submitted). Fifty parental MHC haplotypes were derived from phenotype determinations (the missing two parental haplotypes did not occur in the offspring with the parents being deceased). A significant increase was seen for the C4 haplotype A4,B2 (gene frequency for A4 8/50 = 16 % vs. 5,1 % in normal controls, for B2 8/50 = 16 % vs. 8,5 % in normal controls). When comparison was made within families between the patients and their healthy siblings, the data suggest that MS is more closely associated with C4 A4,B2 (p=0.035) than with HLA-DR2 (p=0.33). The Bf F allele was found in 5/50 parental haplotypes which corresponds to a decrease just above significance. For Gm and alpha 1-antitrypsin polymorphisms no deviations from random distributions could be found. Differences in the serum levels of C2 and C3 (low for C2, elevated for C3) correlated more closely with the zygosity of HLA-DR2 than with MS. In 7 MHC-identical sib-pairs discordant for MS, the healthy sibs displayed no functional deviations of NK activity and IFN production. This observation argues against a genetic deficiency of the NK/IFN system in MS (Zander et al. 1982).

Our results corroborate the hypothesis (Batchelor et al. 1978, Tiwari et al. 1980) that a genetically determined, MHC-linked suscepti-bility for MS exists. Additional determinants, not linked to the MHC, must be postulated.

OUTLINES

The one or more susceptibility genes for MS are now clearly ripe for being focussed on by recombinant DNA technology. But a clue is to have informative families. A bottleneck that hampers rapid advance is the lack of appropriate clinical pedigrees. Overcoming this lack necessarily re-quires an extensive field-work engagement of clinical neurologists. An ad-ditional effort will be made to collect and to preserve genomic material from the families presented here, provided that a neurological clinic can be motivated to cooperate. Within any interdisciplinary medical study there can be no reasonable doubt that the recruitment of informative patients of course must be the clinics' workload and responsibility.

ACKNOWLEDGEMENTS

These studies were supported by Deutsche Forschungsgemeinschaft, Schwerpunkt Multiple Slerose, grants Za 59/2/3/4/5.

Laboratory investigations other than HLA were carried out in cooper-ation with the Institute of Immunology, the Max von Pettenkofer Institute, the Institue for Forensic Medicine, and the Institute for Human Genetics, all at the University of Munich (P. Kaudewitz, G. Riethmüller; J. Abb, F. Deinhardt; L. and J. Jungwirth; S. Weidinger, H. Cleve), the Max Planck Institute for Biochemistry, Martinsried near Munich (C. Nerl, G. Valet), the Institute for Hygiene, University of Cologne (R. Schröder, G. Mauff), and the UCLA Tissue Typing Laboratory (J.L. Tiwari, P.I. Terasaki).

REFERENCES

Batchelor J.R., Compston A., McDonald W.I., 1978 : HLA and multiple sclerosis. Brit. Med. Bull. 34 : 279-284

McDonald W.I., Batchelor J.R., Francis D.A., 1984 : The immunogenetics of
multiple sclerosis. Trends NeuroSci. 7 : 369-371

Schröder R., Zander H., Andreas A., Mauff G., 1983 : Studies on the
association of multiple sclerosis with C2, C4, Bf, C3, C6 and
GLO polymorphisms. Immunobiol. 164 : 160-170

Tiwari J.L., Morton N.E., Lalouel J.M., Terasaki P.I., Zander H., Hawkins
B.R., Cho Y.W., 1980. Multiple sclerosis joint report. In: Histocompatibility Testing 1980, P.I. Terasaki, ed., pp. 687-692

Zander H., Kuntz B., Scholz S., Albert E.D., 1976 : Multiple sclerosis :
analysis for joint segregation with HLA, a family study. In: HLA and
Disease, J. Dausset and A. Svejgaard, eds., INSERM, Paris 1976, 58:91

Zander H., Scholz S., Albert E.D., 1980 : Multiple sclerosis disease
study: HLA-A,B,C,DRw haplotypes in 13 sib-pair double case families
from West Germany. In: Histocompatibility Testing 1980, P.I. Terasaki, ed.; UCLA, Los Angeles 1980; p.947

Zander H., Nerl C., Mauff G., Albert E.D., 1981 : Multiple sclerosis :
Immunogenetic analyses of double case families. In: 12th World
Congress of Neurology, Kyoto, Japan, 1981; Abstracts, Excerpta
Medica, Amsterdam-Oxford-Princeton 1981; pp. 90-91

Zander H., Abb J., Kaudewitz P., Riethmüller G., 1982 : Natural killing
activity and interferon production in multiple sclerosis.
Lancet 1982 i, 280

47

Twin Studies in Multiple Sclerosis

A. HELTBERG

In genetic studies of MS a Mendelian mode of inheritance has not been established, but a higher occurrence of the disease among relatives of patients with MS has been shown. Whether this higher incidence is caused mainly by genetic factors or by environmental factors is not clearly established. The classical method to elucidate whether genetic factors are involved in the etiology of a given disease, and if they are to which extent is the twin method. By this method it is the aim to evaluate how much of the variability observed between different individuals is due to hereditary differences between them, and how much is due to differences in the environments. If the concordance rate for a given disease is significantly higher for monozygotic (mz) than for dizygotic (dz) twin pairs, and intrapair differences of environmental factors can be assumed to be equal for mz and dz twins, this can be taken as evidence for genetic factors to be of importance for the development of the disease.

In order to make genetical conclusions it is of fundamental importance that the material is an unselected, unbiased material derived from a twin population. The most limiting factor for twin studies is the relative rarity of twins. Other limiting factors are the biases that occur in the selection of twin samples and the difficulties which arise because of the interactions between genotype and environment. The twin method offers recognition of the hereditary basis for phenotypic differences, but is not an analysis of the genotype responsible. So the method does not answer the question of which kind of genes are responsible nor what kind of environmental factors are involved. It may also be assumed that the environments in which non-identical twins live are more different than those in which identical twins live, and even prenatal differences may be of importance.

Another basic point in twin studies is the establishment of twin zygosity. The most reliable method for establishing twin zygosity is immunologic typing of genetic systems in blood. Another method is the similarity method. It has been shown that by this method the twin zygosity can be stated with a probability of above 95%.

As stated: to make genetical conclusions it is of fundamental importance that the material is representative being derived from an unselected unbiased twin population. In most countries this has not been easy, and this claim has therefore not been fulfilled in prior twin studies. In 1936 Thums (Thums, 1936) made a twin investigation in which he concluded that MS was a disease mostly caused by environmental factors. The same conclusion was made by Bammer and Schaltenbrand in their investigation from 1960 (Bammer et al., 1960). In the classical study of MacKay and Myrianthopoulos from 1958 and 1966 (MacKay et al., 1958 & 1966) the material was not unselected because of the ascertainment method. However, it was concluded that MS was partly caused by genetic factors probably by an autosomal recessive gene with reduced penetrans (43%), but also environmental factors were necessary. This conclusion was mainly supported by the risk figures of relatives to the twin pairs showing a pattern with higher prevalence in sibs than in parents and children and other relatives. Bobowick (Bobowick et al., 1978) made an investigation of twins which was primarily a discordance analysis of mz pairs. In a later investigation by Williams (Williams et al., 1980) it was mentioned that because of the mode of selection it was not possible to make genetical conclusions, but their results pointed to genetical factors to be of some importance for MS. So no general conclusion concerning genetic factors can be drawn from these investigations. The available reports tell, however, that under the assumption of etiological homogeneity there is no genotype which irrespective of environments always leads to MS. There may perhaps be certain genotypes which are more prone to develop MS, but non-genetic influences will be rather decisive in provoking or preventing the disease. MS could not be due to one single gene only; environmental factors also contribute to the development of the disease. Thus regular dominant, recessive and sex-linked inheritance are ruled out. Two types of genetic determination remain as possibilities. It may be one gene (or a pair of identical recessive genes) with reduced ability to penetrate and determine the phenotype, or it may be a case of more than one gene or a set of genes being responsible, i.e. polygenic inheritance.

The establishment of population-based twin registers (as for instance in Denmark) has helped to facilitate adequate sample selection. In my own study (Heltberg, 1981) the probands were primarily ascertained by a matching of The Danish Twin Register and The Danish MS Register. In this way the material is unselected and derived from a twin population. The Danish Twin Register is covering all like-sexed twin births in Denmark in the period 1870-1930. All twin pairs recorded are followed from birth until a given date or to death without paying attention to the presence or absence of disease or to zygosity. The nationwide Danish MS Register was founded in 1948. Almost all MS patients in contact with the medical profession are reported here. By a combination of these two registers 50 twin pairs were ascertained. 19 were mz and 31 were dz. 19 were male pairs and 31 were female pairs. Where both twins were alive at the time of the investigation, the zygosity diagnosis was based on extended blood group examination, and in the remaining pairs the zygosity diagnosis was based on the similarity method.

4 of the 19 mz pairs and 1 of the 31 dz pairs were concordant for MS. The proband concordance rate for mz twins was 34.8% and for dz twins 6.3%. The heritability estimate is about 0.80. The proband concordance rate in dz twins which is comparable with the recurrence risk of ordinary sibs is similar to risk figures of sibs. The high heritability estimate of about 0.80 suggests that genetic factors are of importance for the development of MS (Heltberg et al., 1982).

HLA determination was performed on 30 probands from 28 MS twin pairs (Heltberg, 1984). 63.3% of MS probands were DR-2 positive as compared to 28.7% in the normal Danish population. This gives a relative risk of 4.4. Of the 28 pairs 13 pairs were mz and 15 pairs were dz. The number and distribution of HLA - DR-2 according to pairs and to probands will be seen on the figure. Also the distribution of HLA - DR-2 positive and HLA - DR-2 negative in the dz pairs will be shown. The conclusions will also ap-

pear from the figure. Also other investigations were **made.** Circulating immune complexes and measle virus antibodies were determined. Investigations
of mixed leucocyte reaction, natural killer cell activity, T-helper/T-sup-
pressor cell quotient and monocyte number were performed (Heltberg et al.,
1985).

In the future it will be highly desirable that new twin series are
collected and studied - maybe especially in low-risk areas - because if
genetic factors are of real importance one might perhaps expect higher concordance rates in mz twins in such areas. If external factors of causative
importance are weak or rare, only those having an unusually sensitive genotype would present the disease, if such predisposing genetic factors
really exist. As twin pairs also are useful for any other purposes than
just genetically oriented analyses it is worth recommending that anyone who
meets a patient with MS who has a twin partner of the same sex, should ar-
range for a full serological zygosity test of both partners. This would be
of tremendous importance to future research (Hauge, 1977).

If we here at this meeting will be able to make concrete plans for
future studies in which participants from different countries can work together, it would be very rewarding.

References:
Bammer, H., Schaltenbrand, G. and Solcher, H., 1960. Zwillingsuntersuchun-
    gen bei Multipler Sklerose. Deutsche Z. Nervenheilkunde, 181: 261-279.
Bobowick, A.R., Kurtzke, J.F., Brody, J.A., Hrubec, Z. and Gillespie, M.,
    1978. Twin study of multiple sclerosis. Neurology, 28: 978-987.
Hauge, M., 1977. The aetiology of MS-genetic aspect. Acta Neurol. Scand.,
    Suppl. 63, vol. 55: 49-53.
Heltberg, A., 1981. Twins with multiple sclerosis. Abstracts of the 12th
    World Congress of Neurology, International Congress Series, Excerpta
    Medica, Abstract no. 173: 548.
Heltberg, A. and Holm, N.V., 1982. Concordance in twins and recurrence in
    sibships in multiple sclerosis. The Lancet, I: 1062.
Heltberg, A., 1984. HLA-determination in twins with multiple sclerosis.In:
    R.E. Gonsette and P. Delmotte (eds.), Immunological and clinical
    aspects of multiple sclerosis. MTP Press Limited, 333-336.
Heltberg, A., Kalland, T., Källén, B. and Nilsson, O., 1985. A study of
    some immunological variables in twins discordant for multiple sclero-
    sis. Accepted for publication in European Neurology (Nov. 1984).
MacKay, R.P. and Myrianthopoulos, N.C., 1958. Multiple sclerosis in twins
    and their relatives. Arch. of Neurol. and Psychiatr., vol.80: 667-674.
MacKay, R.P. and Myrianthopoulos, N.C., 1966. Multiple sclerosis in twins
    and their relatives. Final Report. Arch. of Neurol., vol. 15: 449-462.
Thums, K., 1936. Neurologische Zwillingstudien. Z.ges. Neurol. Psychiat.,
    155: 185-253.
Williams, A., Eldridge, R., McFarland, H., Houff, S., Krebs, H. and McFar-
    lin, D., 1980. Multiple sclerosis in Twins. Neurology, 30: 1139-1147.

MONOZYGOTIC: 13 PAIRS

concordant: 2 pairs   discordant: 11 pairs

DR2+   DR2-   DR2+   DR2-
  2   0   6   5

DIZYGOTIC: 15 PAIRS

concordant: 0 pairs   discordant: 15 pairs

                        DR2+   DR2- ⎫
                          9   6 ⎬ probands
                                         ⎭

MONOZYGOTIC: 15 PROBANDS

DR2+   DR2-
 10   5

DIZYGOTIC: 15 PROBANDS

DR2+   DR2-
  9   6

DIZYGOTIC PAIRS, ALL DISCORDANT FOR MS, BOTH TYPED = 8 PAIRS

	DR2 +/+	DR2 +/-	DR2 -/+	DR2 -/-
MS/not MS	3 pairs	2 pairs	o pairs	3 pairs

Section V
Imaging and
Neurophysiology

48

The Role of Imaging in the Diagnosis of Multiple Sclerosis

W. I. McDONALD

Imaging of lesions of the brain in multiple sclerosis has been
possible since the introduction of gamma scanning but as Young et al.
(1981) have shown, NMR imaging is more sensitive than any other
technique at present available. The NMR Group at the National Hospital
has been investigating the pattern of abnormalities seen in NMR images
of patients with multiple sclerosis, the frequency of multiple lesions
in patients with primary isolated syndromes of the kind seen in multiple
sclerosis (e.g. acute optic neuritis) and the specificity of the changes
for multiple sclerosis. We have used a Picker superconducting NMR
system imaging proton, initially at 0.25 Tesla and subsequently at 0.5
Tesla. Both spin-echo and inversion-recovery sequences were used.
Standard diagnostic criteria have been used in the classification of the
patients.

Clinically definite multiple sclerosis

In keeping with the pathology of multiple sclerosis (Dawson, 1916;
Hallervorden, 1940; Allen 1981) we have found periventricular
abnormalities in 59/60 patients aged 17 to 70 years (mean 38 years).
Discrete white matter changes were seen in almost all.

Control observations

We have not seen regions of altered signal from the periventricular
region in 36/37 apparently healthy individuals aged 19 to 62 years (mean
38 years), although in keeping with the occasional surprise discovery of
the pathological changes of multiple sclerosis at post mortem (Gilbert &
Sadler, 1983; Phadke and Best, 1983) one apparently healthy control

345

subject showed NMR appearances indistinguishable from those of multiple sclerosis. Others have reported altered signals from the periventricular regions in individuals over the age of 60 (Bradley, Waluch, Wycoff and Yadley, 1984).

Isolated acute optic neuritis

Periventricular and/or discrete white matter abnormalities other than in the optic nerves were found in 16 of 25 patients aged 16 to 48 years (mean 32). While the proportion of cases with disseminated abnormalities corresponds with the proportion of cases in the United Kingdom which ultimately develops multiple sclerosis (McDonald, 1983) it is premature in the absence of other evidence indicating that the lesions have also been disseminated in time, to conclude that such cases have multiple sclerosis. About half of 25 patients with symptoms of isolated brainstem lesions also showed abnormalities in the central white matter additional to those in the brainstem.

Vascular disease

(Ormerod et al. 1984) Eighteen patients with evidence of cerebral vascular disease, including cases with late onset epilepsy, stroke, Binswanger's disease, transient global amnesia and haemorrhage (aged 23 to 80 (mean 63) have been scanned. Periventricular abnormalities were found in 17 and discrete lesions in 18. Although the outline of the periventricular abnormalities sometimes appeared to be smoother in the cases with vascular disease than in those with multiple sclerosis the distinction was often impossible on the scan appearances alone.

Cerebellar degeneration

We have studied 11 cases of primary cerebellar degeneration classified according to the criteria of Harding (1984). All showed evidence of cerebellar and/or brainstem atrophy. Three showed periventricular abnormalities.

DISCUSSION

It is clear that as Young et al. (1981) suggested NMR imaging is a very sensitive means of detecting abnormalities in the central nervous system in multiple sclerosis. It is equally clear that while NMR appearances may be highly suggestive of multiple sclerosis they are not in themselves specific for it. The position is precisely as Halliday, Mushin and I expressed it in relation to the role of the visual evoked potential in the diagnosis of multiple sclerosis in 1973: "an ....

abnormality assumes the status of an objective physical sign. It
provides evidence of neurological damage but its exact interpretation
depends on the clinical context." NMR imaging, like the evoked
potential, is not in its present state of development, capable of making
a specific diagnosis in isolation. It is nevertheless useful in a
diagnostic setting, particularly in relation to patients with
insufficient evidence of anatomical dissemination of lesions to permit a
clinically definite diagnosis to be made and in those patients with
symptoms unaccompanied by abnormal physical signs in whom it is
difficult to establish the existence of organic disease of the central
nervous system.

The origin of the abnormal signals in multiple sclerosis is not
known. Oedema is likely to play a part in the acute lesion. In chronic
lesions, the fibrillary astrocytic reaction may be important (McDonald,
1985).

ACKNOWLEDGEMENTS

The NMR Unit at the National Hospital was established with a
generous grant from the Multiple Sclerosis Society of the United Kingdom
and Northern Ireland and the work in it is supported by the Society and
by the Medical Research Council. I am grateful to my colleagues in the
NMR Group at the National Hospitals for permission to quote from
unpublished work: I E C Ormerod, E P G H du Boulay, M M Callanan, A M
Halliday, G Johnson, B E Kendall, S J Logsdail, D G Macmanus, I S
Moseley, M A Ron, P Rudge, K J Zilkha.

REFERENCES

Allen, I.V. (1981) The pathology of multiple sclerosis – fact, fiction
    and hypothesis. Neuropathology and Applied Neurobiology, 7:
    169-182.
Bradley, W.G., Waluch, V., Wycoff, R.R. and Yadley, R.A. 1984.
    Differential diagnosis of periventricular abnormalities in MRI of
    the brain. Abstract in the Third Annual Meeing of the Society of
    Magnetic Resonance in Medicine, August 13-17, New York, 1984.
Dawson, J.W., 1916. The histology of disseminated sclerosis.
    Trans.Roy.Soc.Edinb., 50: 517-740.
Gilbert, J.J. and Sadler, M. 1983. Unsuspected multiple sclerosis.
    Arch.Neurol. 40: 533-536.
Hallervorden, J.,1940. Die Zentralen Entmarkungskrankheiten. Deutsche
    Zeitschrift für Nervenheilkunde,150: 201-239.
Halliday, A.M., McDonald, W.I. and Mushin, J. 1973. Visual evoked
    response in diagnosis of multiple sclerosis. Br.Med.J. 4: 661-664
Harding, A.E. 1984. The hereditary ataxias and related disorders.
    London: Churchill Livingstone.

McDonald, W.I. 1983. Doyne Lecture. The significance of optic neuritis. Trans.Ophthalmol.Soc.U.K.,103: 230-246.
McDonald, W.I. 1985. The mystery of the origin of multiple sclerosis. Brain, in press.
Ormerod,I.E.C.,Roberts, R.C., du Boulay, E.P.G.H., McDonald, W.I., Callanan, M.M., Halliday, A.M., Johnson, G., Kendall, B.E., Logsdail, S.J., Macmanus, D.C., Moseley, I.S., Ron, M.A., Rudge, P. and Zilkha, K.J. 1984. NMR in multiple sclerosis and cerebral vascular disease. Lancet, 2: 1334-1335.
Phadke, J.D. and Best, P.V. 1983. Atypical and clinically silent multiple sclerosis: a report of 12 cases discovered unexpectedly at necropsy. J.Neurol,Neurosurg,Psychiat. 46: 414-420.
Young,I.R., Hall, A.S., Pallis, C.A., Bydder, G.M., Legg, N.J. and Steiner, R.E. 1981. Nuclear magnetic resonance imaging of the brain in multiple sclerosis. Lancet, 2: 1063-1066.

49

Nuclear Resonance Imaging of Multiple Sclerosis Brain Lesions

L. RUMBACH, M. C. CAIRES, C. SCHEIBER, J. M. WARTER, J. CHAMBRON and M. COLLARD

INTRODUCTION

Nuclear magnetic resonance (NMR) imaging of the brain has in late years been developed into a sensitive tool for clearly revealing lesions in white matter, and has thus become important in the study of multiple sclerosis (MS). Here we report preliminary observations made on 49 MS patients in Strasbourg. Our aim has been to describe the NMR-derived morphological signs of this disease, and to evaluate the utility of NMR scans for the diagnosis of MS. (Rumbach et al., 1985).

MATERIAL AND METHODS

Forty-nine patients were examined, 13 men and 36 women, 18 to 60 years of age at the time of the NMR scans, but at variable delays after MS onset, and at different stages of disease progression. NMR examinations were performed with an experimental scanner assembled from Brucker brand components. The resistive magnet of 0.15 Tesla corresponds to a proton resonance frequency of 6 MHz. The multiple spin-echo type sequence we used for signal aquisition is now known to clarify white matter pathology particularly well. Repetition time was 750 msec, and inter-echo time differed : 12 msec for the back-projection technique, 33 msec for the 2-dimensional Fourier transform technique. Four images can be reconstructed from a single cerebral section by the analysis of the first 4 echo groups. On each patient, 4 1-cm sections were imaged in the transverse plane at the level of the lateral ventricles.

RESULTS

Forty-eight of the 49 MS patients presented NMR scans with one or more abnormalities, which we classed as atrophies, parenchymal lesions or periventricular abnormalities.

Atrophies, seen in 23 patients, were of the cortical- subcortical type, and varied in severity, being often more pronounced in subjects displaying a certain intellectual deterioration. Atrophies were always more evident in images of first-group echos, whereas the other classes of abnormalities were seen better on 2nd- and 3rd-echo group images.

Parenchymal lesions of the white matter gave images of variable forms and dimensions : small bright spots, or, more often, the individual or multiple patches we saw in 35 patients. The patches were variably rounded and spread out, with clear-cut edges, and were situated in the white matter of frontal, parietal and occipital cortex, and adjacent to ventricles. Parenchymal lesions differed in intensity in a given section ; some corresponded to x-ray computer tomographic (CT) hypodensities. Since we made few sections on each patient, we did not count NMR parenchymal lesions ; our impression is that they were much more common that CT hypodensities.

Periventricular abnormalities were the most frequent : they were seen in 43 patients and were of 4 distinct patterns. First, strips encircled ventricles. Second, bright thicker streaks appeared along the lateral edges of the ventricles. They extended often to the occipital region as merging bands, thinning towards the occipital cortex. Third, bright crescents capped the frontal and/or occipital horns of the ventricles, usually bilaterally. Fourth, large blotches of various sizes and shapes were seen.

We were unable to correlate the NMR image abnormalities with the various clinical parameters studied ; in particular, specific image patterns were not associated with the stage of MS progression, or with the state of the blood-brain barrier.

DISCUSSION

The NMR signal amplitude which controls the luminosity of a point image depends on proton density, weighted by the mean relaxation times T_1

and T_2 of the tissues. Their increase in degenerative lesions of white matter is the origin of a contrast with healthy tissue stronger than that seen in CT scans, and explains the greater sensitivity of NMR images. The findings of Young et al., (1981), that NMR imaging was more sensitive for the study of white matter pathology, has since been amply confirmed.

The imaging method and the signal aquisition sequence used are very important, for they determine image contrast. The spin-echo sequence yields more information than other techniques, and the analysis of late echos increases its sensitivity. The spin-echo sequence we used gave an optimal contrast between normal cerebral structures and characteristic MS abnormalities. Late-echo images arrive when the relaxation constants of white matter and CSF cross : at that point, they have the same intensity, the ventricles are invisible, and the periventricular areas are more clearly seen. The relaxation times of pathological tissues then remain higher than those of normal tissues.

It is the general opinion that NMR abnormalities reflect demyelination lesions. Neuropathological examinations show the juxta- and periventricular localisation of the lesions, and Stewart et al., (1984) have observed that post-mortem NMR scans of brain section from an MS patient showed luminous abnormalities at demyelinated areas. The image luminosity corresponds to a longer relaxation time, which reflects a higher tissular water content and a modified lipid composition. The quantitative analysis of the relaxation constants, especially T_2 for transverse relaxation, opens the way to tissular physiological investigations, notably of the nature of the edema and the degree of demyelination.

The diagnostic valve of NMR abnormalities is not yet clear. In the subjects we report on the image sensitivity was 98 %, but the population included only clinically defind MS patients, and the proportion of MS was abnormally high. In 264 examinations performed in 1984 (including the 49 MS), we found periventricular abnormalities in 40 non-MS patients. Thirty-seven of the 40 clearly had other diseases(cerebral tumors, vascular pathology, encephalitis, etc.,) and the last 3 had pyramidal syndromes still undiagnosed. We thus consider it necessary to extend NMR examination to a larger population, in order to evaluate specific abnormalities as criteria of MS diagnosis.

ACKNOWLEDGMENT

Text translated from the French by Sarah Dejours.

REFERENCES

Rumbach, L., Caires, M.C., Scheiber, C., Warter, J.M., Chambron, J. and
    Collard, M., 1985. L'imagerie par résonance magnétique dans la sclé-
    rose en plaques. Société Française de Neurologie, Paris - Communica-
    tion orale.
Stewart, W.A., Hall, L.D., Berry, K. and Paty, D.W., 1984. Correlation
    between NMR scan and brain slice date in multiple sclerosis. Lancet,
    2 : 412.
Young, I.R., Hall, A.S., Pallis, C.A., Legg, N.J., Bydder, G.M. and
    Steiner, R.I., 1981. Nuclear magnetic resonance imaging of the brain
    in multiple sclerosis. Lancet, 2 : 1063-1066.

50

Neurophysiological Studies in Demyelination and Remyelination

T. A. SEARS

Through its symptoms and signs Multiple Sclerosis challenges the neurophysiologist with many basic problems whose solution should enhance understanding of the disease process itself, even, perhaps, its aetiology, as well as offer those suffering from its effects the prospect of symptomatic relief. But this panacea eludes us still despite considerable biophysical advances in our understanding of the pathophysiology of demyelination over the last 20 years. Why should this be so? As a disease of white matter M.S. shows clinical manifestations which are understood most simply as being due to conduction block, or conduction vulnerability, at sites of demyelination. Presuming that axon continuity is retained distal to the plaques, then an ideal therapy would be based simply on restoring an adequate safety factor for transmission through the demyelinated regions. But since this has yet to be achieved without unwarranted side effects, pragmatism must rule. Thus the treatment of spasticity, for example, is based on that used for 'upper' motoneurone lesions of quite different aetiology, such as stroke, tumour or trauma, in which, by contrast, there would be an irreversible degeneration of fibres (descending or ascending systems) since intrinsic neurones in general do not regenerate their axons (cf. Barron, 1983) although many have the capacity to do so (Richardson, Issa & Aguayo, 1984).

The physiological abnormalities can be summarized as slowing of conduction velocity, impaired ability to transmit trains of impulses and most drastic of all, total conduction block (see Sears & Bostock, 1981; Waxman, 1982; Bray, Aquayo & Rasminsky 1982). The amyelinated or thinly myelinated fibres of the dystrophic mouse have been shown to be sites for ephaptic cross-talk, where impulses in one fibre may excite an adjacent fibre, and of ectopic impulse generation (Rasminsky, 1980). These properties provide a satisfactory explanation for 'positive' symptoms in M.S. such as focal epilepsy, paraesthesae or other central sensory syndromes,

353

such as trigeminal neuralagia where pain may be evoked by
minimal peripheral stimuli. Similarly, Smith & McDonald
(1982) have demonstrated that the focal lesion induced by
lysophosphatidyl choline is both a site of ectopic impulse
generation and of enhanced local mechanosensitivity, thus
giving an explanation of Lhermitte's phenomenon induced by
neck flexion.

As summarized in Sears & Bostock (1981) there is now
clear evidence that the internodal axon membrane beneath the
myelin sheath is electrically excitable and is able to
support continuous conduction through a region of
demyelination. However, this property does not pre-exist,
since with <u>acute</u> demyelination there is no evidence in the
internodal axon of the specific inward current which
indicates the presence there of Na channels. Such
excitability takes about 6-7 days to develop, probably
reflecting in part the time course of the particular
pathological process of diphtheria toxin induced
demyelination since with the lysolecithin lesion foci of
internodal inward currents were detected at 4 days. Thus it
is reasonable to suppose that in the case of paranodal
demyelination, the development of electrical excitability at
the widened (or widening) nodes of Ranvier is a recovery
mechanism that offsets the deleterious effect that the
increase in electrical capacity of the widened node has on
the safety factor of transmission. Although continuous
conduction is potentially capable of maintaining nervous
transmission though a 'plaque', the problem remains that the
last <u>normal</u> node of Ranvier may be unable to generate
sufficient outward current at demyelinated axon to excite
electrically excitable membrane. An 'ideal' drug should
simply prolong the duration of the action potential at a
normal node of Ranvier (cf. Bostock, Sherratt & Sears, 1978).
One drug that does this most effectively in an experimental
model is scorpion venom, but clinically usable drugs with
this action have yet to be developed. The normal nodal
membrane lacks K+ channels, so that alternative drugs like 4-
aminopyridine, which blocks K+ channels, can only prolong
action potentials in demyelinated axons where <u>pre-existing</u> K+
channels are exposed. Although this can help secure
tranmission through a region of demyelination, side effects
can be expected, since presynaptic action potentials are also
prolonged in duration (Konishi & Sears, 1984) leading to
enhanced transmitter release and the posibility of
unwarranted side effects (Sears & Bostock, 1981). Results
with 4-AP that should encourage further research along these
lines were however obtained by Jones, et al (1983) without
adverse side effects on patients with (labile visual
symptoms, but not in those with stable spinal lesions. In
this regard it is unreasonable to suppose that chronic
spasticity would be quickly reversed if conduction were
restored in the relevant axons since the 'spastic' element
itself has an insidious evolution, dependent, as it must be
on a variety of mechanisms (cf. Kirkwood, Sears & Westgaard
1984; Mendell, 1984).

The recent imporant finding that trains of impulses induce a membrane hyperpolarization which contributes to blocking of demyelinated fibres by raising their threshold (Bostock & Grafe, 1984) means that future pharmacological approaches to symptomatic therapy are likely to involve drug cocktails which act on different channels and pumps in nerve membranes that display infinitely more heterogeneity in properties then suspected a decade ago. Equally important is that different experimental models of M.S. should be comprehensively studied so as to ensure that the clinical signs are caused by CNS lesions and not due to peripheral nerve (e.g. D.R. ganglion) lesions as recently demonstrated for acute EAE in the rabbit (Pender & Sears, 1984).

References

BARRON, (1983). Axon reaction and central nervous system regeneration. In: Frederick, J. Seil (Ed.) Nerve, Organ, and Tissue regeneration: Research perspectives. pp. 3-36. New York. Academic Press.

BOSTOCK, H. & GRAFE, P. (1984). Demyelinated rat spinal root fibres fail to transmit long-lasting trains of impulses because of hyperpolarization. J.Physiol. 357, 27P.

BOSTOCK, H., SHERRATT, R.M. & SEARS, T.A. (1978). Overcoming conduction failure in demyelinated nerve fibres by prolonging action potentials. Nature 274, 385-387.

BRAY, G.M., RASMINSKY, M. & AGUAYO, A.J. (1981). Interactions between axons and their sheath cells. Annual Review Neuroscience 4, 127-162.

JONES, R.E., HERON, J.R., FOSTER, D.H. SNELGAR, R.S. & MASON, R.J. (1983). Effects of 4-aminopyridine in patients with multiple sclerosis. J.Neurol.Sci. 60, 353-362.

KIRKWOOD, P.A., SEARS, T.A., & WESTGAARD, R.H. (1984). Restoration of function in external intercostal motoneurones of the cat following partial central deafferentation. J.Physiol. 350, 225-25.

KONISHI, T. & SEARS, T.A. (1984). Electrical activity of mouse nerve terminals. Proc.R.Soc.Lond. B. 222, 115-120.

MENDELL, L.M. (1984). Modifiability of spinal synapses. Physiological Reviews, 64, 160-324.

PENDER, M.P. & SEARS, T.A. (1984). The pathophysiology of acute experimental allergic encephalomyelitis in the rabbit. Brain 107, 699-726.

RASMINSKY, M. (1980). Ephaptic transmission between single nerve fibres in the spinal nerve roots of dystrophic mice. J.Physiol. 305, 151-169.

RICHARDSON, P.M. ISSA, V.M.K. & AGUAYO, A.J. (1984). Regenration of long spinal axons in the rat. J.Neurocytology 13, 165-182.

SEARS, T.A. & BOSTOCK H.(1981). Conduction failure in demyelination: Is it inevitable? In: Demyelinating Disease: Basic and Clinical Electrophysiology, Raven Press, New York.

SMITH, K.J. & McDONALD, W.I. (1982). Spontaneous and evoked electrical discharges from a central demyelinating lesion. J.Neurol.Sci. 55, 39-47.

WAXMAN, S.G. (1982). Membranes, myelin, and the pathophysiology of multiple sclerosis. New England Journal of Medicine 306, 1529-1533.

51

Horizontal Eye-Movement Abnormalities in Multiple Sclerosis and Optic Neuritis

E. A. C. M. SANDERS and J. P. H. REULEN

INTRODUCTION

The development and application of objective non-invasive techniques
for the monitoring of neurological function or disease activity is of increasing interest to clinicians, in particular, as diagnostic aids for
the detection of diseases in which diagnosis is difficult, of which multiple sclerosis (MS) is perhaps most important.
The diagnosis of MS rests on objective evidence concerning the presence
of at least two lesions in the central nervous system (Schumacher et al.,
1965). On the basis of the clinical evidence, MS in a given patient may
be classified as definite, probable or possible (McAlpine et al., 1972).
Various invasive and non-invasive methods for the detection of subclinical lesions are currently available to increase certainty and
reliability of the clinical diagnosis, and to provide additional support
for the diagnosis in a monosymptomatic or early state of the disease. A
few studies on oculomotor recording have been published (Mastaglia et al.,
1979; Sharpe et al., 1981; Reulen et al., 1983). They all concluded
that oculomotor examination is potentially most usefull for the detection
of subclinical lesions of the oculomotor system of MS patients. As far as

we know only Tackmann et al. (1980) combined a number of non-invasive
electrophysiological tests to detect the diagnostical value of his eye
movement recording method.

In the present study, abnormal oculomotor test results will be compared with the results of three other electrophysiological diagnostical
techniques:
1. Auditory brainstem evoked response (ABER);
2. Somatosensory evoked response (SSER);
3. Blink reflex.
This in order to find out which contribution to the diagnosis of MS is
obtained by the eye-movement test.

PATIENTS

All patients were examined during a period lasting one year. The
patients' material comprised 89 MS and 25 ON patients. The MS patients
were classified according to the clinical criteria of McAlpine et al.
(1965) into definite (n=31, mean age 48 years, mean duration of disease
14,5 year, mean Kurtzke DSS-score 6,7), probable (n=31, mean age 41, mean
duration of disease 7,5 years, mean Kurtzke DSS-score 3,7) and possible
(n=27, mean age 37 years, mean duration of disease 5,1 years, mean
Kurtzke DSS-score 1,6).

METHODS

The horizontal saccadic and smooth pursuit eye-movement signals
(ENG) were recorded by the method developed and described by Reulen et al.
(1983, 1985). The auditory brainstem evoked responses (ABER) and somatosensory evoked responses (SSER) were recorded with an averaging method.
The interpretation of the SSER was based on the differences of latencies
between the N14-N20 peaks only (Sanders et al., 1984a+b). The latency of
the blink reflex was measured using the method described by Ongerboer de
Visser and Goor (1974) and Kimura (1975). Statistical analysis was performed by the wilcoxon Chisquare or Kendall tau B and tau C tests.

RESULTS

Abnormal prolongation of saccadic latency was found in 80 percent of
the definite, 55 percent of the probable and 24 percent of the possible
MS patients. In total 49 of the 89 (55 percent) showed abnormally pro-

longed mean saccadic latencies. Eight of the ON patients (32 percent) showed an abnormal mean saccadic reaction delay (Table 1).

Table 1 Incidence ( ) of different ENG-abnormalities in 89 Multiple Sclerosis and 25 Optic Neuritis patients

Electrophysiological eye movement disorders	Definite n=31	Probable n=31	Possible n=27	Total n=89	ON n=25	Overall n=114
Saccadic latency	80	58	30	57	24	50
Saccadic velocity	65	13	22	34	4	27
ENG/INO	61	13	22	33	4	26
Saccadic accuracy	32	29	18	27	-	21
Smooth pursuit	77	52	37	55	20	47
Total eye movement abnormalities	84	80	63	76	36	68

A high incidence of internuclear ophthalmoplegia (INO) was found among clinically definite MS patients (53 percent) as compared with 17 percent and 15 percent in the possible group. One patient with ON showed a bilateral INO on oculomotor testing. The number of subclinical INO's found among multiple sclerosis was high in all categories (definite 60 percent, probable 60 percent, possible and ON 100 percent).

The incidence of abnormal pursuit eye-movements decreases successively from the definite (76 percent) through the probable (52 percent) to the possible (28 percent) categories of MS patients. Three ON patients showed cogwheel pursuit abnormalities without any other oculomotor disturbancy.

The ABER, SSER and blink reflex recordings all gave statistically the highest percentage of positive abnormal results in the clinically definite group (Table 2).

Table 2 Percentage electrophysiological disorders in 89 Multiple Sclerosis and 25 Optic Neuritis patients

Test	Definite n=31 .	Probable n=31	Possible n=27	Total n=89	ON n=25	Overall n=114
ABER	84	74	59	73	32	64
SSER N14-N20	97	68	41	70	20	59
Blink reflex	81	65	56	67	12	55
ENG (total)	84	80	63	76	36	68
Total	100	97	81	93	44	83

The significant associations between the various tests and the recorded eye-movement disorders are presented in Table 3. One correlation not shown in this table was that found between clinical INO and the first response of the blink reflex (R1, $p < 0.05$). When subclinical INO's were included, bringing the total number up to 29, the association with R1-blink-reflex abnormalities remained significant ($p < 0.005$). An association between overall blink-reflex disorders and clinically as well as subclinically (ENG) detected INO's was not found however. Of the ENG parameters, the saccadic accuracy abnormalities did not cor-relate with any of the "brainstem tests" (ABER, blink reflex, INO, SSER, saccadic latency).

Table 3

Association between eye movement disorders and different electrophysiological abnormalities

		SSER N14-N20		Blink reflex		ENG/INO		Smooth pursuit	
		+	−	+	−	+	−	+	−
Increased	sacc. latency	39	12	40	11	24	27	37	14
Normal	sacc. latency	26	12	20	18	5	33	12	26
		p=0.001		p=0.02		p=0.02		p=0.001	

		SSER N14-N20		Blink reflex		Saccadic Accuracy	
		+	−	+	−	+	−
Abnormal	smooth pursuit	39	10	38	11	20	29
Normal	smooth pursuit	23	7	22	18	4	36
		p=0.04		p=0.04		p=0.0025	

p = level of significance of the two parameters considered
+ test result abnormal
− test result normal

Table 4

Increase yield of detected electrophysiological abnormalities by combining two or more tests

Combination of electro-physiological tests	Multiple sclerosis n = 89	Optic neuritis n = 25	Total n = 114
	%	%	%
ENG	76	36	68
ABER	73	32	64
SSER N14-N20	69	20	59
Blink reflex BR	67	12	55
ENG + ABER	92	40	81
ENG + SSER N14-N20	88	40	77
SSER N14-N20 + ABER	87	36	75
SSER N14-N20 + BR	87	28	74
ABER + BR	83	36	73
ENG + BR	82	32	71
ENG + ABER + SSER N14-N20	93	44	83
ENG + SSER N14-N20 + BR	93	40	82
ABER + ENG + BR	92	40	81
ABER + SSER N14-N20 + BR	91	40	80
ABER + SSER N14-N20 + ENG + BR	93	44	83

As compared to the other three tests the ENG-test revealed the highest percentage of clinical and subclinical disorders: 100 resp. 69%; ABER 83 resp. 66%; blink reflex 81 resp. 58% and SSER N14-20 85 resp. 51%. The yield of detected electrophysiological abnormalities increased when 2 or more tests were combined (Table 4). The combination of ENG and ABER tests revealed a total of 82 (92%) abnormalities. The addition of a third test or the combination of all four tests provided essentially no greater yield.

DISCUSSION AND CONCLUSION

As mentioned in the Introduction, detection of two CNS lesions is considered mandatory for the diagnosis of MS. Now it goes without saying that these two lesions will not always occur at the same time. In the interest of early detection of MS, it is thus highly desirable to have simple, non-invasive screening tests which can be applied to patients who already show one symptom, indicating the possibility of MS, in order to allow the second (subclinical) symptoms - if present - to be detected without having to wait for it too, to reach the clinical stage.

The ENG-test as applied in the present study reveals most symptomatic and asymptomatic lesions in the central nervous system. The ENG test happens to be the one which is least dependent on parameters, such as the patients age, disease duration or disability, hence the ENG-test is the most suitable one as a diagnostic tool, especially in early stages of MS. The yield of detected electrophysiological abnormalities increases when two or more tests are combined. Addition of a third test only yielded 1% of new information for MS and 4% for the ON patients while the combination of all 4 tests did not increase the information yield any further.

The numbers of electrophysiological abnormalities detected in our 25 ON patients is of the same order as that reported by Feasby and Ebers (1982). Our overall data indicate the presence of one or more electrophysiological abnormalities in 11 ON patients, adding strength to the supposition that ON may be regarded as a possible early sign of MS (Sanders et al., 1984a+b). Only a prospective study of this ON patient group may give an answer to the question whether these ON patients really run a higher risk to develop MS in the future.

REFERENCES

Feasby, F.E. and Ebers, G.C., 1982. Risk of Multiple sclerosis in isolated optic neuritis. The Can. J. Neurol. Sci., 9 (2), abstract.

Kimura, J., 1975. Electrically elicited blink reflex in the diagnosis of multiple sclerosis. Review of 260 patients over a seven-year period. Brain, 98: 583-598.

Mastaglia, F.L., Black, J.L. and Collins, D.W.K., 1979. Quantitative studies of saccadic and pursuit eye movement in multiple sclerosis. Brain, 102: 817-834.

McAlpine, D., Lumsden, C.E. and Acheson, E.D., 1965. Multiple sclerosis. A reappraisal. Livingstone, Edinburgh-London.

Ongerboer de Visser, B.W. and Goor, C., 1974. Electromyographic and reflex study in idiopathic and symptomatic trigeminal neuralgias:

latency of the jaw and blink reflex. J. Neurol. Neurosurg. Psych., 37: 1225-1230.

Reulen, J.P.H., Sanders, E.A.C.M. and Hogenhuis, L.A.H., 1983. Eye movement disorders in multiple sclerosis and optic neuritis. Brain, 106: 121-140.

Reulen, J.P.H., van Heuningen, R., Tiesinga, G. and Bos, J.E., 1985. A computerized eye-movement processor for clinical application. Submitted.

Sanders, E.A.C.M., Reulen, J.P.H. and Hogenhuis, L.A.H., 1984a. Central nervous system involvement in optic neuritis. J. Neurol. Neurosurg. Psych., 47: 241-249.

Sanders, E.A.C.M., Volkers, A.C.W., van de Poel, J.C. and van Lith, G.H. M., 1984b. Spatial contrast sensitivity function in optic neuritis. Neuro-ophthalmology, 4: 255-259.

Sanders, E.A.C.M., Reulen, J.P.H., Hogenhuis, L.A.H. and van de Velde, J., 1985. Brainstem involvement in multiple sclerosis, a clinical and electrophysiological study. Acta Neurol. Scand., 71: 54-61.

Schumacher, G.A., Beebe, G., Kibler, R.F., Kurland, L.T., Kurtzke, J.F., McDowell, F., Nagler, B., Sibley, W.A., Tourtellotte, W.W. and Willmon, T.L., 1965. Problems of experimental trials of therapy in multiple sclerosis. Ann. N.Y. Acad. Sci., 122: 522-568.

Sharpe, J.A., Goldberg, H.J., Lo, A.W. and Herishanu, Y.O., 1981. Visual-vestibular interaction in multiple sclerosis. Neurology, 31: 427-433.

Tackmann, W., Strenge, H., Barth, R. and Sojka-Raytscheff, A., 1980. Evaluation of various brain structures in multiple sclerosis with multimodality evoked potentials, blink reflex and nystagmography. J. Neurol., 224: 33-46.

52

The Vestibulo-Ocular Reflex in Multiple Sclerosis

P. L. M. HUYGEN, E. J. J. M. THEUNISSEN and O. R. HOMMES

INTRODUCTION

It is well-known that a large proportion of patients with MS may have some
type of vestibular disorder with dizziness as a possible symptom from a
relatively early stage of the disease. For a review, we refer to a previous paper on this subject (Huygen, 1983). Since this previous study, we
learnt more about normal and abnormal rotatory responses and therefore we
decided to study the vestibulo-ocular reflex (VOR) again in an entirely
new group of patients. A more thorough vestibular analysis is now attempted. Optomotor responses were also examined; the correlation with the VOR
findings has been also considered in the previous report. The results of
the VS tests comprise only the first examination as far as the incidences
of the various types of response are concerned. This avoids ambiguity of
results, since a considerable variation of responses with time may be
found, which will be also dealt with. The differential diagnosis will be
discussed.

MATERIAL AND METHODS

Velocity steps (VS) of $90^{\circ}/s$ were performed after constant rotation, in
clockwise and counterclockwise direction. Such VS elicits a postrotatory
nystagmus response with exponentially decaying slow phase velocity (SPV).
The patient was seated on a rotatory chair (Tönnies) in total darkness
with eyes open and auditory (non-oriented) communication, to keep him
alert, with the head 30° in anteflexion to place the horizontal semicirc-

ular canals in the earth-horizontal plane of rotation. Nystagmus was measured with dc-electro-nystagmography and analyzed as previously reported
(Huygen, 1979; 1983). Details of ocular motor tests can be found in the
latter report. Calibration of horizontal eye movement was done before the
start of each rotation. The response parameters relevant to vestibular
diagnosis are: V, initial velocity ($^{\circ}$/s) of SPV of postrotatory nystagmus;
T, the time constant (s), i.e. the time needed to let SPV decay from V to
0.37V and G, which is the product VT ($^{\circ}$), designated by others as 'low-
frequency gain' (Baloh et al., 1984). Asymmetry is measured by the direct-
ional preponderance (DP) values: $DP(X) = 100\% (X_r - X_l)/(X_r + X_l)$, in which X
denotes a general variable name and the subscripts r and l right- and
left-beating nystagmus. The normal values established in a group of 20
normal subjects were used: $V = 30-65^{\circ}$/s, $T = 11-26s$, $G = 485-1135^{\circ}$;
$DP(V) = \pm 28\%$, $DP(T) = \pm 25\%$ and $DP(G) = \pm 22\%$ (Theunissen et al., 1985). For
the findings in each nystagmus direction a special notation is used, which
is called a 'response pattern' or 'VTG pattern'. The following is an ill-
ustrative example: V-T0G+; 0 indicates a normal value, - a significant low
and + a significant high value. Such patterns are useful in vestibular
diagnosis (Huygen & Nicolasen, 1985). The patients were 130 consecutive
patients, able to sit upright, fixed with a safety belt if necessary, in
whom VS tests in 2 directions were completed. They have been selected
afterwards on the diagnosis definite MS, absence of concomitant other diseases and hearing disorders and not taking drugs that might influence the
VOR.

RESULTS

From Table I it appears that abnormal (overall) types of VOR response
were found in 94 patients, i.e. 72% (Table Ia). The designations of abnormal response types are explained in this table. Five of the patients
with normal responses had a significant DP, of the DP(G) type in all cases
(Table Ib), which increases the total number of patients with abnormal VOR
to 99, i.e. 76%.

There was no significant preferent combination of response and DP
types. Examples of various types of VS responses are shown in Figs 1-2.
The occurrence of a very short time constant in the Vh or Vm types of
response (see Table Ia for explanation) such as shown in Fig.1C (i.e. 3s)
appeared to be strongly associated with the presence of ocular motor def-

Table   I: No. and % of patients by overall response type (a) or DP type
           (b). The overall response type is the response type per pat-
           ient, i.e. the result of the combination of 2 single response
           types, 1 for each nystagmus direction. The symbols h, H, m
           and ? are introduced and explained in the line headings of
           Table Ia. In Table III they appear as indicated and in Table
           IVa and in the text the corresponding response types are ind-
           icated as Vh, VH, Vm and V? As is clear from Table III, the
           pattern code for the single response type h contains - signs
           only, that for the H type + signs only and that for the m type
           both - and + signs (apart from 0). This also holds for the ov-
           erall response types, but in addition the m overall type may
           consist of 1 h and 1 H type of single responses. Examples of
           all response types are shown in Figs 1-2 and an example of a
           DP(T)+DP(G) type is shown in Figs 2A-B.

Table Ia		
Overall response type	no. of patients	%
normal (n)	36	28
hyporeactive (h)	12	9
hyperreactive (H)	58	45
mixed (m)	18	14
indeterminate (?)	6	5
Total	130	100

Table Ib	
DP type	no. of patients
DP(V)	1
DP(T)	2
DP(G)	10^a
DP(V)+DP(G)	1
DP(T)+DP(G)	10
Total	24,i.e.18%

a) including 5 patients with
   bilateral normal response

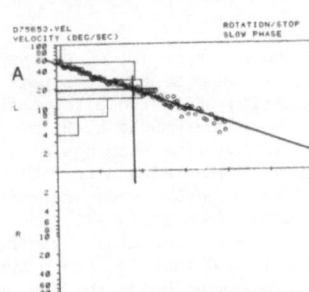
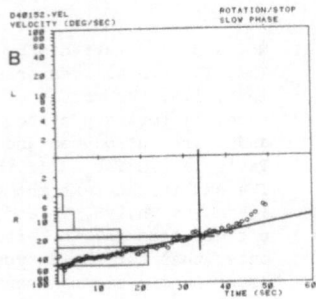
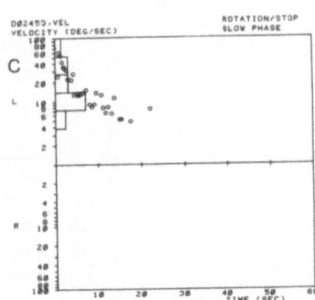
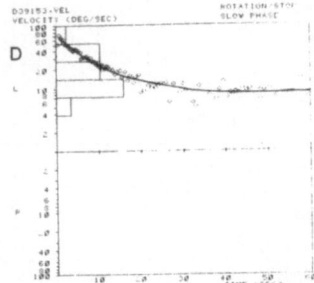

Fig.1. Four different types of VS responses in 4 different patients.
In each panel the computer plot is shown of SPV (of each analyzed nystagmus beat in °/s on a logarithmic scale, R and L indicating the direction of
the fast phase of nystagmus) against the time (s) after stopping the rotation. The regression lines were fitted by eye and V and T (time at SPV =
0.37V) can be read from the scales at the intersection points with the
drawn horizontal and vertical lines. The histograms are designed for fac-
ilitating the detection of left-right asymmetry; they can be ignored here.
The response patterns are: A, VOTOGO (n type in Table I); B, VOT+G+ (VH);
C, V+T-G- (Vm); D, V+T?G? (V? type). The patterns in C and D have interesting features. In C, T is extremely short (3s), probably due to ocular
motor disturbance. The curved course of SPV shown in panel D was presumably caused by summation of the usual exponentially decaying component and a
static offset component. This effect occurs if SPV is plotted on a logarithmic scale and spontaneous nystagmus is present. It then occurs in the
direction of spontaneous nystagmus only (see Fig.1 of Huygen & Nicolasen,
1985). The difference in the present case is that this curvature was shown
symmetrically in two directions in absence of nystagmus without rotatory
stimulation. Such response behaviour is typical of release from inhibition
and thus consistent with the concept of VH.

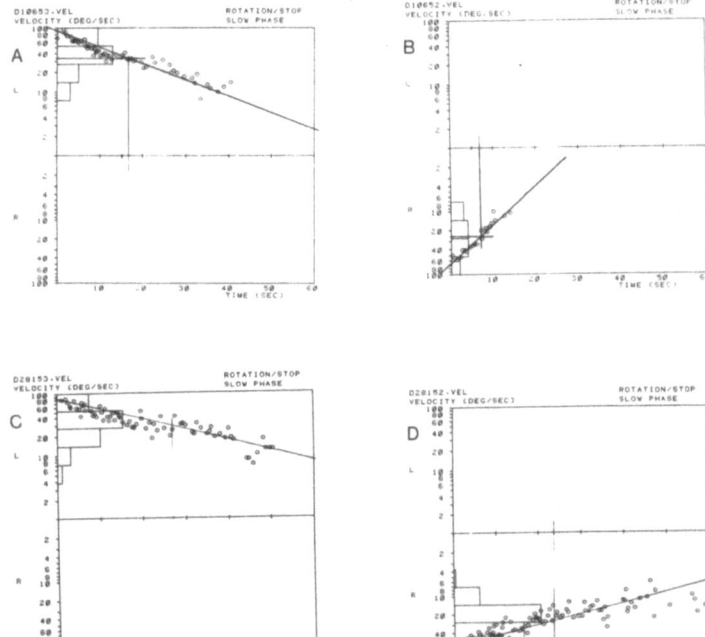

Fig.2. The variability of the VS responses of a patient during follow-up.
A-B, exam 1, right- and left-beating responses. The response patterns are
V+T0G+ (A) and VOT-G- (B); DP(T) and DP(G) are significant. C-D, exam 2,
14 months later. The patterns are now V+T+G+ (C) and VOTOG+ (D) and DP
values are within normal limits. It is clear that the right-beating response (B, D) changed more than the left-beating response (A, C). The response in B is of the Vh type, the others are of the VH type. The combination of a (single response) VH type (A) in one and a Vh type (B) in the
other direction constitutes another overall Vm type of response in this
patient at exam 1 (see definition in Table I).

icits such as gaze nystagmus, slowing or dysmetria of saccades and/or defective smooth pursuit and optokinetic nystagmus. Such deficits were present in about 80% of the patients with Vh or Vm overall response types,
which is exceptionally high.

All (3) response parameters could be evaluated in both nystagmus directions in 250 VS tests. In Table II the frequencies of normal and significant low or high values of each parameter are presented with their prob-
abilities. The frequencies of significant high and low values were generally significantly higher than expected (250 x 0.025), except for low V,

Table II: Incidence and probability (in parentheses) of
           parameter values being within normal limits (0),
           significantly low (-) or high (+), both at 5%
           level, for V, T and G for both nystagmus dir-
           ections combined.

	V	T	G
-	2	41	24
	(0.008)	(0.164)	(0.096)
0	148	180	143
	(0.592)	(0.720)	(0.572)
+	100	29	83
	(0.400)	(0.116)	(0.332)
Total	250	250	250
	(1)	(1)	(1)

which had a significantly low frequency (Poisson statistics). Table III is
a survey of the frequencies of all the VTG patterns found with an indication to which type of single response (defined similar to the overall types
in Table Ia) they belonged. Some of the most frequent patterns are illustrated in Figs 1-2. It is clear from Table III that of the primary response parameters (V and T), V is most often involved in the VH patterns.

Table III: Frequencies of the various VTG patterns of the single responses (N=260) in 130 patients. If the column heading is placed directly behind the line heading, the notation of the corresponding VTG pattern will appear. The response type is indicated for each pattern (see codes in Table I) and it is shown by the + and - signs in superscript whether the frequency is significantly high or low (according to Poisson statistics or chi-square test) as tested against the expected frequency (not shown) calculated with the data of Table II. Examples of response patterns are shown in Figs 1-2.

	G0	G-	G+	G?
V0T0	$97n^+$	$4\bar{h}$	$12\bar{H}$	
V0T-	$7h$	$9n^+$	0^-	
V0T+	$4H$		$14H^+$	
V-T0		$1h$		
V-T-				
V-T+			$1m$	
V+T0	$19\bar{H}$	0^-	$47H^+$	
V+T-	$16m$	$10m^+$	0^-	
V+T+	0^-		$9H^+$	
V+T?				$10?$

Total of types:	n	h	H	m	?
	97	21	105	27	10
(%)	(37)	(8)	(40)	(10)	(4)

The transitions that occurred between the overall response types during follow-up are presented in Table IVa. There was much variability, which is also clear from the fact that transitions occurred between responses with and without significant DP and among the various DP types (Table IVb). Only the VH response type was maintained significantly often. The combined proportion of responses of the Vh and VH types increased (from 0.50 to 0.64) at the cost of the other types.

Table IV: Transitions between overall response types (a) and DP
types (b) among 44 repetition-tests (2 months - 2 years
apart) in 34 patients. See Table I for symbols. +,
significantly high frequency (chi-square test or Poisson statistics). Fig.2 shows an example of the shift
from a Vm to a VH type and disappearance of DP(T)+DP(G)
type.

Table IVa

Overall response type

	after				
Before	Vn	Vh	VH	Vm	V?
Vn	4		3	2	1
Vh		2	1		
VH	3		15$^+$	1	
Vm		3	2	4	
V?		1	1	1	

Table IVb

DP type

	after			
Before	no	T	G	T+G
no	35	3	1	
T	1			
G	2			
T+G	1			1

DISCUSSION

Most of the response types were consistent with VH. The properties of the
Vm and Vh types are not quite clear. T- is a component common to these
types. It was striking that the time constant was very short (about 3s,
see Fig.1C) in some patients, even shorter that the primary afferent time
constant of the VOR in primates (5-6s, see Willson & Melvill Jones, 1979).
This finding appeared to be strongly associated with the presence of
ocular motor deficits. We have seen the concomitant appearance of T- type
and ocular motor dysfunction in some patients as well as a corresponding
lateralization of both these features. The presumed deficit is a faulty
central integration.

In a previous study on rats with experimental allergic encephalomyelitis (EAE) as a model of demyelinating disease, the major findings were an
abnormal VOR in all animals with a significant increase in time constant

(Huygen & Brinkman, 1984). The responses in the affected animals changed from normal to VH within one day (Brinkman & Huygen, 1984). This makes it unlikely, that the increase of T could have been due to vestibular dishabituation, as previously suggested in the case of patients (Huygen, 1983). Although, in general, cerebellar or brain stem dysfunctions are viewed as possible causes of VH, the occurrence of VH in the EAE rats, in the light of evidence presented by others for this animal model, seems to favour a brain stem lesion, presumably involving the vestibular nuclei and/or commissure (see previous reports for references).

The differential diagnosis of abnormal VS responses comprises ear disease, posterior fossa disease and the hyperventilation syndrome (HVS) (Huygen & Nicolasen, 1985). The occurrence of types of VH involving V+T0 or V0T+ patterns in patients with ear disease makes clear that an ear inspection and audiogram are obligatory in combination with VS tests, which is generally true. Keeping this in mind, the exclusion of such causes of VH should not be too difficult. More problematic is the exclusion of other possible causes of VH. The exclusion of cerebellar disease not due to MS may be troublesome for obvious reasons. Quantitatively more important is the HVS, which we have found in 75% of patients with VH, with exclusion of other possible causes. On the other hand, a similar high percentage (77%) was found for VH in patients with proven HVS without other disorders (Theunissen et al., 1985). It was also found that patients with MS and VH may have ventilatory characteristics typical of a HVS. Patients with HVS having VH show response patterns similar to those found in MS (Huygen & Nicolasen, 1985). When taking the medical history of the patient, the possibility of HVS with its broad spectrum of symptoms and signs, should be kept in mind if VH is found.

REFERENCES

Baloh, R.W., Hess, K., Honrubia, V. and Yee, R.D. 1984. Low and high frequency sinusoidal testing in patients with peripheral vestibular lesions. Acta Otolaryngol., Suppl. 406: 189-193.
Brinkman, C.J.J. and Hüygen, P.L.M. 1984. Physiological abnormalities in experimental allergic encephalomyelitis (EAE) II. Acta Neurol. Scand., 70: 155-159.
Huygen, P.L.M. 1979. Nystagmometry. ORL 41: 206-220.
Huygen, P.L.M. 1983. Vestibular hyperreactivity in patients with multiple sclerosis. Adv. Oto-Rhino-Laryngol., Vol.30 (Karger, Basel), pp.141-149.
Huygen, P.L.M. and Brinkman, C.J.J. 1984. Physiological abnormalities in experimental allergic encephalomyelitis (EAE) I. Acta Otolaryngol., Suppl. 406: 154-160.

Huygen, P.L.M. and Nicolasen, M.G.M. 1985. The diagnostic value of veloc-
ity step responses. ORL, accepted for publication.
Theunissen, E.J.J.M., Huygen, P.L.M. and Folgering, H.Th. 1985. Vestibul-
ar hyperreactivity and hyperventilation. Submitted for publication.
Wilson, V.J. and Melvill Jones, G. 1979. Mammalian vestibular physiology.
Plenum Press, New York.

53

New Possibilities in the Diagnosis of Multiple Sclerosis by Accurate Registration of Eye Movements with the DMI Method

L. J. BOUR and J. DE VETH

It has been known since long that multiple sclerosis very often is accompanied by deficient eye movements. With respect to saccadic eye movements several pathological phenomena can be observed and in many patients a so called internuclear ophthalmoplegia (INO) becomes manifest (Cogan et al., 1950; Baloh et al., 1978; Reulen et al., 1983). Due to the reduction of eye velocity of the adducting eye and the "overshoot" of the contralateral eye in INO, maximum velocities lie outside the normal standard deviation of the main sequence (Bahill et al., 1975). Abducens paresis or even paralysis of the eyes in MS can occur, cerebellar dysfunction can cause dysmetria of saccades (Selhorst et al., 1976). Some cases also show oscillatory eye movements (opsoclonus) or saccadic overshoots (Zee and Robinson, 1979). With respect to the tracking eye movements in MS the ratio between eye velocity and target velocity of the smooth component is reduced, especially for vertical pursuit (Baloh et al., 1978). Asymmetries can be observed between leftward and rightward or upward and downward pursuit. Furthermore, due to the reduced gain, tracking will become saccadic. As a last deficit the gaze evoked nystagmus is mentioned here, which is thought to be caused by impaired functioning of the neural integrator (Zee et al., 1980).

Most of the eye movement research in MS has been performed with EOG since it is non-invasive, cheap and can be used routinely in the clinic. However, the EOG method has many drawbacks due to the large amount of artifacts. Due to the unfavourable S/N ratio of EOG, saccades smaller than 2 degrees cannot be reliably measured. Furthermore, slow eye movements cannot be distinguished from EOG drift. Another serious artifact is variability in EOG gain during an experiment. Schlag et al. (1983) reports that a new calibration is necessary after time intervals. We measured (see Results) that even within 1 second this gain can change a few percent. Moreover, the EOG signal is a filtered version of the actual eye movement (see Results). Vertical eye movements measured with EOG are completely unreliable and disrupted by eye blinks.

We report here results obtained with the double magnetic induction (DMI) method which is much more accurate than the EOG method. This DMI method has the advantage with respect to the classical electromagnetic method, that is more adapted to clinical use and experimenters who use already the classical electromagnetic method with a search coil have to perform only slight modifications to change over to DMI. Results obtained with DMI and EOG both will be compared and the specific advantages of the use of the DMI method in MS will be discussed.

METHOD

Eye movements of the subject's eye were measured with the DMI method described by Bour et al. (1984). With this method horizontal as well as vertical eye position are detected indirectly by determining the strength of the induced secondary magnetic field of a metallic ring on the subject's eye (Fig. 1) caused by an alternating primary magnetic field. The secondary

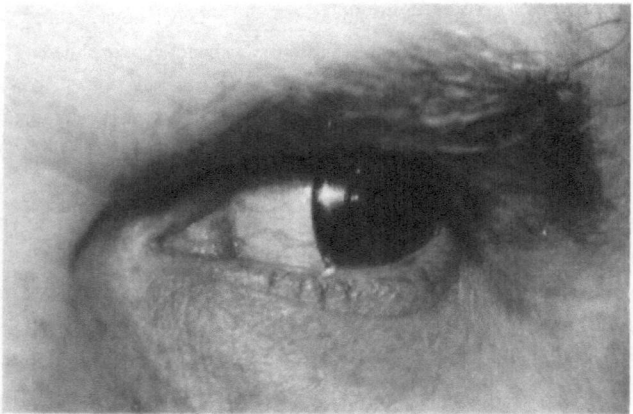

FIGURE 1   Close-up of the human eye with the metallic ring placed on the sclera.

induced field is picked up by a detection coil placed in front of the eye without the need of connecting wires. The use of a metallic ring instead of a search coil (classical method) has considerable advantages. There are no vulnerable connecting wires, irritation by the ring is minimal and visual acuity remains good. Within the -10,10 degrees range the method does not deviate from linearity more than 0.1 degree and its accuracy is 3'. Beyond this range the data are corrected for nonlinearities. The subject's head was stabilized by a chin rest and a tie around the head in order to reduce drift. An extra drift compensation was performed electrically by subtraction of a certain amount of the quadrature signal from the in-phase signal. Normally drifts are smaller than 0.25 degree. Eye position signals were low-pass filtered (- 3 dB at 150 Hz), FM-recorded on tape (Bell & Howell) and afterwards digitized with a sample frequency of 500 Hz and stored in the computer (PDP 11/34). In order to measure EOG Beckman electrodes were used and the amplified signals (1000x) were low-pass filtered and handled in the same was as the DMI signals.

RESULTS AND DISCUSSION

Figure 2 shows saccadic eye movements of a normal subject measured simultaneously with the DMI method and the EOG method. The subject was asked to track a target that succesively jumped from 15 degrees eccentricity at the left to 15 degrees at the right and vice versa. The figure shows clearly that in adduction EOG shows an overshoot of about 10% of the final amplitude after 400 ms. It can also be observed that the second corrective saccades, with an amplitude of about 2 degrees, are seen in the DMI recordings but not in the EOG signals.

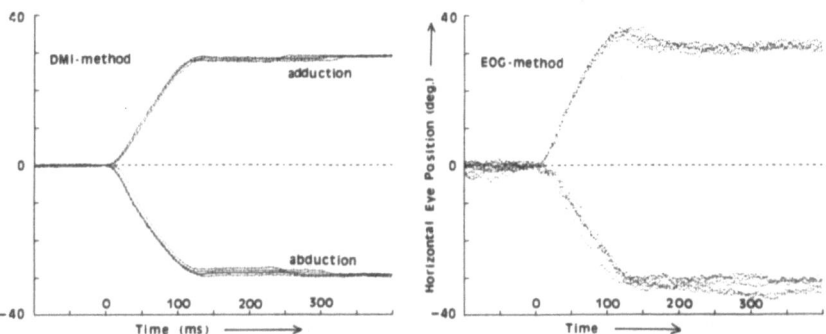

FIGURE 2   Saccadic eye movements in a normal subject measured simultaneously with the DMI method and the EOG method. For further explanation see text.

The left panel at the top of Fig. 3 again shows the eye position signals of Fig. 2 (DMI), but now in the top panel at the right the velocity
profiles of these saccades are shown. The two figures at the bottom of Fig.
3 demonstrate for one saccade the difference between the velocity profiles
calculated from the DMI and EOG signals (same algorithm). For this adducting eye movement (left eye) maximum velocities of EOG are too high and
strongly perturbed by noise.

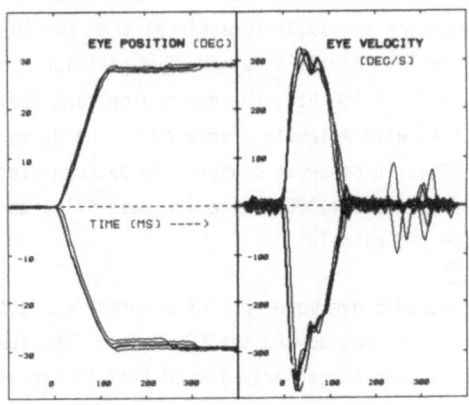

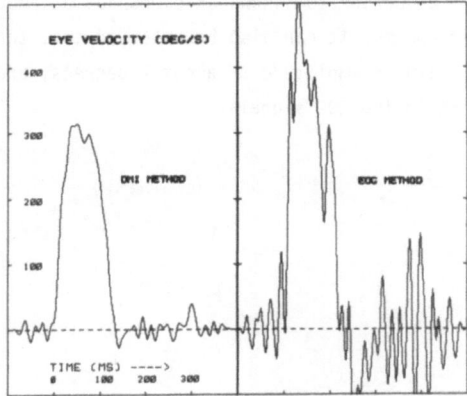

FIGURE 3   Velocity profiles calculated from the DMI-recordings (top
figure) and a comparison between a velocity profile computed
from DMI and from EOG signals (bottom figures).

In MS patients saccadic as well as pursuit eye movements were measured with the DMI method. The Figures 4, 5, 6 and 7 show some examples of
DMI eye movement registrations, that cannot be obtained with EOG and they
emphasize that the diagnosis of MS by means of eye movements can be extended to an earlier stage by virtue of the sensitivity of the method.

Figure 4 shows the velocity profiles of the left eye of an MS patient
with an INO. The patient was asked to track a target that succesively
jumped from 10 degrees at the left to 10 degrees at the right and vice
versa. Changes in the shape of the position signal can be appreciated
more clearly from these velocity profiles and maximum velocity can be used
as a quantitative parameter in the diagnosis of MS (van Munster et al.,
this book).

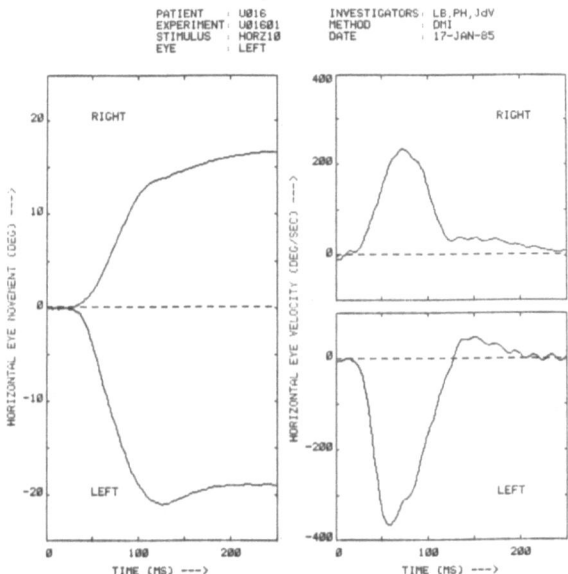

FIGURE 4   Saccadic eye movements and velocity profiles of a MS patient
            with a bilateral INO (only the left eye is shown).

Figure 5 shows the test of the velocity ratio (see Introduction). Horizontal and vertical eye movements were measured in a patient with juvenile MS (aged 11). This patient had to pursue a small circular target that moved with a continuous velocity of 10 ^{0}/s between -10 degrees and 10 degrees horizontal or vertical positions. The traces at the top and the bottom represent the horizontal and vertical pursuit, respectively. In two traces the actual eye movement and the averaged horizontal eye velocity are shown. The Tables under the two traces represent the average velocity ratio of the cumulative smooth part of the eye tracking. Values of zero and 1 mean no and optimal tracking, respectively. The patient has an impaired horizontal pursuit from left to right and vertical pursuit is also subnormal.

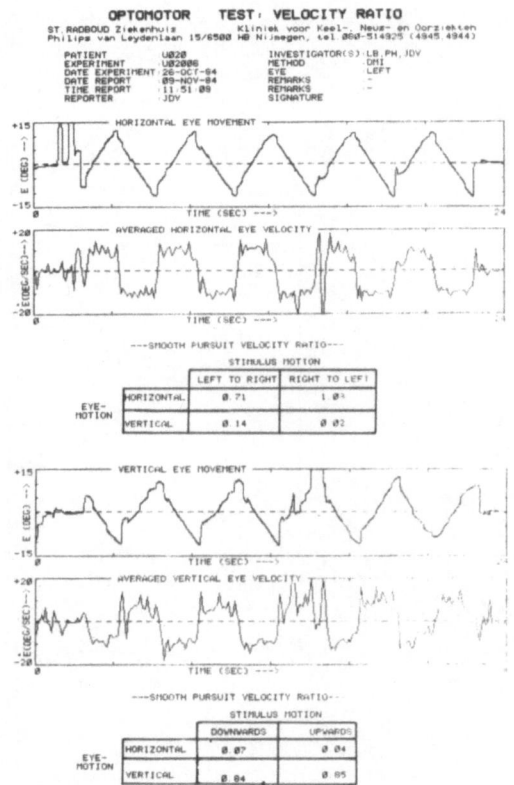

FIGURE 5   Optomotor test of the velocity ratio obtained in a patient with juvenile MS. For further explanation see text.

Figure 6 shows two different eye movement deficiencies in the same MS patient. At the top of Figure 6 a small burst of oscillatory activity during pursuit is shown. At the bottom of Fig. 6 a hypermetric saccade and two corrective saccades afterwards are shown. At this stage of disease the extent of hypermetry is still limited.

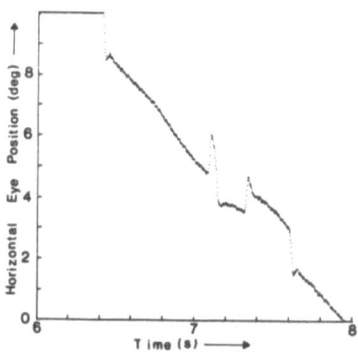

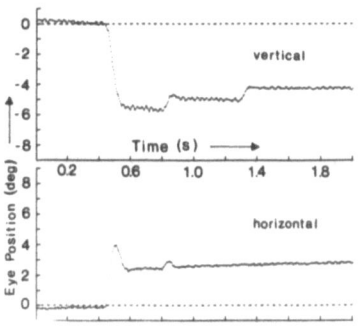

FIGURE 6   Oscillatory behaviour during pursuit (top figure) and hypermetria (bottom figure) in the same MS patient.

As a last result Fig. 7 shows at the right a reconstruction of the netto motoneuron activity pertaining the saccadic eye movements that are shown at the left (same saccades as in Fig. 4). By an inverse method these "pulse step" signals can be reconstructed (van Opstal et al., 1985). A prerequisite for this procedure are low noise registrations such as can be obtained with the DMI method. A first inspection of this reconstructed signal learns that mainly the pulse is affected by the demyelination of the MLF (medial lateral fasciculus) in MS.

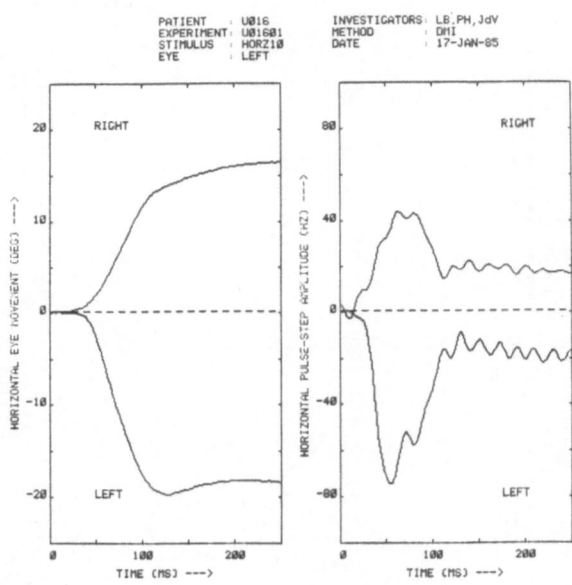

FIGURE 7   Saccades and pulse step reconstruction of the left eye of a MS patient with a bilateral INO. For further explanation see text.

ACKNOWLEDGEMENTS

This work was performed in collaboration with the Department of Oto-rhino-laryngology and the Department of Neurology of the Radboud University Hospital at Nijmegen.

REFERENCES

Bahill, A.P., Clark, M.R. and Stark, L., 1975. The main sequence: a tool
  for studying eye movements. Math. Biosci., 24: 191-204.
Baloh, R.W., Yee, R.D. and Honrubia, V., 1978. Internuclear Ophthalmoplegia. II pursuit, optokinetic nystagmus and vestibulo-oculo reflex. Arch.
  Neurol., 35: 490-493.
Bour, L.J., Gisbergen van, J.A.M., Bruijns, J. and Ottes, F.P., 1984. The
  double magnetic induction method for measuring eye movement - results
  in monkey and man. IEEE Trans. Biom. Eng.., BME-31, 5: 419-427.
Cogan, D.G., Kubik, C.S. and Smith, W.L., 1950. Unilateral internuclear
  ophthalmoplegia. Arch. Ophthalm., 44: 783-796.
Munster van, E.T.L., Huygen, P.L.M., Bour, L.J. and Hommes, O.R., 1985.
  A parametric atudy of saccadic eye movements in follow-up of normals
  and MS patients. This book.
Opstal van, A.J., Gisbergen van, J.A.M. and Eggermont, J.J., 1985.
  Reconstruction of neural control signals for saccades based on an inverse method. Vis. Res., in press.
Reulen, J.P.H., Sanders, E.A.C.M. and Hogenhuis, L.A.H., 1983. Eye movement disorders in multiple sclerosis and optic neuritis. Brain, 106:
  121-140.
Schlag, J., Merker, B. and Schlag-Rey, M., 1983. Comparison of EOG and
  search coil techniques in long-term measurements of eye position in
  alert monkey and cat. Vis. Res., 23: 1025-1030.
Selhorst, J.B., Stark, L., Ochs, A.L. and Hoyt, W.F., 1976. Disorders in
  cerebellar ocular motor control. I Saccadic overshoot dysmetria, an
  oculographic, control system and clinico-anatomic analysis. Brain,
  99: 497-508.
Zee, D.S. and Robinson, S.A., 1979. A hypothetical explanation of saccadic
  oscillations. Annal. Neurol., 5: 405-414.
Zee, D.S., Leigh R.J. and Mathieu-Millaire, F., 1980. Cerebellar control
  of ocular gaze stability. Annal. Neurol., 7: 37-40.

54

A Parametric Study of Saccadic Eye Movements in Follow-up of Normals and Multiple Sclerosis Patients

E. T. L. VAN MUNSTER, P. L. M. HUYGEN, L. J. BOUR and O. R. HOMMES

INTRODUCTION

The study of saccades in MS is worthwhile, since so many of the patients, at some stage of the disease, have or develop some form of saccade pathology. The saccade test is an easy test, feasible in almost any patient and completed in a few minutes. Saccadic slowing may be found in relation to internuclear ophthalmoplegia (INO) and other types of ocular motor pathology. Although parametric studies of saccadic slowing in MS have been performed before with electro-oculography (EOG) (for review see Leigh and Zee, 1983), attempts to define objective oculomotor scores and correlate them with clinical scores, which was the aim of the present study, have not been made before, as far as we know. For the study of follow-up, especially for evaluating the results of attempted treatment, the introduction of useful objective scores would be favourable.

MATERIAL AND METHODS

Horizontal saccades were elicited by jumps of a visual target over 20 deg. For bedridden patients the target was displayed at the ceiling. The horizontal movement of each eye was measured with dc-EOG. A wide-band system (0-100 Hz) was used with monocular leads from both canthi of

each eye. A ground electrode was attached to the forehead and a vertical
lead served as a blink detector. The signal was sampled at 250 Hz (2
channels, one for each eye) for subsequent computer analysis. This analysis was performed with automatic detection of on- and offsets of primary
(i.e. non-corrective) saccades in each eye position signal separately,
followed by interactive checking on unsuitable or disturbed saccades
(e.g. coinciding with eyeblinks). Calibration was done interactively with
a programme in which a videocursor was used to identify the ontarget
parts of the eye position signal. A differentiation algorithm (Usui and
Amidror, 1982) was used to obtain saccade velocity profiles. Four sets
of output data (for adduction and abduction of each eye) were obtained,
each containing mean and SD of saccade amplitude (A) and maximum velocity
(V) of all selected (i.e. 3-13) saccades.

74 Patients with definite MS and 15 subjects with normal eye movements (i.e. ENT patients) were measured twice at intervals of 3-55 months.
During this interval the patients received immunosuppressive therapy in
the form of intensive immunosuppression (IIS) with 400 mg cyclophosphamide and 100 mg prednison daily for 20 days and/or chronic immunosuppression (CIS) with 100 mg cyclophosphamide and 10-50 mg prednison daily for
at least 1 year.

The parameter V/A (s^{-1}) was selected on account of a previous study
on the metrics of normal and disturbed saccades. Values equal to or smaller than 16.2 s-1 or equal to or greater than 26.4 s^{-1} indicate pathology
(both at 2.5% tail probability). This previous study also showed that the
(4) values of V/A for adduction and abduction of both eyes could be
pooled in the normal subjects. Although the absolute values of A and V
for ad- en abduction differ from each other, the relative differences
between ad- and abduction were equal for both parameters.

In the study of the normal subjects a very suitable parameter for
follow-up evaluation appeared to be the sequential relative difference
(SRD) of V/A: SRD = (V/A before -V/A after)/(V/A before +V/A after). "Before" and "after" means before and after immunosuppression. SRD has a
normal distribution with mean and SD leading to 95% confidence limits at
+/-0.08 (exclusive).

Oculomotor scores 1, 2, pattern change score A and pattern shift
score B are defined as shown in Fig. 1 and 2. The "combination score" (C)
is the sum of the scores A and B, which are more or less complementary.

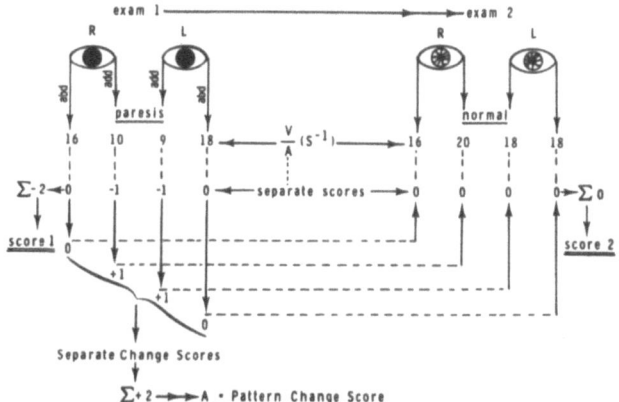

<u>Fig. 1:</u>   Definitions of the oculomotor scores 1 and 2 and the
        pattern change score (A). The change of bilateral
slowing of adduction (INO) at exam 1 back to normal saccades
at exam 2 is depicted. A significant low V/A value leads to a
separate score of -1 (normal 0). Scores 1 and 2 are the sums
of the 4 corresponding separate scores. The separate change
scores indicate the numerical difference between two corresponding separate scores at exam 1 and 2 (+1 is improvement,
-1 is deterioration). The pattern change score (A) is the sum
of the separate change scores. The pattern codes (not shown
here) are obtained by reading the separate scores whilst
omitting the digits 1 and retaining the signs and zeros which
are combined in one character string: e.g. the oculomotor
score at exam 1 in our example is 0--0.

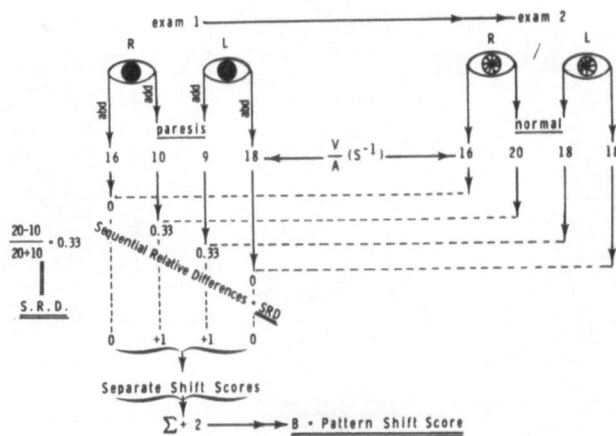

Fig. 2:   Definition of the sequential relative difference
          (SRD) and the pattern shift score (B). The obser-
vations and V/A values are the same as in Fig. 1. The separate
shift scores are assigned after the SRD value of each saccade
has been calculated as illustrated. The separate shift score
+1 denotes a significant increase (SRD > 0.08); -1 denotes a
significant decrease in V/A value (SRD < -0.08). The pattern
shift score (B) is the sum of the 4 separate shift scores.
The pattern shift code (not shown) is defined similar to the
other pattern codes.

A minus sign of such a score indicates pathology or deterioration, depending on whether the score pertains to an oculomotor status (at exam 1 or exam 2) or a status change (from exam 1 to exam 2). Alternative scores were also derived, which were based on the assumption that a significant low value of V/A does not necessarily indicates saccadic slowing if the saccade concerned is hypermetric (overshoot). Exclusion of Hypermetria leads to the definition of "ex patterns" and the "ex scores" 1, 2, A and C, indicated as 1 ex, 2 ex, A ex, C ex. The ex patterns conform with the clinical diagnosis of oculomotor pathology: e.g. the pattern code 0--0 (see example in Fig. 1) indicates bilateral INO, where the original oculomotor pattern code may have been --- if including the significant low V/A values of the overshooting (abducting) saccades.

The scores DSS (disability status score), FS (functional system) and BS (brain stem score as part of FS) of the scoring system of Kurtzke (1970)   were used. The shifts in these scores are symbolized by S (DSS), S (FS) and S (BS); a minus sign indicates improvement: e.g. DSS_1 = 7 (severe invalidation) becomes DSS_2 = 5 (less deterioration), so the shift will be: S (DSS) = -2, i.e. improvement.

RESULTS

Important pattern shifts and pattern changes are presented in Table 1. For each pattern shift the expected frequency was calculated and tested against the frequency found (by using Poisson statistics and tables). Some frequencies found appear to be significantly high (indicated by the affixed + sign in Table 1). It appeared from the pattern shifts (related to significant values of the SRD), that the frequencies of slowing of unilateral adduction, conjugate gaze and all saccades were significantly higher than expected. The same holds for the frequencies of speeding up of bilateral abduction, conjugate gaze, monocular and all saccades. It can be seen that these findings were not always related to the findings apparent from the pattern changes (pertaining to the change in V/A status of each saccade) with inclusion (in) or exclusion (ex) of significant low values of V/A associated with hypermetria. In particular, the clinical picture apparent from the latter (ex) pattern change did not confirm the high incidences of patterns associated with slowing. The relatively high incidence of speeding up patterns was confirmed except for the monocular pattern.

TABLE I   Number of cases found in important categories of shift patterns compared with pattern changes including (in) or excluding (ex) hypermetria.

Category	Pattern code(s)		Pattern shift found	expected	Pattern change in	ex
Unilateral						
- adduction: slowing	00-0	0-00	7+	(3.17)	0	2
speeding up	00+0	0+00	5	(3.17)	3	3
- abduction: slowing	000-	-000	4	(3.17)	6	2
speeding up	000+	+000	3	(3.17)	5	5
Bilateral						
- adduction: slowing	0--0	0-0	0	(0.04)	1	1
speeding up	0++0	0+0	0	(0.04)	0	1
- abduction: speeding up	+00+	+00	1+	(0.04)	2	2
Conjugate						
- gaze: slowing	0-0-	-0-0	2+	(0.08)	0	0
speeding up	0+0+	+0+0	4+	(0.08)	4	3
Monocular speeding up	00++	++00	2+	(0.08)	0	0
Overall slowing	----		3+	(0.00)	0	0
speeding up	++++		3+	(0.00)	2	2

The cross-correlations of the parameters as defined before were calculated from cross-tables such as presented in Table II. Only the cases with significant individual change in saccade pathology were included in the calculation of the presented coefficients. Part of the correlation matrix is shown in Table III. Oculomotor scores (1 or 2) were significantly correlated with the clinical scores (1 or 2), but not with the shifts in clinical scores. The scores related to changes in saccade pathology, i.e. the scores A, B and C were strongly cross-correlated. Score B was significantly correlated with the shifts in clinical scores and so was score C; this does not hold for score A. It is worth of note that the significance as indicated was maintained if the relevant coefficients were calculated for the whole patient sample (n=74). In Table IV the scores 1, 2, A and C have been recalculated with exclusion of hypermetria as outlined above. Although the scores 1 ex and 2 ex still show significant correlations with the clinical scores (but lower now than for scores 1 and 2), the derived score C ex is no longer significantly correlated with the shifts in clinical scores. This means that correction for hypermetria in the pattern change score (A, which becomes A ex) causes the loss of significance of some relevant cross-correlations.

TABLE II   Cross-table of pattern shift score (B) and S (DSS) with correlation coefficient for the patients with significant individual change in saccade pathology (n=47).

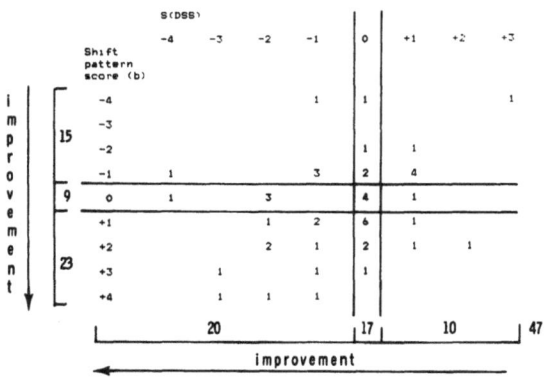

Correlation coefficient: r = -0.31 (p < 0.05)

TABLE III   Part of the correlation matrix. Significant correlation
coefficients are underlined (n=47, p< 0.05).

	Score 1	Score 2	Score A	Score B	Score C
DSS1	-0.35				
FS1	-0.42				
BS1	-0.43				
Score 2	0.64				
DSS2		-0.42			
FS2		-0.54			
BS2		-0.64			
Score A	-0.35	0.50			
Score B	-0.03	0.53	0.68		
Score C	-0.18	0.56	0.88	0.95	
S(DSS)	-0.07	-0.24	-0.21	-0.31	-0.30
S(FS)	0.03	-0.18	-0.26	-0.34	-0.33
S(BS)	0.10	-0.11	-0.24	-0.31	-0.30

TABLE IV   Same part of the correlation matrix as in Table III with scores 1, 2, A and C replaced by the ex scores, i.e. these scores were recalculated with exclusion of pathology scores associated with hypermetria. Score B is the same as in Table II and is repeated for clarity.

	Score 1_{ex}	Score 2_{ex}	Score A_{ex}	Score B	Score C_{ex}
DSS1	-0.27				
FS1	-0.32				
BS1	-0.39				
Score 2_{ex}	0.91				
DSS2		-0.39			
FS2		-0.46			
BS2		-0.42			
Score A_{ex}	-0.63	0.38			
Score B	-0.18	-0.03	0.62		
Score C_{ex}	-0.43	0.44	0.84	0.82	
S(DSS)	-0.05	-0.07	-0.14	-0.31	-0.13
S(FS)	0.01	0.03	-0.21	-0.34	-0.22
S(BS)	0.16	0.10	-0.25	-0.31	-0.23

DISCUSSION

As far as we know, this is the first report on significant correlations between objective neurophysiological scores and clinical scores.

It seems difficult to exclude the possible influence of variations in factors such as alertness and fatigue, in the case of saccadic slowing as well as apparent speeding up. It must be realized that on the basis of chance alone slowing may be detected in a number of cases, as indicated in Table I. This is especially true for shifts in 1 saccade only.

Although score A correlated significantly with score B and C it did not with any of the shifts in clinical scores. Significant cross-correlations were found between the shifts in clinical scores and score B. This also holds for score C, but not for score C ex, i.e. if significant low values of V/A of separate saccades associated with hypermetria were excluded. There is no doubt that this effect is caused by the fact that the ex pattern changes are more conservative, as stipulated in presenting Table I, and thus yield lower scores. Score B is the most practical score, which is directly derived from test-retest measurements (SRD). Score C seems redundant. The SRD is a parameter with a nicely distribution with mean zero and a small SD indicating that the parameter V/A has relatively little test-retest variability, i.e. it is a parameter particularly suited for studying follow up.

REFERENCES

Kurtzke, J.F., 1970. Neurologic impairment in multiple sclerosis and the disability status scale. Acta Neurol. Scand., 46: 493-512.
Leigh, R.J. and Zee, D.S., 1983. The neurology of eye movements. Davis, Philadelphia.
Usui, S. and Amidror, I., 1982. Digital low pass differentiation for biological signal processing. IEEE Trans. Biomed. Eng. BME, 29 (no. 10): 686-693.

55

Visual Evoked Responses in Definite and Suspected Multiple Sclerosis. Comparison of Them to Cerebrospinal Fluid Oligoclonal Bands

I. MILONAS

Since introduction of visual evoked responses (VER) in clinical practice by Halliday et al in 1972 the use of this technique has been spread all over the world and has been widely recognized as a standard method of clinical testing. VER was the first technique to be used and cortical and subcortical somatosensory responses (Small et al.,1977, Chiappa, 1980, Aminoff, 1984) and brainsted auditory potentials (Chiapa, 1980, Stockard et al.,1980) were followed and have now also been widely used in the diagnosis of multiple sclerosis (MS).

The main target of evoked potential (EP) technique is to reveal clinically silent lesions and so contribute in diagnosis of MS showing the disseminated nature of the disease.

When evoked responses are used to patients with MS the percentage of abnormal responses must be given in relation to an organ or system which does not present any clinical manifestation. It is expected for instance that if an eye with optic neuritis is investigated VEP will be delayed but this does not reveal a new lesion, it simply confirms the clinical diagnosis of optic neuritis, but does not add any new element supporting the diagnosis of a demyelinating disease. On the contrary if VEPs are abnormal in a patient with a cord syndrome and with no symptoms or signs from his optic system this finding is highly significant for the diagnosis of MS.

The existense of oligoclonal bands in the gamma globulin region of cerebrospinal fluid (CSF) is considered one of the most sensitive laboratory tests for the diagnosis of MS (Thompson et al 1979). Oligoclonal bands are detected very rarely (9%) in other neurological diseases mainly, in infectious diseases of the nervous system (Hutchinson et al.,1983).

The above mentioned techniques (VERs and CSF oligoclonal bands) were studied in patients with MS for assessing the efficiency of them in the diagnosis of demyelinating disease.

MATERIAL AND METHODS

Two groups of patients with MS were evaluated; one group with the diagnosis of clinically definite MS (53 patients) and one with the diagnosis of suspected MS (17 patients) according to the criteria of McDonald and Halliday (1977). In these two groups VEPs were recorded and agarose gel electrophoresis was performed on their CSF.

VEPs were recorded with a silver disc electrode placed 5cm above the inion with a mid-frontal reference electrode. The patient was sitted in a distance of 1m from the stimulator. The stimulus was a black and white chequerboard pattern (dimensions 2.4X2.4cm) reversing at a frequency of once or twice per second using a revearsal pattern TV stimulator ST10 sensor (dimensions 35X28cm). Responses were amplified, averaged and recorded using the Medelec Sensor equipment. 256 responses were averaged for each eye and regarded as abnormal if the major positive peak (P100) was seen after a latency bigger than 115ms (normal mean+3SD) or if there was a latency difference greater than 7ms between the two eyes. There was a 25% stimulus delay in the recording.

Agarose gel electrophoresis was performed on concentrated CSF using the panagel electrophoresis system of Millipore Corporation (Johnson et al. 1977). The appearance of two or more bands in the γ-globulin region was considered as abnormal finding.

RESULTS

Delayed VERs were found in 48 out of 53 patients with definite MS (90.5%). In the same group CSF oligoclonal bands were seen in 46 patients (86.8%).

In twelve of the above patients which had abnormal VERs and oligoclonal bands the two methods were repeated one month later while the patients were under treatment with steroids and the findings were almost the same. Delayed VERs as well as the presence of oligoclonal bands were seen again and with no significant changes from the first investigations.

Only four of the patients with suspected MS from the total of 17 had delayed VERs (23,5%) while in the same group six had oligoclonal bands in their CSF (36%).

DISCUSSION

Delayed VEPs were obtained in 90.5% of the patients with definite MS and this percentage is similar to that in most of the reports reviewed by Halliday (1978). These abnormal findings were seen in patients having a history of visual impairment as well as in patients with no such history and of course it was much more valuable in the second category. Only one patient with history of visual impairment had normal VEPs and this finding has been reported by other too (Walsh et al.,1982).

Oligoclonal bands in the γ-globulin region were seen in 86.8% of the patients with definite MS a percentage which is similar to that of abnormal VERs. The same values are given in other papers (Walsh et al.,1982, Thomson et al., 1983).

From the 53 patients with clinically definite MS 52 had either abnormal VERs or existence of oligoclonal bands in their CSF or more frequently both. So in 98% of these patients the diagnosis of MS was confirmed by one or both of the above techniques.

In 12 patients of the above group with definite MS the two investigations were repeated one month later while the patients were receiving steroids and 10 of them had shown a significant improvement of their clinical status. In spite of this no appreciable changes were seen in their VERs or the pattern of oligoclonal bands, and this supports the view that the above techniques remain abnormal even if there is remission of the demyelinating disease.

In contrast with the impressingly high positive finding in clinically definite MS in the suspected form of the disease the two used techniques were low. So only 4 patients of this group had delayed VERs (23,5%) and only 6 patients had oligoclonal bands in their CSF (36%). Low percentages for this form of MS are given by Walsh et al (1982) but the values are lower in delayed VERs (15%) and higher in the existence of oligoclonal bands (55%). Nine totaly patients from the 17 of this group with suspected MS had abnormal one or both techniques and so the percentage of abnormal tests was increased to 52,9%.

Comparing the findings of the two groups we can see the great difference in the results between the group with definite MS and that with suspected. This difference shows the need for more precise methods which could help the clinicians in the difficult cases of suspected MS. Some trials for evaluating other components of the VER or their amplitude proved not to be succesful. So although the EPs gave a great impact in the diagnosis of MS and their doubtless usefulness in the clinical practice has been emphasized by many investigators (Halliday 1981a, Halliday 1981b, Chiappa 1980) their most detailed evaluation is needed.

The combination of VEPs with the other EPs and with the study of oligoclonal bands contribute greatly in the correct diagnosis of MS but there are still cases in which the diagnosis of demyelinating disease remains uncertain.

REFERENCES

Aminoff, M.J., 1984. The clinical role of somatosensory evoked potential studies: A clinical appraisal. Muscle and Nerve 7, pp. 345-354.
Chiappa K., 1980. Pattern shift visual, brainsted auditory and short latency somatosensory evoked potentials in MS.Neurology,30(2), 110.
Halliday, A.M., McDonald,W.I., Mushin, J. 1972. Delayed visual evoked responses in optic neuritis, Lancet. pp. 982-985.
Halliday, A.M.,1978. New developments in the clinical application of evoked potentials. In:Cobb W.A., Van Duijn H.(eds) Contemporary Clinical Neurophysiology. Elsevier, Amsterdam. pp.105-121.
Halliday, A.M., 1981a. Visual evoked potentials in Demyelinating Disease. In Waxman and Ritchie (eds): Demyelinating Disease: Basis and Clinical Electrophysiology. Raven Press. New York. pp.201-215.
Halliday, A.M., 1981b. How useful are evoked potentials in clinical diagnosis. In Henry (ed):Current Clinical Neurophysiology. Elsevier, North Holland. pp. 555-569.
Hutchinson, M., Martin, E.A., Maguire, P., Glynn, D., Mansfield, M., Feighery, C., 1983. Visual evoked responses and immunoglobulin abnormalities in the diagnosis of MS. Acta Neurol.Scand. 68:90-95.
Johnson, K., Arrigo, S.C., Nelson, B.J., 1977. Agarose electrophoresis of CSF in MS. Neurolgoy (Minneap.) 27:273-277.
McDonald, W.I., Halliday, A.M., 1977. Diagnosis and classification of multiple sclerosis. Br.Med.Bull. 33:4-8.

Small, D., Matthews, W., Small, M., 1977. Subcortical somatosensory evoked potentials in MS. Electroencephal.Clin.Neurophysiol. 43:536.

Stockard, J.J., Stockard, J.E., Sharbrough, F., 1980. Brainstem auditory evoked potentials in neurology: Methodology, interpretation, clinical application. In: Electrodiagnosis in clinical neurology (M.Aminoff ed.) Churchill Livingstone, N.York. pp. 370-413.

Thompson, E., Kaufmann, P., Shortman, R., Rudge, P., McDonald, I., 1979. Oligoclonal immunoglobulins and plasma cells in spinal fluid of patients with MS. Br.Med.J., 1:16-17.

Thompson, E., Kaufmann, P., Rudge, P., 1983. Sequential changes in oligoclonal patterns during the course of MS. J.Neurol.Neurosurg.Psych. 46:547-550.

Walsh, J.C., Garrick, R., Cameron, J., McLeod, J.G., 1982. Evoked potential changes in clinically definite MS: a two years follow up study. J.Neurol.Neurosurg.Psychiat. 45:494-500.

Index

ABER (auditory brainstem evoked response)
  358-60
ABR (auditory brain stem response)
  pathology and course parameters   95-99
Active demyelinating lesions   131-39
Actuarial analysis   19, 22
Age at onset   17-20, 25-27
Albumin   233,242,245
Alpha-fetoprotein   9
Animal studies   290-92
Annual relapse rate (ARR)   45
AntiGalC antibodies
    affinity purification of   268
    as probe for basic research   269
    immunological detection of 268
    in clinical research   269
    preparation of   267
Antigen-presenting cells (APC)   144,
  199, 200
Anti-lymphocyte serum (ALS)   49-53
Antipyretics   8
Anti-viral antibodies   262
Astrocytes   133, 149, 155, 160,
  189-90, 199-206
Auditory brainstem evoke response (ABER)
  358-60
Auditory brainstem response (ABR)   95-99
Autoimmune disease   9, 109
Autoimmune encephalitogenesis   185-93
Autoimmune mechanisms   185, 292

Azathioprine   50, 51
    clinical assessment   61-70
    clinical course with   66
    complications   59
    daily dosage   65
    immunosuppression   55-59
    long-term experience with   56-59
    material and methods   65
    versus placebo   67

B-cells   123, 233
B-lymphocytes   131, 168, 169
Blink reflex   358-60
Blood brain barrier (BBB)   188, 199,
    283-87
    pathology of   284-85
    permeability in MS plague   285
Blood-brain-cerebrospinal fluid system
    283
Blood serum, cytotoxic antibodies in
    195-98
Bout   90
Bout frequency   92
Brain lesions. See NMR imaging
Brain sections, oligoclonal pattern of IgG
    251-56

Cancer risk   47
Central nervous system (CNS)   109
    autoimmune disease   185, 202
    immune reactions   123, 199
    immunological capacity   105, 106
    inflammatory reactions   167, 203
    myelin lipids in   209
    myelin proteins in   210
    oligoclonal response   236-37
    pathological process inside lesions
    205
Central nervous tissues   145, 159
Cerebella degeneration   346
Cerebral grey matter   145
Cerebral white matter   144, 145
Cerebrospinal fluid   (CSF)
    alterations in   15
    cloning of lymphoid cells from
        167-74
    cytology   30
    cytotoxic bodies in   195-98
    IgA levels in   234

Cerebrospinal fluid (CSF) (cont)
    IgM levels in   235
    immunoglobulin levels   163,
        217-23, 231
    in diagnostic criteria   11, 86
    lymphocyte subsets in   141-42
    myelin constituent recovery   214
    oligoclonal bands   393-96
    T-cells in   123-30
    viral antibodies in   163
    see also Blood-brain-cerebrospinal
        fluid system
Charcot's triad   3
Childbirth   9, 10
Chi-square test   16
Circulating immune complexes (CIC)
    271-75
Cisternographic pictures   225, 226
Clinical course. See Course
Clinical features   3
Clinical studies   3-12
    history   3
Clinical trials   13-14
Complement factors   271-75
Computer analysis   16
Computer programs   6
Con-A-induced suppression of MLR   116,
    117, 119
Corticosteroids   51
Course   6, 7, 19, 231-39
    and HLA system   315-21
    basic parameters   90-91
    intermittent   43
    progressive   43
    types of   15, 91
Cyclophosphamide (CY) immunosuppression
    45-48, 77-78
Cytotoxic antibodies in sera and CSF
    195-98

Deficit score   92
Demyelination   111, 112, 143, 213,
    257, 286, 289, 290
    neurophysiological studies
        353-56
    of central nervous tissue   159
d'Este, Augustus   3
Diagnostic categories   85-87
    Göteborg incidence material   87
    paraclinical methods   85-86
Diagnostic classification   11, 87
Diagnostic criteria   11, 85, 310, 357
Dietary fats consumption   71
Dietary therapy   71-79

Differential diagnoses   86
Disability data   41-44
Disability distribution   6
Disability status scores (DSS) 5,
    41-44, 68, 69, 72-74, 82
Dissemination in space   15
Dissemination in time   15
Double case families   333-36
Double magnetic induction (DMI)
    method   374

Electro-oculography (EOG) 373-76, 383
Emotional difficulties   8
ENG-test   360-61
Environmental factors   295, 310
Environmental Status Scale (ESS)
    31, 36-37, 43
Epidemiological studies   305-14
Equine antiglobuline antibodies   50,
    51, 52
Ethnic factors   295, 298
Etiological study   295-303
Evoked potential (EP) technique   393
Expanded Disability Status Scale (EDSS)
    31-33, 226
Experimental allergic encephalomyelitis
    (EAE)   109-13, 285, 290, 370
Extracellular space (ECS)   283
Eye movement deficiencies   357-62,
    373-81
Eye movement research   373

False negative rate   13
False positive rate   13
Frequency of disturbances   5
Frequency of symptoms   4
Functional outcome   22, 25
Functional system scale   5

Galactocerebroside   112
Galactosylceramide (GC) antigenicity
    267-70
        immunolocalization of   269
Genetic markers   30
Gestational processes   8
Glial fibrillary acidic protein (GFAP)
    144, 147, 161, 199
Göteborg incidence material   87

Haplotypic associations   318
Haplotypic frequencies   319, 320

Heat effects   8
Histological abnormalities   163-66
HLA antigens
    and clinical course   315-21
    Barbagia, Sardinia   329-32
    Benelux   323-28
    double case families   333-36
    phenotypic frequencies   317
HLA determination, twin studies   339
HLA-genes   143, 149
HLA markers   315-21
HLA-specific human cells   265
HLA system   143

Ia-positive cells   144, 145, 147, 148, 149
Ia-presenting cells   143-51
IgA index   237
IgA levels   233, 234, 241-50
IgA secreting cells   234
IgG index   226, 237, 241, 258
IgG levels   163, 232-33, 241-56
IgG producing cells in CSF   232-33
IgG synthesis 257-66
IgM index   237, 244, 246
IgM levels   235, 241-50
IgM producing cells   235
Illness severity score   6
Imaging   345-48
Immune complexes (IC)   225-29, 261,
    271-75
Immune function   103
Immune reactions   123, 199
Immune response   103-5, 123, 143, 257
Immune system   103-7, 156, 291
    regulation of   106
Immunogenetic markers   333
Immunoglobulin abnormalities   241-50
Immunoglobulin indices   246-48
Immunoglobulin synthesis   243
Immunoglobulins   217-23, 231-39
Immunohistological methods   143
Immunological abnormalities   163-66
Immunological function   199-206
Immunological parameters   9
Immunopathological mechanisms   185
Immunoregulation   103
Immunosuppression
    anti-lymphocyte serum (ALS)   49-53
    azathioprine   55-59
    cyclophosphamide (CY)   45-48, 77-78
    linoleic acid   77
Incapacity data   41-44
Incapacity Status Scale (ISS)   5, 31,
    36, 43, 226

Incidence study   305-14
Infections   8
Inflammatory demyelination   111
Inflammatory reactions   137, 167
In-patients, comparative study   31-40
Interferon   175-81, 201, 334
Interleukin-2 (Il-2)   175-81
Internuclear ophthalmoplegia (INO)   359,
    373
Intrathecal gamma globulin production   86
Isofocusing (IEF) spectrum   163-64
Isolated acute optic neuritis   346

Kappa/lambda ratio   233
Kappa light chains   233
Kurtzke disability score. See Disability
    status scores

Lambda light chains   233
Linoleic acid   71, 75-78
Lumbar puncture data   24, 30
Lymphocyte isolation   116
Lymphocyte subsets   141-42
Lymphocytes   143, 145, 156, 172
    natural cytotoxic activity in vitro
        175-83
Lymphocytotoxic antibodies (LCA)   195
Lymphocytotoxins   195
Lymphoid cells, cloning of   167-74

Macrophages   143, 147
    in active demyelinating lesions
        131-39
Major histocompatibility complex (MHC)
    199, 200
Mann Whitney U Tests   73
Migrating bout   91
Migration effects   295, 297-301
Minimal Record of Disability (MRD)
    31
Monoclonal antibodies   153, 154, 156
    against oligodendrocytes   159-62
Mononuclear pleocytosis   237
Myasthenia gravis   9
Myelin
    biochemistry   209-15
    comparison between CNS and PNS   213
Myelin assembly   213
Myelin associated glycoprotein (MAG)
    212
Myelin basic protein (MBP)   109, 200,
    202, 210, 211, 277-81, 290

Myelin basic protein (MBP) (cont)
    determination in cerebrospinal
      fluid and serum   279-80
    fragments of   278-79
    preparation of   278-79
    purification of   278
Myelin degradation   213
Myelin enzymes   212
Myelin lipids   209
Müller, R.   3
Multiple sclerosis   11
    definite   11, 16, 90, 95, 345
    possible   11, 16, 87-88, 95
    postmortem diagnosis   90
    probable   11, 16, 88-90
    questionable   87
    registration   85-87
    suspected   95
    target in   106
    two stage process   225-29
    verified   90

Natural killer (NK) cells   175-83
Natural killing (NK) activity   334
Neurological rating scale   6
NMR imaging   345-52

O-antibodies   159-62
Oculomotor examination   357-62
Oculomotor tests   384, 385
Oligoclonal bands   393-96
Oligoclonal pattern   241, 246-48, 251-56
Oligoclonal response   236-37
Oligodendrocyte differentiation   154-56
Oligodendrocyte heterogeneity   155
Oligodendrocyte structure and function
  153-58
Oligodendrocytes, monoclonal antibodies
  against   159-62
Onset   16-19
    age at   17-20, 25-27
    mode of   28
    progression   29
    progressive   17, 18, 24
    remittent   24
    symptomatology at   8, 16-19
Optomotor test   378
Outcome index   27-29
Out-patients, comparative study   31-40

Peripheral blood, T-cells in   123-30
Periventricular abnormalities   345

406   INDEX

Phenotyped association   318
Phenotypic frequencies   317, 318
Plaque histology   164, 165
Polyphasic bout   91
Poser, Ch.M.   11
Predictors   8
Prednisone   50
Pregnancy   50
Prevalence investigations   306, 307
Primary demyelination   111
Problem profile   38
Prognosis   6-8
    factors affecting   22-24
Progression index   9, 10, 33, 34, 38
Prolonged bout   91
Protein antigen   191
Proteolipid protein (PLP)   210
Pseudobout   90
PWM-Ig synthesis   116, 119

Relapse scores   75, 76
Relapses   21, 104
    chronology of   19
    interval between   22, 24, 28, 29
Remittent phase   19, 21, 22, 24, 28, 29
Remittent-progressive cases   19, 24, 29
Remyelination, neurophysiological
    studies   353-56
Residence area   8
Rheumatoid arthritis   9

Saccadic eye movements   373-81, 383-92
Sequential relative difference (SRD)
    386
Serum lipids assessment   72
Sib-pair double case method   333
Socioeconomic scale   5
Somatosensory evoked response (SSER)
    358-60
Steady progress   91, 92
Steroids   49
Subacute demyelinating (SDE) disease
    290
Subacute sclerosing panencephalitis (SSPE)
    brain   164, 171
Symptomatology
    at onset   8, 16-19
    present   3, 5
    survey on   3, 4

T-cell funtions in vitro   117, 119
T-cell subsets   115-22

T-cell subsets (cont)
    in active demyelinating lesions   131-39
    in blood   117
    in CSF   117
    monoclonal-antibody defined   117
    phenotyping   116
T-cells   105, 110, 123-30, 167, 171, 172,
    189-90, 199-204, 265
    antigen-reactive   128-29
    autoaggressive   187-88
    helper activity   127-28
    proliferative response   124
    TET-activated   125
T-lymphocytes   131, 135, 137, 168, 265
    autoaggressive   188
    cloning of   169
    MBP specific   186
    potentially autoimmune   186-87
T-tests   32
Temperature changes   8
Therapy trials   13-14
Transfer factor (TF) treatment   81-83
Trauma   8
Twin studies   337-41

Vaccinations   8
Variance analysis   16
Vascular disease   346
Velocity ratio   378
Vestulo-ocular reflex (VOR)   363-72
Viral antibodies   263, 289
Virological studies   290
Virus infection   289-92
Visual evoked responses (VER)   393-97

Wallerian degeneration   213, 214
Wilcoxon-Mann-Whitney tests   32

Xenogeneic cell-mediated lympholysis (CML)
    116, 119
Xenogeneic T-cell mediated cytotoxicity
    120